Practical Guide to
Ovulation Induction

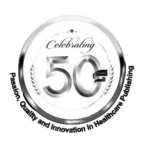

Practical Guide to Ovulation Induction

Chaitanya Nagori MD DGO
Director
Dr. Nagori's Institute for Infertility and IVF
Ahmedabad, Gujarat, India

Sonal Panchal MD
Ultrasound Consultant
Dr. Nagori's Institute for Infertility and IVF
Ahmedabad, Gujarat, India

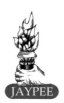

JAYPEE BROTHERS MEDICAL PUBLISHERS
The Health Sciences Publisher
New Delhi | London | Panama

Jaypee Brothers Medical Publishers (P) Ltd

Headquarters

Jaypee Brothers Medical Publishers (P) Ltd
4838/24, Ansari Road, Daryaganj
New Delhi 110 002, India
Phone: +91-11-43574357
Fax: +91-11-43574314
E-mail: jaypee@jaypeebrothers.com

Overseas Offices

JP Medical Ltd
83 Victoria Street, London
SW1H 0HW (UK)
Phone: +44 20 3170 8910
Fax: +44 (0)20 3008 6180
E-mail: info@jpmedpub.com

Jaypee-Highlights Medical Publishers Inc
City of Knowledge, Bld. 235, 2nd Floor
Clayton, Panama City, Panama
Phone: +1 507-301-0496
Fax: +1 507-301-0499
E-mail: cservice@jphmedical.com

Jaypee Brothers Medical Publishers (P) Ltd
Bhotahity, Kathmandu, Nepal
Phone: +977-9741283608
E-mail: kathmandu@jaypeebrothers.com

Website: www.jaypeebrothers.com
Website: www.jaypeedigital.com

Practical Guide to Ovulation Induction

First Edition: **2019**

ISBN 978-93-5270-861-1

Printed at: Samrat Offset Pvt. Ltd.

Ovulation induction is one of the most crucial step in the success of ART. Its concept has been changing since the inception of fertility treatment. With the invention of gonadotropins, the ovulation induction protocols have revolutionized. But these are still in a dynamic phase. New understanding of the complicated reproductive physiology every leads to modifications in these protocols to make it more and more effective and also to increase the safety levels to maximum. The most recent concept is individualizing the stimulation protocols depending on the individual case scenario. In this book, we have tried to cover all the possible alternatives of ovulation induction protocols, correlating with different clinical conditions and have tried to compare the pros and cons of each. We hope this book would be a complete and a concise guide for the infertility practitioners to have more precise and clear concepts about different protocols of ovulation induction in patients with different clinical conditions.

Chaitanya Nagori
Sonal Panchal

Contents

1 Physiology of Ovulation

Chaitanya Nagori, Sonal Panchal

INTRODUCTION

Ovulation is a very complex phenomenon and its clear understanding is essential to understand the abnormalities of the same. Ovulation will be discussed here under following heads:

- Physiology of ovulation
- Endocrinal control of ovulation
- Tests to detect ovulation
- Causes of anovulation.

PHYSIOLOGY OF OVULATION

Introduction

Detailed understanding of physiology of ovulation is very essential to manage ovulation dysfunction, which is one of the important causes of fertility problems. Ovulation occurs from the ovaries. Each oocyte is surrounded by a number of cells to create a *follicle*. When the menstrual cycle begins one, or maybe even a few, primary oocytes begin to grow larger and the follicle cells increase in number and cause the follicle to grow larger too. Usually, some of the developing oocytes will degenerate and only leave one follicle that will mature, but every once in a while two, or even more, follicles will mature. As a follicle reaches maturity, the primary oocyte completes its first meiotic division and becomes a secondary oocyte. Very soon after that the follicle ruptures, and the secondary oocyte is released into the fallopian tube, even though the second meiotic division has not occurred yet. The release of a secondary oocyte from the ovaries is called ovulation.[1]

During intrauterine life of a woman, there are 7 million oogonia that reduce to only 1 million at the time of birth.[2]

This number is further reduced to only 300–400 thousands at the menarche. At the time of menopause, only 1,500 ova are available. During reproductive age only 400 ova reach up to ovulation, i.e. only 0.1% of the total available ova at menarche, reach up to ovulation and 99.9% become atretic.[3]

Ovulation occurs once in a month in majority of the normal women. It is the result of the integrated and synchronized succession of hormonal action and morphological changes in hypothalamus, pituitary and ovary. Autocrine and paracrine factors also take part in ovulation induction. So neuroendocrine complex system regulates ovulation and menstrual cycle.

Figure 1.1 explains the influence of different hormones on ovaries and endometrium. Grossly the gonadotropin-releasing hormones (GnRHs) released from the hypothalamus, control the gonadotropin [luteinizing hormone (LH) or follicle-stimulating hormone (FSH)] secretion from the pituitary and these gonadotropins finally control the estrogen and progesterone secretion from the ovaries. These steroids are responsible for the cyclical changes in ovaries and uterus. The entire control system is thus called hypothalamic-pituitary-ovarian axis. This hypothalamic-pituitary-ovarian axis should be intact and synchronized for normal ovulation (Fig. 1.2).

ROLE OF INDIVIDUAL HORMONE AND ITS CLINICAL APPLICATION

Gonadotropin-releasing Hormone

A decapeptide is synthesized and secreted from the neuronal endings in anterior and mediobasal part of the hypothalamus. It is released from hypothalamus and acts on the pituitary. GnRH traverses through hypothalamic-hypophyseal portal system. This is a compact blood vessel system and so it is not detected in circulation and it releases FSH and LH from the pituitary. Its secretion is pulsatile in nature and stimulates pituitary to secrete more LH than FSH. It is always correlated with LH pulse. Each pulse is of 60–90 minutes. It is chiefly influenced by ovarian steroids.

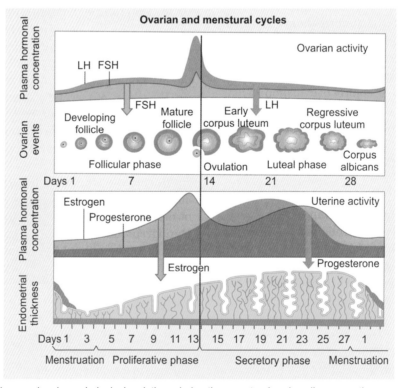

Fig. 1.1: Hormonal and morphological variations during the menstrual cycle—diagrammatic representation.[4]
(LH: luteinizing hormone; FSH: follicle-stimulating hormone).

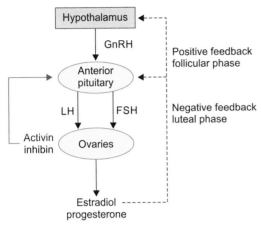

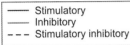

Fig. 1.2: Diagrammatic representation of hypothalamic-pituitary-ovarian (HPO) axis.[5] (GnRH: gonadotropin-releasing hormone; LH: luteinizing hormone; FSH: follicle-stimulating hormone).

Opiates, catecholamines and neuro-peptides, all have an influence on GnRH secretion. There is enormous release of GnRH before the LH surge and then under the effect of progesterone, the frequency of the GnRH pulse decreases to only one in 8–12 hours.[6] GnRH is suppressed by inhibitory factors till puberty.

Clinical Application for Ovulation Induction

- It is used for ovulation induction in hypogonadotropic hypogonadism. But unfortunately it is not yet widely available.
- GnRH agonist (GnRHa) can be used for downregulation in in vitro fertilization (IVF).
- GnRHa as short protocol is used for endogenous FSH and LH surge for ovulation induction.
- GnRHa is used for ovulation trigger to elicit endogenous LH surge.
- GnRH antagonist is used for prevention of LH surge in intrauterine insemination (IUI) and IVF cycles.

Follicle-stimulating Hormone

Follicle-stimulating hormone is secreted from anterior pituitary. FSH secretion is controlled by the feedback system though estradiol (E2) and progesterone. When corpus luteum undergoes atresia or regression just before the menstruation, the FSH secretion increases markedly. It acts on the preantral and antral follicles and helps in recruitment and stimulation of the graafian follicle to make it dominant. It also enhances the conversion of androgens to estrogen though the pathway of aromatase enzyme. Secretion of FSH is governed by estrogen. It frees the oocyte from follicular attachment and converts plasminogen into plasmin. It helps in development of LH receptors for ovulation and for the luteal phase action. It has a definite minimum value, below which it is not sensed by the follicles. This is called FSH threshold. This value is different for every individual. Second peak of FSH is in the midcycle. It has been observed in animals that this second peak of FSH is must for successful ovulation. If this peak is absent, it may cause luteinized unruptured follicle (LUF). But its role in human is not clear. This is so because in humans when surrogate trigger is used in form of LH or human chorionic gonadotropin (hCG), it acts successfully even in absence of FSH. Though the second FSH surge may select the follicles for the next cycle.

Clinical Application

- It is responsible for LH expression after the follicle size of 10–12 mm. This means FSH rescues the follicle to maturity. So there is no need to increase the dose of FSH for follicular growth after 10–12 mm size. Instead supplementation of LH will grow the follicle.[7]

- Follicle-stimulating hormone secretion decreases during periovulatory period because of progesterone, but bioactivity is highest during this period.
- Granulosa cells have androgen receptors. Androgen acts on the immature cells and potentiates action of FSH, e.g. aromatase inhibitor that increases androgen and dehydroepiandrosterone (DHEA) also potentiates the action of FSH.
- Only 1% of the LH receptors are required for folliculogenesis and so in spite of downregulation with GnRHa in long protocol, the follicle continues to grow.
- Follicle-stimulating hormone can stimulate paracrine signal that sustains thecal androgen synthesis. So FSH is capable of ovarian androgen synthesis.[7]

Luteinizing Hormone

Luteinizing hormone is another hormone secreted from anterior pituitary. In the first half of the cycle, its level is low and secretion is pulsatile. High levels of LH are detrimental to ova. This can be explained by the LH threshold and LH ceiling concept.

Luteinizing hormone ceiling and LH threshold:[8] Figure 1.3 indicates that threshold level, i.e. certain minimum amount is required for growth of follicle. But if the level goes beyond a certain level, it hampers the growth of the follicle. This is known as ceiling effect and that level of LH is called the LH ceiling level. So LH level required for follicle maturation should be between the threshold and the ceiling level. This is known as LH window[9] (Fig. 1.4).

Luteinizing hormone causes luteinization of granulosa cells. LH acts on theca cells to produce androgen. With the rising estrogen levels with developing follicle, when the FSH gets a negative feedback, LH gets a positive feedback. LH permits final maturation of follicle forming secondary oocyte and first polar body. It causes disruption of cumulus-oocyte complex and rupture of the follicle. LH surge should be between 14 hours and 27 hours after E2 peak for ovum maturation for rupture and LH surge lasts for 48–50 hours. The two-cell-two hormone theory explains the role of LH in ovarian steroidogenesis[10,11] (Fig. 1.5).

Both the gonadotropins—FSH and LH as well as both the cells, i.e. granulosa cells and theca cells are required for maturation of ova. LH stimulates theca cells to produce androgen from cholesterol. Androgen from theca cells go to granulosa cells where under the influence

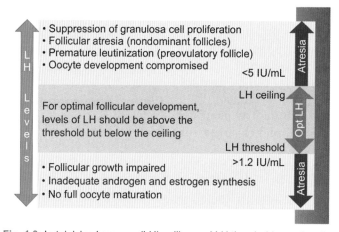

Fig. 1.3: Luteinizing hormone (LH) ceiling and LH threshold—explanation.

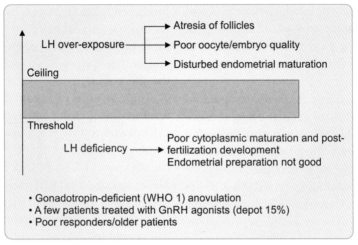

Fig. 1.4: The concept of luteinizing hormone (LH) window.

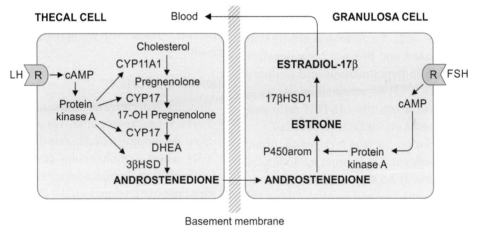

Basement membrane

Fig. 1.5: Diagrammatic explanation of two-cell-two gonadotropin theory.

of FSH, androgen is converted into estrogen by aromatase activity. So both gonadotropins and both the cells are required for folliculogenesis.

Clinical Application

- *Luteinizing hormone in clomiphene citrate cycle*: Clomiphene citrate stimulates FSH and LH from the hypothalamus. This LH may reach the ceiling level especially in polycystic ovarian syndrome (PCOS) and is detrimental

to ova. The level of LH is therefore checked on day 8–10 of the cycle and if it is more than 10–12 IU/mL, it is less likely that clomiphene can give pregnancy as the follicle quality deteriorates due to high LH.[12]

- *Luteinizing hormone in PCOS*: There is tonically high level of LH that causes abnormal oocyte maturation. There is also premature luteinization that decreases implantation because of progesterone secretion. So chronic low-dose protocol and antagonist protocol in PCOS gives very good pregnancy rate. High level of LH causing ceiling effect is clearly seen in PCOS.

- *Luteinizing hormone in downregulated cycle*: In a downregulated cycle, there is low level of LH. When it reaches below the threshold level, the growth of the follicle is hampered. Low level of LH causes poor luteal conversion and so luteal phase defect (LPD) is very common. To compensate this loss, hCG works very well as luteal support but ovarian hyperstimulation syndrome (OHSS) should be kept in mind in PCOS patients.
- *Luteinizing hormone and ovarian drilling*: By drilling, we are destroying stroma, i.e. theca cells. So androgen production is decreased and this will have negative feedback to hypothalamus and pituitary to decrease LH secretion. This decrease in LH will revert the LH/FSH ratio and spontaneous ovulation is established.
- *Luteinizing hormone in hypogonadotropic hypogonadism*: LH is must for follicular development as it is discussed in two-cell-two gonadotropin theory. Without LH follicular growth is present but estrogen level is low.
- *Luteinizing hormone in poor responder*: In poor responder rather than increasing dose of FSH, LH or hCG can be added for rescue of the follicle after 10 mm size. Here LH receptors have developed and it can rescue the follicular growth. But dose of more than 150 IU can have a LH ceiling effect.

Estrogen

It is secreted by granulosa cells of the follicles under the influence of FSH as explained in the two-cell-two hormone theory. It is also produced from androgen by aromatization as discussed earlier. This means for the production of estrogen, androgen is essential and androgen is produced in theca cells under the effect of LH.

High level of estrogen causes negative feedback mechanism and decreases FSH and LH. But when estrogen reaches to certain peak, it causes positive feedback mechanism and causes rise of FSH and LH. This rise causes LH peak and second FSH peak (surge). But LH peak is more intense than FSH peak.

Estrogen prepares the endometrium and is essential for development of progesterone receptors. Estrogen concentration is at their lowest at menstruation and rises to maximum at the preovulatory phase. Following ovulation, the estrogen level falls and then again rises in the luteal phase with the activity of corpus luteum.

Clinical Application

- Because of negative feedback mechanism, FSH level decreases after rise of estrogen from developing follicle. This decrease in FSH causes monofollicular development of the follicle. Letrozole does not abolish this negative feedback unlike clomiphene citrate and so letrozole gives monofollicular development.
- Exogenous estrogen is given for preparation of endometrium in premature ovarian failure (POF) patients.

Other Factors

Inhibin (Fig. 1.6)

Inhibin is also produced by granulosa cells. It has two dimers, inhibin A and inhibin B and both differ in their secretion pattern. Inhibin B rises in follicular phase and is inhibitory to FSH (similar to estrogen). Inhibin A rises in periovulatory period and luteal phase.

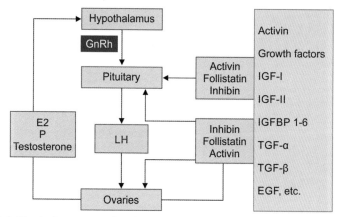

Fig. 1.6: Fine tuning system of HPO axis (short loop and long loop feedback systems).

Clinical application: Inhibin B is assessed for measuring ovarian reserve but anti-Müllerian hormone (AMH) and antral follicle count (AFC) are more reliable.

Activin and Follistatin (Fig. 1.6)

These increase secretion and promotes action of FSH, and lead to follicular growth and inhibit androgen production. Follistatin being an activin-binding protein, and neutralizes activin bioactivity.

Growth Factors

Insulin-like growth factor (IGF), IGF-2, IGF-binding protein (BP) 1–6, transforming growth factor (TGF), TGF-α, TGF-β, epithelial growth factor (EGF), etc. are the growth factors for the follicle growth. Activity of IGFs can be counteracted by IGF-BPs. Receptors to these are present in ovaries and promote androgen production. All these factors passively help the growth of the follicle (Fig. 1.6).

Ovulation

Ovulation occurs after 34–36 hours of onset of LH surge. Onset of LH surge correlates with perifollicular blood flows. Pre-LH surge perifollicular resistance index (RI) between 0.4

and 0.48 and peak systolic velocity (PSV) of 10 cm/sec are the indicators of a mature follicle on Doppler ultrasound[13] (Fig. 1.7). Ovulation occurs 10–12 hours after LH peak (Fig. 1.8). Estrogen peak initiates LH peak and ovulation occurs after 24–26 hours of estrogen peak. Inhibitory activities are high before and after ovulation. But it is important to remember that apart from these hormones, normal levels of prolactin, thyroid and androgen are also essential for normal ovulation.

Human chorionic gonadotropin plays a major role in inducing influx of blood within follicles. Follicular PSV rises markedly with the rise in the LH levels at the time of preovulatory LH surge.[15] Because of this physiology, when PSV of the follicle is high, it means that the follicle is likely to rupture early, IUI should be done earlier than the conventional protocol of 34–38 hours.

Progesterone

Luteinizing hormone induces the secretion of progesterone from luteinized granulosa cells (Fig. 1.9). Progesterone rises before ovulation and this rise is because of rise of FSH. It has a triggering role for high GnRH which may give LH surge. It helps in increasing

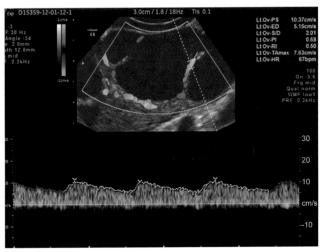

Fig. 1.7: Color and pulse Doppler ultrasound image of a mature follicle.

proteolytic enzymes for rupture. Progesterone production from corpus luteum keeps on rising till the midluteal period (7–8 days postovulation), when its level is at its peak. Rising progesterone has a negative feedback on the pituitary gonadotropins and decreases the frequency of LH pulse. During this phase, FSH is synthesized but not secreted. It is stored for release when corpus luteum fails and estrogen and progesterone levels decrease markedly. Decrease in LH causes demise of corpus luteum and decrease in progesterone secretion towards the end of the cycle, just before menstruation.

Progesterone prepares endometrium for implantation by expressing genes needed for implantation. hCG of pregnancy rescues corpus luteum and progesterone secretion is maintained till the trophoblastic and placental hormones take over.

Clinical Application

- Preparation of endometrium occurs with progesterone along with estrogen in POF patients.

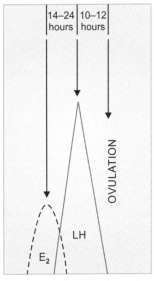

Fig. 1.8: Estradiol (E2) and LH fluctuations around ovulation.[14]

- Human chorionic gonadotropin can be used to rescue corpus luteum as a luteal phase support.
- Luteal support with progesterone is given to the patients at high risk of LPD, especially those on agonist cycles and antagonist cycles.

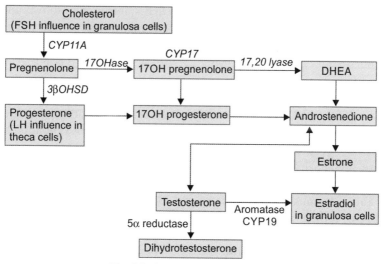

Fig. 1.9: Ovarian steroids genesis.[6]

CLINICOPATHOLOGY OF OVULATION

Introduction

For the diagnosis of ovulatory dysfunction, it is extremely important to advice for precise investigations depending on the history of the patient. It helps the clinician to reach to the correct diagnosis. Unnecessary investigations may give no relevant information but may create more confusions.

Profiles and packages are useless in infertility and are expensive in clinical practice. In infertility management, specific investigations are required at specific times for correct interpretation. So one has to be very precise when requesting for investigations. The routinely required investigations for infertility and assisted reproductive techniques (ART) are discussed here.

Serum Follicle-stimulating Hormone

- *Day 2–3 serum FSH and serum LH for diagnosis of PCOS*: High LH indicates anovulation and it is very evident from

the history. Therefore, ratio of LH/FSH is not required for diagnosis of PCOS. Both high LH and PCOS can be diagnosed by an ultrasound scan done on day 2–3 of the menstrual cycle.

- *Serum FSH for diagnosis of menopause*: FSH of greater than 40 IU/mL indicates ovarian failure. Oral contraceptive (OC) pills can be used to induce withdrawal bleed in these patients to confirm menopause. When the patient does not have a withdrawal bleed after giving progesterone for 3–5 days, it indicates she is menopausal. Ultrasound shows hardly any follicles and ovaries are small.

- *Follicle-stimulating hormone for assessment of ovarian reserve*: Day 2–3 FSH is done to know the ovarian reserve and also to predict the possibility of pregnancy. Higher the FSH, lesser is the chance for development of good quality follicles/ova, thus resulting in a lesser chance to achieve conception. FSH of less than 8 IU/mL is considered normal. Between 8 IU/mL and 12 IU/mL FSH, the values are considered high. But when these values are greater than 12 IU/mL, there is very little chance of retrieving good quality ova and therefore decreased chance of achieving pregnancy. Chances of pregnancy beyond FSH level of 15 IU/mL is rare.[16] Though currently age, AFC and AMH are used for assessment of ovarian reserve and thought to be much more accurate and reliable for the purpose, than FSH. Utility of FSH as a marker for ovarian reserve has significantly reduced. This is because, AFC indicates the number of follicle available in that cycle for recruitment, whereas serum FSH level gives overall impression about the availability of the ova.

If the patient with low ovarian reserve is given DHEA for 3 months, the AFC may rise, but the FSH still remains high. In these cases, it would be worthwhile to initiate ovulation induction. AFC thus may be a better marker for patient counseling too. Moreover, repeated FSH assessment is of no significance, because it is the highest level of FSH that acts as the decision maker for the possibility of pregnancy. AFC is so far considered the most feasible and reliable parameter for assessment of ovarian reserve.[17,18]

- *Low FSH*: Less than 5 IU indicates pituitary or hypothalamic cause for anovulation.

Serum Luteinizing Hormone

- *Serum LH for PCOS*: Day 2/3 serum level of LH is not required for the diagnosis of PCOS. In PCOS, LH is high and this can be clinically judged by anovulation or oligo-ovulation resulting in delayed menstrual cycles. High LH, leads to high androgen can be diagnosed by high stromal volume.[19,20]
- *Serum LH on day 8–10 in clomiphene citrate cycle*: Clomiphene citrate stimulates hypothalamus to secrete both FSH and LH as it blocks estrogen receptors. This high

LH is detrimental to ova and gives poor pregnancy rate in spite of good ovulation rate. Therefore, when LH is more than 10–12 IU/mL on day 8–10 of a clomiphene cycle, the subsequent cycles should not be continued with clomiphene citrate, instead the ovulation induction should then be done with gonadotropins in these patients. This is more common scenario in PCOS patients.

- *Serum LH in downregulated cycle*: In downregulated patients on long protocol, the LH on day 2–3 of the treatment cycle should be between 0.5 IU and 2 IU to confirm the adequacy of downregulation. Actually 0.1 IU/mL LH is sufficient for the development of follicle and so assessment of LH levels at this phase of cycle is questionable.
- Serum LH less than 5 IU/L indicates pituitary or hypothalamic cause for anovulation, especially with low FSH.

Serum Estradiol

- *Follicular maturity*: When the follicle is mature, serum E2 will be 150 pg/mL/follicle. If E2 is normal and endometrium is poor, it is a local cause for poor endometrium. But if the E2 level is low, the endometrium is usually poor, and may grow to normal when E2 level rises. Using color Doppler for the assessment of follicular quality can be a useful tool for the same because the flow parameters of the follicle can be correlated with the functional maturity of the follicle which indirectly indicates E2 levels. So E2 can differentiate between the causes of poor endometrium.
- *For poor responder*: In IVF cycles, E2 is assessed on day 2 of the cycle to confirm downregulation. If it is greater than 80 pg/mL, it indicates a possibility of poor

response to stimulation. This high E2 is because of high FSH that is present in poor responders and causes early recruitment of the follicle.

- *To assess ovarian suppression*: In long agonist protocol IVF cycles, GnRHa is started from day 21 of the previous cycle. This downregulates pituitary and FSH and LH levels become very low. This also leads to low E2 levels (30–50 pg/mL). The stimulation is started only thereafter. If E2 level is more than 50 pg/mL, it is advisable to continue downregulation for 1 day or 2 days more before starting the stimulation. In patients on OC pills, E2 should be checked after 12–14 days after starting OC pills.

- *For suspected risk of hyperstimulation*: In IUI cycles or in non-IVF gonadotropin cycles, hyperstimulation is suspected if E2 is more than 1,600 pg/mL on the day of trigger. This is common in PCOS patients. In IVF cycles, if E2 is more than 4,000 pg/mL on the day of trigger, hyperstimulation is suspected. Now with chronic low-dose protocol in IUI cycles and ultrasound-based scoring systems for deciding the stimulation protocols,[21,22] extremely low OHSS rates are claimed. Though in IVF cycles with antagonist protocol and agonist trigger, OHSS can be almost completely prevented. Therefore, the strategy in PCOS patients should be antagonist protocol with agonist trigger.

Ovarian hyperstimulation syndrome can also be predicted by calculating the ovarian volume. If total ovarian volume of both the ovaries together is more than approximately 180 cc, OHSS should be suspected,[23] whereas if it is less than approximately 110 cc the risk of OHSS is extremely low. We depend more on ovarian volume than on the E2 levels and withhold hCG trigger when combined ovarian volume of two ovaries is more than 180 cc.

Serum Progesterone

Progesterone is chiefly secreted by corpus luteum in 2nd half of the cycle. Otherwise it is an intermediate hormone for other steroid hormones during their production after conversion from cholesterol.

Normal values:

- Follicular phase : 1 ng/mL
- LH surge   : 1–2 ng/mL
- Ovulation   : 3 ng/mL

Midluteal serum progesterone, i.e. a week before menstruation is approximately 10 ng/mL. A level of greater than 3 ng/mL indicates ovulation. Therefore, if only ovulation is to be documented, repeated ultrasound scans are not required. In the same way, endometrial biopsy is not required to confirm secretory changes in endometrium and serum progesterone estimation suffices for the same.

Ultrasound with color Doppler is a better modality to assess the secretory phase of the cycle. It can diagnose luteal phase problems viz. LPD/LUF. So it is an inevitable conclusion that random serum progesterone has little value beyond documenting ovulation.

17-Hydroxyprogesterone

This investigation is done in all patients with hirsutism. It is increased due to 21-hydroxylase deficiency. Because of 21-hydroxylase deficiency in patients of heterogeneous carrier, late onset of congenital adrenal hyperplasia is observed. 17-hydroxyprogesterone (17-OHP) is weak androgen and manifests as hirsutism, acne, clitoral enlargement and menstrual irregularity at puberty.

Normal level of 17-OHP is less than 200 ng/dL. Whenever the level is between 200 ng/dL and 800 ng/dL, one should get the adrenocorticotropic hormone (ACTH) levels assessed in serum. Level of greater than 800 ng/dL is diagnostic of 21-hydroxylase deficiency. These patients are treated with dexamethasone 0.5 mg daily at bedtime.

Serum Testosterone

Normal value of serum testosterone is 20–80 ng/dL. Its normal production is 0.2–0.3 mg/day. Out of this 80% binds to sex hormone-binding globulin (SHBG) and 19% to albumin. Only 1% is free testosterone. Testosterone may be high in patients with PCOS and tumors. Tumor is suspected if there is sudden onset of symptoms due to increased testosterone. PCOS patients show gradual rise in testosterone levels. Routine estimation of serum testosterone is not required, as it does not change the line of treatment.

Androgens and their sources have been shown in Table 1.1.

Serum Dehydroepiandrosterone Sulfate

Dehydroepiandrosterone sulfate (DHEA-S) is exclusively secreted from adrenal glands. The normal value is 350 ng/dL. It increases with hyperprolactinemia. In patients with PCOS, prolactin and DHEA-S are a little high and do

TABLE 1.1: Androgens and their sources.

Hormone	Source
Testosterone	50% Peripheral conversion 25% Ovary 25% Adrenal
Androstenedione	50% Ovary 50% Adrenal
DHEA	90% Adrenal 10% Ovary
DHA	100% Adrenal

(DHEA: dehydroepiandrosterone; DHA: dehydroandrosterone)

not require any specific treatment except the treatment of PCOS. This rise is secondary to estrogen because of anovulation.

Whenever DHEA-S is very high, it is due to adrenal tumor. DHEA-S greater than 700 µg/dL is accepted as a marker for adrenal dysfunction. This is rarely found and does not change the management. And ultrasound is a better guide to diagnose adrenal tumor. Serum testosterone and ultrasound suffices to rule out adrenal tumors. If 17-OHP is normal, there is no need to search for adrenal enzyme defect. Therefore, routine testing of DHEA-S is not required.

Inhibin A and B

Inhibin B is predominantly secreted by antral follicles. Low day 3 inhibin B level less than 45 pg/mL indicates poor response to superovulation and patient is less likely to conceive. Same thing can be judged by serum FSH, serum AMH or AFC and so routine use of inhibin B estimation is not justified. Inhibin A is secreted from preovulatory follicles. Both inhibin A and B are secreted from granulosa cells and regulate FSH by negative feedback mechanism. Routine estimation of inhibin A does not add any information to change the management of the patient.

Serum Anti-Müllerian Hormone

It is a member of TGF. It is produced from granulosa cells of small antral follicles. The expression of AMH is localized in granulosa cells of primary preantral and small antral follicles and has important role in human folliculogenesis. AMH expression in follicle decreases in antral follicle greater than 8 mm in size. It is now well established that serum AMH concentrations reflect the number of preantral and small antral follicles in the ovary, this would account for raised AMH levels found in both polycystic ovarian morphology (PCOM) and PCOS.[24] In follicles undergoing atresia and in corpus luteum also, the AMH expression is completely lost.[11] AMH levels in women are low until the age of 8, rise rapidly until puberty and decline steadily from the age of 25 until menopause, when AMH production ceases.

Physiology of Anti-Müllerian Hormone

Anti-Müllerian hormone has an inhibiting role in the ovary, contributing to follicular arrest.[19] It lowers the sensitivity of follicles to FSH, which is required for normal folliculogenesis. In vitro studies have shown that the action of FSH in promoting follicular growth is counteracted by AMH.[25] It has a steady level throughout the cycle except for a slight dip just after LH peak.[26]

Though some investigators have recorded cyclical fluctuations in AMH with rapid decrease in early luteal phase.[27] This can be correlated with the follicular atresia before recruitment in the late luteal phase.

It can predict ovarian response. It can predict menopause by low levels. High AMH is very high in PCOS, and it predicts OHSS.

Anti-Müllerian hormone values and its interpretation for ovarian response have been shown in Table 1.2.

Anti-Müllerian Hormone and PCOS

The reported property of AMH to counteract the actions of FSH imply that the high

TABLE 1.2: Anti-Müllerian hormone values and ovarian response.

Ovarian fertility potential	pmol/L	ng/mL
Optimal fertility	28.6–48.5	4.0–6.8
Satisfactory fertility	15.7–28.6	2.2–4.0
Low fertility	2.2–15.7	0.3–2.2
Very low/undetectable	0.0–2.2	0.0–0.3
High level	48.5	6.8

production of AMH by polycystic ovary may have an important role in the pathophysiology of the syndrome.[28] In anovulatory PCOS, the failure of follicle development is due to an intrinsic inhibition of FSH action and that this inhibition is due to an intrinsic inhibition of FSH action and due to the high concentration of AMH.[29]

Increased ovarian stromal blood flow in PCOS may be because of over expression of vascular endothelial growth factor (VEGF) that modulates the permeability of theca cells and increased IGF-1[30,31] which in turn enhances gonadotropin-stimulated steroid production in granulosa cells and theca cells resulting in increased ovarian androgen production and subsequently increased AMH production.[32]

Anti-Müllerian hormone levels are two to three times higher in PCOS, than in healthy controls.[33] This has been attributed not only to increased number of antral follicles but also to higher production of AMH per follicle in patients with PCOS as compared to size-matched counterparts from normal ovary.[34] In addition, a positive correlation between AMH and both LH and testosterone serum concentrations in PCOS has been reported.[35]

Each individual follicle in women with PCOS produces significantly more AMH than its size-matched counterpart from a patient with normal ovary.[34] Moreover, it has also been shown that metformin administration in PCOS patients is associated with reduction in AMH concentration in follicle and serum, suggesting that the measurement of AMH can be used to evaluate the treatment efficacy with insulin sensitizers.[36]

Anti-Müllerian Hormone and IVF

In IVF patients, serum AMH value can predict the response of ovary and so it is useful for counseling the patient. When calculated optimal AMH cutoff of less than 1.26 ng/mL was used to predict responses to controlled ovarian stimulation (COS), it was found to have a 97% sensitivity for predicting poor responses (<4 oocytes retrieved) and 98% accuracy in predicting a normal COS response.[37]

Nelson et al. suggested the AMH-based strategy for deciding the COS protocol.[38]

But we have found AFC as equally effective and more precise for prediction of ovarian response. With extremely low-serum AMH levels, moderate, but reasonable pregnancy and live birth rates are still possible. Extremely low AMH levels do not seem to represent an appropriate marker for withholding fertility treatment. Younger women are likely to have better pregnancy rates than their older counterparts with equally low AMH.[39] Constant AMH and inhibin B levels suggest that neither AMH nor inhibin B is an accurate marker of ovarian response after low-dose gonadotropins ovulation induction in patients with PCOS.[40] Mashiach et al. have also shown a relationship between follicular fluid AMH concentrations and the quality of embryos in patients with PCOS.[41]

All these references indicate that routine use of AMH does not help in managing non-ART patients. Only 1–2 mature follicles are required for superovulation with IUI and AMH will not help us in change the line of treatment. Poor responding ovary or low reserve ovary can be very precisely diagnosed by ultrasound. Serum AMH estimation is indicated in:[42]

- Predicting both over and under response in COS
- Determining the most appropriate treatment regimen
- Pretreatment counseling for couples to make an appropriate and informed choice
- Predicting long-term fertility
- Predicting the age of menopause

- Predicting ovarian aging prior to or following chemotherapy/surgery
- Screening for polycystic ovaries.

Clinical Applications of AMH, Apart from Fertility Assessment

- To confirm presence of testicular tissue in children with low testosterone levels.
- Differential diagnosis of intersex disorders.
- In patients with bilateral nonpalpable gonads.
- Females with granulosa cell tumors.
- The inhibitory effect of AMH on folliculo-genesis may in future be used for hormonal contraception.

Insulin Resistance

Now it has been proved that in patients of PCOS there is high androgen because of increased insulin level and insulin resistance. It indicates the severity of PCOS. Clinically waist circumference of 35 inches or 90 cm is predictive of abnormal endocrinology and metabolic function.

There are various methods to diagnose insulin resistance. But 2-hour glucose and insulin response is the one of the most reliable ones.

Two-hour glucose tolerance test (75 gm of glucose):

- Normal   : <140 mg/dL
- Impaired   : 140–190 mg/dL
- Noninsulin-dependent diabetes mellitus   : ≥200 mg/dL

Two-hour insulin response:

- Insulin resistance very likely   : 100–150 µU/mL
- Insulin resistance   : 151–300 µU/mL
- Severe insulin resistance   : >300 µU/mL

In clinical practice, patients with high insulin resistance are the ones who have tonically high LH levels require ovarian drilling. Alternatively they may also be benefitted by GnRH antagonist. Antagonist decreases LH levels, prevents premature luteinization and improves oocyte quality.

Patients who do not want immediate pregnancy are the patients in whom insulin sensitizer alone is the recommended line of treatment. It has been proved beyond doubts that insulin sensitizers do not have any direct effect on ovulation induction, though when given for 3–6 months, the improved insulin sensitivity, improved the hormonal milieu of PCOS patient, thus improving the chance of spontaneous ovulation and conception.

Three-dimensional (3D) ultrasound is a novel way to diagnose insulin resistance, based on assessment of stromal volume.[43] But when volume ultrasound is unavailable, 2-hour glucose and 2-hour insulin test is the best alternative.

So for chronic anovulation only three investigations are required:
1. Serum prolactin
2. Serum TSH
3. Insulin resistance.

Serum Prolactin

Prolactin is the hormone secreted by anterior pituitary and is regulated by prolactin inhibitory factor that is secreted from hypothalamus.
- Normal level of prolactin is 10–25 ng/mL.
- In microadenoma, it is between 100 ng/mL and 200 ng/mL.
- In macroadenoma, it is greater than 200 ng/mL.
- Immunoassay for prolactin does not reflect its bioassay levels always.
- Many a times patients have no symptoms in spite of high prolactin level because of presence of macromolecules which are big prolactin molecules that account for 10–12% of hyperprolactin in a symptomatically normal patient.

Galactorrhea with Normal Prolactin Levels

Patients with galactorrhea present with normal serum prolactin levels. This may be mucoid discharge and not actual galactorrhea. Any discharge therefore from the breast should be seen under microscope. If it contains fat globules, only then it is galactorrhea.

When ovulation induction is done, in many patients estrogen leads to rise in prolactin levels in first half of the menstrual cycle. These patients have night spikes of high prolactin level and are known as spikers. This is transient hyperprolactinemia. The clinical presentation is poor endometrium in spite of good follicles. This condition is difficult to diagnose, but bromocriptine can be given in a dose of 1.25 mg twice a day, in these patients in first half of the cycle. It is a therapeutic test. If endometrium improves, it is continued in the subsequent cycle, otherwise it is stopped. Apart from bad oocyte quality, the spikers also have a high chance of LPD.

As discussed earlier, marginally high prolactin levels are also found in PCOS patients due to high estrogen and high DHEA-S. In these cases, bromocriptine or cabergoline is not required, PCOS is to be treated and this corrects hyperprolactinemia.

DIAGNOSIS OF OVULATION

Detection of ovulation is extremely important to decide the further line of treatment in patients for treatment of infertility. There are various tests to detect ovulation and current status of each test is discussed here.

Clinical Presentation

- Regular menstrual cycle (24–35 days) is in favor of ovulation. Any type of irregularity, beyond the limits (24–35 days), strongly indicates anovulation or dysovulation.

- *"Mittelschmerz"*: This is a mid-cycle pain in an ovulatory cycle because of contraction of smooth muscles surrounding the follicle about 12–24 hours prior to ovulation. This contraction helps the follicle to rupture and ovulation occurs.
- *Cervical mucus feel*: Patient feels watery discharge at the introitus which becomes thin and copious prior to ovulation. This indicates a mature follicle and not ovulation.
- Pregnancy is the only surest sign of ovulation.
- Painful menstruation is also an indicator of the previous cycle being ovulatory.

Basal Body Temperature

The principle of basal body temperature (BBT) measurement is that progesterone secretion after ovulation raises the body temperature. BBT is between 97°F and 98°F during the follicular phase. After ovulation, it starts rising and goes high by 0.4–0.8°F, as the progesterone rises. BBT is at its lowest just before ovulation which is known as nadir. The temperature falls before the period or when progesterone level decreases due to regressing corpus luteum. The rise in temperature persists, in case the patient conceives and patient feels her body temperature as much as low-grade fever. This is because of persistent and high levels of progesterone from the corpus luteum of pregnancy, stimulated by hCG.

Method

Basal body temperature is taken before rising from bed, with glass thermometer placed in oral cavity. The calibration on thermometer is 96–100°F. The change pattern in thermometer is known as biphasic pattern. The next period in normal cycle starts after 12 days of rise in temperature if pregnancy does not occur. It is a low cost, noninvasive and simple method and indicates abnormalities of follicular and luteal phase. But the temperature may be altered with smoking and disturbed sleep. It may be stressful for the patient to take temperature daily. There may not be shift in temperature in spite of ovulation and in this case, only after a few days of ovulation it may be diagnosed. This is not clinically useful. BBT is not commonly used in clinical practice.

Midcycle LH Surge Diagnosed by LH Kit

Luteinizing hormone surge occurs for 48–50 hours. LH has short half-life. LH rise can be detected by urinary LH kits. When the threshold level of 40 mIU/mL is crossed, test becomes positive on the kit and the color is seen. The intensity of the color increases as LH level increases. LH level normally starts rising early in the morning and may be misinterpreted as negative if urine is tested in the morning as it appears in the urine after 6–8 hours. Therefore, LH assessment in the afternoon is more reliable.

The test is done daily. But doing it twice daily decreases the false negatives. Too much of fluid intake is avoided few hours before the test to prevent dilution of the urine and LH in urine.

Ovulation occurs 20 hours ±6 hours after detection of urinary LH surge.[44-47] Patient is advised intercourse for 2 days following detection of LH surge as these days are the most fertile ones. If artificial insemination of donor (AID) is planned, it should also be done for 2 days. The specificity and sensitivity for LH surge are 90% and 96% respectively and if test is done twice a day, sensitivity reaches to 99%.[47]

So LH detection kits are noninvasive, self-monitored and indicate fertile period, so it is useful clinically for planning timed intercourse, IUI and AID. It can diagnose abnormality of follicular phase and luteal phase. But the disadvantage is that it is tedious, may be false negative and restricts patients from fluid intake. False positive results may occur with OC pills, clomiphene citrate, hCG, human menopausal gonadotropin (hMG) and danazol. But easy availability of ultrasound has reduced the utility of LH kits.

Endometrial Biopsy

It was used to document secretory changes in the endometrium after ovulation. Endometrial biopsy differentiates follicular phase from secretory phase. An experienced pathologist can date the endometrium after ovulation. Two days out of phase endometrium is regarded as LPD.[48] This test is not as preferred as ultrasound or serum progesterone levels as it is inaccurate and highly invasive.

Luteal Serum Progesterone Levels

Progesterone level is below 1 ng/mL during follicular phase. Before ovulation it rises up to 1–2 ng/mL. The peak reaches after a week of ovulation. Level more than 3 ng/mL indicates ovulation. Normally on 7th postovulatory day, progesterone level is greater than 10 ng/mL.[49] Serum progesterone level is only used to document ovulation as it is simple, fairly accurate, noninvasive and reliable.

Daily assessment of progesterone for diagnosis of LPD is not used as is inconclusive and multiple levels are required for accuracy.

Estrogen

Clinically estrogen peak will give copious mucus discharge and when dried on a slide will show a "fern" pattern. Before ovulation it shows tertiary branches. Normal preovulatory mucus strand can be stretched to 8–10 cm between two ends of artery forceps. Both these tests indicate high estrogen level, mostly due to mature follicle but do not indicate ovulation.

Ultrasound

A follicle that is of greater than 10 mm in diameter, grows at a rate of 2–3 mm/day has no internal echogenicity and has thin (pencil line like) walls is not only more likely to become the leading follicle but will also give mature healthy ovum. The growing follicle can be assessed by transvaginal sonography. A mature follicle is 16–18 mm, has thin walls, regular round shape and no echogenicity in the lumen. When functionally mature, on color Doppler, the follicle shows blood vessels covering at least three-fourths of the follicular circumference (see Fig. 1.7). On pulse Doppler, these blood vessels show an RI of 0.4–0.48[13] and PSV of greater than 10 cm/sec. The endometrium starts appearing multilayered on ultrasound as early as mid-proliferative phase with rising estrogen. On transvaginal scan, endometrial thickness of 6 mm is considered minimum that is required on the day of ovulation or on the day of hCG trigger for a successful outcome, although 8 mm is generally considered optimum.[50] Segmental uterine artery perfusion demonstrates significant correlation with hormonal and histological markers of uterine receptivity, reaching the highest sensitivity for subendometrial blood flow.[51]

Endometrial vessels on pulse Doppler if have RI of less than 0.6, it have been reported to be a good prognostic factor for implantation.[52] Rupture of the follicle is documented as disappearance of the follicle and it may be replaced by a cystic structure with thick shaggy walls and echogenicity in the lumen. But it is known to have variable appearances (Fig. 1.10) like ground glass echogenicity in lumen or lace-like echogenicities. This structure is known as corpus luteum.

Corpus luteum can be seen as low resistance vascular structure with thick walls and internal echogenicities (Fig. 1.11).

Secretory changes are seen in the endometrium in the form of echogenicity of the endometrium which starts from outside in the early luteal phase, proceeding to the central line making a ring sign of the endometrium.[53] Posterior wall of the uterus also appears more echogenic in this phase due to acoustic enhancement by the endometrium due to fluid accumulation (Fig. 1.12).

Serial ultrasound for documenting ovulation should not be done if intervention like ovulation trigger or IUI is not planned. Whether ovulation has occurred or not can be known by postovulatory serum progesterone level only.

Summarizing Diagnosis of Ovulation

- Clinical history suggests ovulation in most cases.
- Basal body temperature is inconclusive and not used routinely.
- Urinary LH kit is useful only for patients who cannot visit clinic off and on. It is not very commonly used.
- Serum progesterone greater than 3 ng/mL postovulatory indicates ovulation and is a most reliable means to document ovulation.
- Daily ultrasound for just confirming that ovulation has occurred or not is not required unless some intervention is intended.
- Endometrial biopsy is not required to assess the secretory phase changes.
- Fern pattern and spinnbarkeit test indicate high estrogen level and not ovulation.

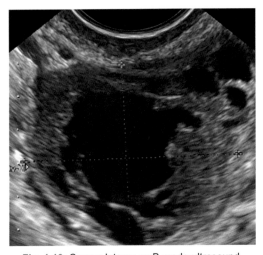

Fig. 1.10: Corpus luteum on B-mode ultrasound.

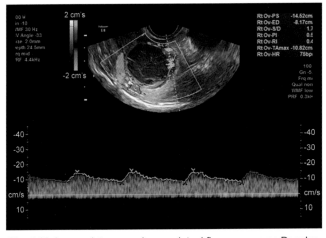

Fig. 1.11: Low resistance pericorpus luteal flow as seen on Doppler.

CAUSES OF ANOVULATION (FIG. 1.13)

Introduction

The incidence of infertility is 15–17% after 1 year of unprotected intercourse. After 2nd year, only 7–8% of couples remain infertile. After 2.5 years almost 7% will still remain infertile. Out of these infertile couples, in 20–40%, anovulation or oligo-ovulation is the causative factor.

The classification of causes of anovulation is very well described by the World Health Organization (WHO). It is classified as:

- WHO group I: Hypothalamic-pituitary failure
- WHO group II: Hypothalamic-pituitary dysfunction
- WHO group III: Ovarian failure
- WHO group IV: Hyperprolactinemia
- WHO group V: Outflow defects (not associated with anovulation).

Hypothalamic-Pituitary Failure (WHO Group I)

It is also known as hypogonadotropic hypogonadism. In this situation, gonadotropin

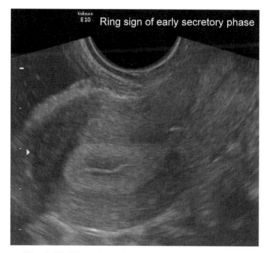

Fig. 1.12: Ring sign of secretory endometrium as seen on B-mode ultrasound.

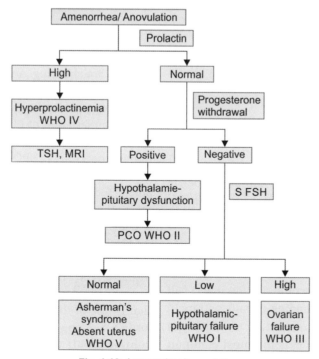

Fig. 1.13: Amenorrhea/anovulation.

(FSH and LH) concentrations are so low that follicle is not stimulated and therefore there is extremely low estrogen level. These patients have anovulation and amenorrhea.

Hypothalamic Causes

- *Anorexia nervosa*: It is weight related. It may be due to crash diet or frank anorexia nervosa.
- *Stress*: It may be stress-related anovulation and amenorrhea. Severe exercises like marathon running can cause amenorrhea.
- *Kallmann syndrome*: It is associated with anosmia.
- Craniopharyngioma.
- Debilitating systemic diseases.
- Idiopathic.

Pituitary Causes

- Hypophysectomy.
- Severe postpartum hemorrhage (PPH) causing Sheehan's syndrome.
- Radiotherapy for pituitary tumors.

In these conditions, GnRH replacement therapy is very useful. But gonadotropins are usually given for ovulation induction.

Hypothalamic-Pituitary Dysfunction (WHO Group II)

As contrast to WHO group I, in patients of this group, FSH is present that stimulates follicle and so estrogen is also present. Clinically this condition presents as oligo-ovulation or anovulation causing amenorrhea. As endogenous estrogen is present in these patients, 5 days of oral progesterone (10 mg hydroxyprogesterone acetate daily) will give withdrawal bleeding usually within 10 days and this is confirmatory of WHO type II anovulation. PCOS is the most common condition amongst WHO group II. Diagnosis of PCOS is made by Rotterdam criteria (2003). These are as follows:

- Oligo-ovulation/anovulation
- Clinical and/or biochemical hyperandrogenism
- Polycystic ovaries on ultrasound.

Any two of these above mentioned three criteria establishes the diagnosis of PCOS. These criteria are defined as mentioned below:

- *Oligo-ovulation/anovulation*: Oligo-ovulation is ovulation occurring once in 35–180 days. Anovulation is defined as no ovulation in 6 consecutive months.
- *Hyperandrogenism: clinical or biochemical*: Clinical signs include hirsutism, acne, alopecia (male type) and female virilization. Biochemical indicators include raised total testosterone, androstenedione and free androgen index.
- *Polycystic ovaries on ultrasound*: Presence of 12 or more follicles in either ovary, 2–9 mm in size and/or ovarian volume greater than 10 cc. The new cut off for follicle number is 20 per ovary.

Though the concepts on the number of follicles and ovarian volume for the diagnosis of PCOS are changing. An average value of 26 or more follicles per ovary is a reliable threshold for detecting polycystic ovaries in women with frank manifestation of PCOS. Sensitivity and specificity for diagnosis of PCOS for follicle number per ovary (FNPO) (26) were 85% and 94% and for ovarian volume (10 cc) were 81% and 84%. But the same study has also quoted that the lower follicle threshold may be required to detect milder variants of the syndrome.[54]

Hyperinsulinemia and high androgen levels are very useful for diagnosis. Postprandial insulin levels (2 hours after 75 g of glucose) are increased in patients with insulin resistance that is one of the major diagnostic features for PCOS. Along with this, increased stromal volume on 3D ultrasound is diagnostic of PCOS. Management includes lifestyle changes, oral ovulogens, gonadotropins and ovarian drilling.

Ovarian Failure (WHO Group III)

This group presents with high FSH along with low estrogen and amenorrhea. The patient will have symptoms of hypoestrinism. Physiologically this condition is found with the onset of menopause. But menopause may set in prematurely.

Causes of Ovarian Failure

- Menopause (>40 years of age)
- Premature menopause (<40 years of age):
  - Familial tendency
  - Autoimmune disease
  - Chemotherapy
  - Radiotherapy
  - Infections like tuberculosis
  - Idiopathic.
- Chromosomal—Turner's syndrome.

Diagnosis is confirmed by high FSH greater than 25 IU/mL with extremely low AMH. The only available treatment option to achieve a pregnancy in these patients is ovum donation. Hormone replacement therapy (HRT) is required in these patients, to support their physiological needs.

Hyperprolactinemia (WHO Group IV)

Anovulation because of hyperprolactinemia is present when prolactin levels are double the upper normal limits. This leads to anovulation. Marginally high prolactin levels do not require any treatment as it does not lead to anovulation. Mildly high prolactin levels are found in PCOS but in these cases no therapy is required to decrease prolactin levels. Prolactin is regulated by "prolactin-inhibiting factor", dopamine. Therefore, any hypothalamic lesion or drugs suppressing hypothalamic activity will increase prolactin level and LH will be low.

Outflow Defects (WHO Group V)

- *Primary:* Imperforate hymen, absent uterus.
- *Secondary:* Asherman's syndrome.

So chiefly three tests: (1) progesterone withdrawal bleeding, (2) serum prolactin and (3) serum FSH level assessment can give accurate diagnosis of anovulation for the management.

CARRY HOME MESSAGE

- In all patients of anovulation/amenorrhea, always assess the prolactin levels as the first investigation to exclude hyperprolactinemia. (WHO IV)
- Progesterone withdrawal bleeding indicates presence of endogenous estrogen and diagnosis of hypothalamic-pituitary dysfunction. (WHO II)
- Low FSH indicates hypogonadotropic hypogonadism. (WHO I)
- High FSH indicates ovarian failure. (WHO III)
- Normal FSH with no withdrawal bleed indicates absent uterus or outflow tract obstruction or Asherman's syndrome. (WHO V)
- Clinical examination:
  - Patient's height and weight are assessed for calculation of body mass index (BMI). (BMI = weight in kg/height^2 in meters.) Normal BMI is 20–25, less than 20 is considered underweight and more than 30 is considered frank obesity. These values are decided according to the western standards, but may differ marginally for the Indian standards. Anovulation is common in patients with abnormal BMI.
  - With obesity, PCOS must be considered, which is characterized by hirsutism and/or acne, acanthosis nigricans, dark

discoloration of skin in axilla and neck and waist circumference more than 35 inches or 90 cm. But it is important to remember here that these features will be seen only in full blown PCOS and there is a much larger percentage of infertile population that has silent forms or milder forms of PCOS.

– Body mass index less than 20 may be seen in thin lean PCOS, malnourishment or anorexia nervosa. Causes of primary amenorrhea and ovarian failures must also be ruled out by excluding the clinical presentation of estrogen deficiencies.

REFERENCES

1. Oogenesis: how the female reproductive system produces eggs, Chapter 16. CLEP Biology: Study Guide and Test Prep/Science Courses. Instructor: Joshua Anderson.
2. Lobo RA. Early ovarian ageing: a hypothesis. What is early ovarian ageing? Hum Reprod. 2003;18(9):1762-4.
3. Gilbert SF. The number of ova therefore decides the reserve of the ovary. In: Gilbert SF (Ed). Developmental Biology, 6th edition. Sunderland (MA): Sinauer Associates; 2000.
4. Chaudhary S, Deshpande A. Physiology of ovulation. In: Deshpande H (Ed). Practical Management of Ovulation Induction. New Delhi: Jaypee Brothers Medical Publishers (P) Ltd; 2016. p. 15
5. Chaudhary S, Deshpande A. Physiology of ovulation. In: Deshpande H (Ed). Practical Management of Ovulation Induction. New Delhi: Jaypee Brothers Medical Publishers (P) Ltd; 2016. p. 7.
6. Homburg R. Ovulation Induction and Controlled Ovarian Stimulation. Switzerland: Springer International Publishing; 2014. pp. 7-23.
7. Hiller SG. Current concepts of the roles of follicle stimulating hormone and luteinizing hormone in folliculogenesis. Hum Reprod. 1994;9:188-91.
8. Balasch J, Fabregues F. Is luteinizing hormone needed for optimal ovulation induction? Curr Opin Obstet Gynecol. 2002;14(3):265-74.
9. Shoham Z. The clinical therapeutic window for luteinizing hormone in controlled ovarian stimulation. Fertil Steril. 2002;14:265-74.
10. Kobayashi M, Nakano R, Ooshima A. Immunohistochemical localization of pituitary gonadotropins and gonadal steroids confirms the two cells two gonadotropins hypothesis of steroidogenesis in the human ovary. J Endocrinol. 1990;126:483-8.
11. Yamoto M, Shima K, Nakano R. Gonadotropin receptors in human ovarian follicles and corpora lutea throughout the menstrual cycle. Horm Res. 1992;37 Suppl 1:5-11.
12. Hughes E, Collins J, Vandekerckhove P. Gonadotropin-releasing hormone analogue as an adjunct to gonadotropin therapy for clomiphene-resistant polycystic ovarian syndrome. Cochrane Database Syst Rev. 2000;(2):CD000097.
13. Kupesic S, Kurjak A. Uterine and ovarian perfusion during the periovulatory period assessed by transvaginal colour Doppler. Fertil Steril. 1993;3:439-43.
14. Regulation of menstrual cycle. In: Speroff L, Fritz MA (Eds). Clinical Gynecologic Endocrinology and Infertility. Baltimore: Lippincott, Williams and Wilkins; 2012. p. 213.
15. Bourne T, Jurkovic D, Waterstone J, et al. Intrafollicular blood flow during human ovulation. Ultrasound Obstet Gynecol. 1991;1:53-9.
16. Scott RT, Hofmann GE. Prognostic assessment of ovarian reserve. Fertil Steril. 1995;63:1.
17. Krishnakumar J, Agarwal A, Nambiar D, et al. Comparison of antral follicle count, anti-Mullerian hormone and day 2 follicle-stimulating hormone as predictor of ovarian response and clinical pregnancy rate in patient with an abnormal ovarian reserve test. Int J Reprod Contracept Obstet Gynecol. 2016;5(8):2762-7.
18. Panchal S, Nagori CB. Comparison of anti-Mullerian hormone and antral follicle count for assessment of ovarian reserve. JHRS. 2012;5(3):274-8.

19. Jonard S, Robert Y, Dewailly D. Revisint the ovarian volume as diagnostic criterion for polycystic ovaries. Hum Reprod. 2005;20:2893-8.
20. Balen A, Conway G, Homburg R, et al. Polycystic Ovary Syndrome: A Guide to Clinical Management. Boca Raton: Taylor and Francis Group; 2007.
21. Panchal S, Nagori CB. Ultrasound based decision making on stimulation protocol for superovulated IUI cycles. IJIFM. 2016;7(1):7-13.
22. Panchal S, Nagori CB. Ultrasound Based decision making on stimulation protocol in IVF. DSJUOG. 2016;10(3):330-7.
23. Oyesanya OA, Parsons JH, Collins WP, et al. Total ovarian volume before human chorionic gonadotropin administration for ovulation induction may predict the hyperstimulation. Hum Reprod. 1995;10:3211-2.
24. Fanchin R, Maria SL, Righini C, et al. Serum AMH is more strongly related to ovarian follicle status that serum inhibin B, oestradiol, FSH and LH on the day 3. Hum Reprod. 2003;18:323-7.
25. Durlinger AL, Gruijters MJ, Kramer P, et al. Anti-Mullerian hormone attenuates the effect of FSH on follicle development in the mouse ovary. Endocrinology. 2001;142:4891-9.
26. La Marca A, Stabile G, Artenisio AC, et al. Serum anti-Mullerian hormone throughout the human menstrual cycle. Hum Reprod. 2006;21(12):3103-7.
27. Streuli J, Fraisse T, Chapron C, et al. Clinical uses of anti-Mullerian hormone assays: pitfalls and promises. Fertil Steril. 2009;91(1):226-30.
28. Pellat L, Rice S, Mason HD. Anti-Mullerian hormone and polycystic ovarian syndrome: a mountain too high? Reproduction. 2010;139:825-33.
29. Pellat L, Rice S, Dilaver N, et al. Anti-Mullerian hormone reduces follicle sensitivity to follicle-stimulating hormone in human granulosa cells. Fertil Steril. 2011;96:1246-51.
30. El Behery MM, Diab AE, Mowafy H, et al. Effect of laparoscopic ovarian drilling on vascular endothelial growth factor and ovarian stromal blood flow using three-dimensional power Doppler. Intern J Gynecol Obstet. 2011;112:119-21.
31. Abd El, Aal DE, Mohamed SA, et al. Vascular endothelial growth factor and insulin like growth factor 1 in polycystic ovary syndrome and their relation to ovarian blood flow. Eur J Obstet Gynecol Reprod Biol. 2005;118:219-24.
32. Willis D, Mason H, Gilling-Smith C, et al. Modulation by insulin of follicle-stimulating hormone and luteinizing hormone actions in human granulosa cells of normal and polycystic ovaries. J Clin Endocrinol Metab. 1996;81:302-9.
33. Pigny P, Merlen E, Robert Y, et al. Elevated serum level of anti-Mullerian hormone in patients with polycystic ovary syndrome: relationship to the ovarian follicle excess and to the follicular arrest. J Clin Endocrinol Metab. 2003;88:5957-62.
34. Pellat L, Hanna L, Brincat M, et al. Granulosa cell production of anti-Mullerian hormone is increased in polycystic ovaries. J Clin Endocrinol Metab. 2007;92:240-5.
35. Carlsen SH, Vanky E, Fleming R. Anti-Mullerian hormone concentrations in androgen suppressed women with polycystic ovary syndrome. Hum Reprod. 2009;24:1732-8.
36. Piltonen T, Morin-Papunen L, Koivunen R, et al. Serum anti-Mullerian hormone levels remain high until late reproductive age and decrease during metformin therapy in women with polycystic ovary syndrome. Hum Reprod. 2005;20(7):1820-6.
37. Gnoth C, Schuring AN, Friol K, et al. Relevance of anti-Mullerian hormone measurement in a routine IVF program. Hum Reprod. 2008;23:1359-65.
38. Nelson SM, Yates RW, Lyall H, et al. Anti-Mullerian hormone-based approach to controlled ovarian stimulation for assisted conception. Hum Reprod. 2009;24:867-75.
39. Weghofer A, Dietrich W, Barad DH, et al. Live birth chances in women with extremely low serum anti-Mullerian hormone levels. Hum Reprod. 2011;26(70):1905-9.
40. Fong SL, Schippe I, de Jong FH, et al. Serum anti-Mullerian hormone and inhibin B concentrations are not useful predictors of ovarian response during ovulation induction treatment with rFSH in women with polycystic ovary syndrome. Fertil Steril. 2011;96(2):459-63.

41. Mashiach R, Amit A, Hasson J, et al. Follicular fluid levels of anti-Mullerian hormone as a predictor of oocyte maturation, fertilization rate, and embryonic development in patients with polycystic ovarian syndrome. Fertil Steril. 2010;93(7):2299-302.

42. Loh JS, Maheshwari A. Anti-Mullerian Hormone—is it a crystal ball for predicting ovarian ageing? Human Reprod. 2011;26(11): 2925-32.

43. Panchal S, Nagori CB. Correlation of ovarian and stromal volumes to fasting and postprandial insulin levels in polycystic ovarian syndrome patients. Int J Infertil Fetal Med. 2014;5(1):12-4.

44. Filicori M, Butler JP, Crowley WF. Neuroendocrine regulation of the corpus luteum in the human. Evidence for pulsatile progesterone secretion. J Clin Invest. 1984;73:1638-47.

45. Syrop CH, Hammond MG. Diurnal variations in midluteal serum progesterone measurements. Fertil Steril. 1987;47:67-70.

46. Jordan J, Craig K, Clifton DK, et al. Luteal phase defect: the sensitivity and specificity of diagnostic methods in common clinical use. Fertil Steril. 1994;62:54-62.

47. Miller PB, Soules MR. The usefulness of a urinary LH kit ovulation prediction during menstrual cycles of normal women. Obstet Gynecol. 1996;87:13-7.

48. Duggan MA, Brashert P, Ostor A, et al. The accuracy and interobserver reproducibility of endometrial dating. Pathology. 2001;33:292-7.

49. Wathen NC, Perry L, Lilford RJ, et al. Interpretation of single progesterone measurement in diagnosis of anovulation and defective luteal phase: observations on analysis of the normal range. Br Med J. 1984;288:7-9.

50. Dickey RP, Olar TT, Taylor SN, et al. Relationship of biochemical pregnancy to preovulatory endometrial thickness and pattern in patients undergoing ovulation induction. Hum Reprod. 1993;8:327-30.

51. Kupesic S, Kurjak A. Prediction of IVF outcome by three-dimensional ultrasound. Hum Reprod. 2002;17:950-5.

52. Kupesic S, Bekavac I, Bjelos D, et al. Assessment of endometrial receptivity by transvaginal colour Doppler and three-dimensional power Doppler ultrasonography in patients undergoing in vitro fertilization procedures. J Ultrasound Med. 2001;20(2):125-34.

53. Bald R, Hackeloer BJ. Ultraschall-darstellung verschiendener endometrium for men. In: Otto R. Jan FX (Eds). Ultraschalldiagnostik 1982. Stuttgart: Thieme; 1983. pp. 187.

54. Lujan ME, Jarrett BY, Brooks ED, et al. Updated ultrasound criteria for polycystic ovary syndrome: reliable thresholds for elevated follicle population and ovarian volume. Hum Reprod. 2013;28(5):1361-8.

2   Assessing Ovarian Reserve

Chaitanya Nagori

INTRODUCTION

Assessment of the ovarian reserve is necessary to decide the line of treatment amongst various assisted reproductive technologies (ART) available. Late marriages, career oriented women, and delay in obstetric career are the factors responsible for decrease in ovarian reserve in the fertility desiring females. Knowledge regarding ovarian reserve can change the management of individual patient stimulation protocols are adjusted, treatments may be refused, advanced or postponed accordingly.[1]

PHYSIOLOGY

The number of ova in the female fetus at 20 weeks of intrauterine age is 6–7 millions and is decreased to approximately 2 million at birth. At puberty the number decreases to approximately 3–4 lacs. Fertility decreases after the age of 30 years when numbers of follicles are as low as approximately 25,000 only. After the age of 35 years, the prevalence of infertility sharply increases and when the woman reaches the age of 40 years, approximately only 8,000 ova are available for recruitment. After the age of 45 years, 99% of women are expected to be infertile.[2] Antral follicle count (AFC) showed the best correlation with women's age and declined linearly at a rate of 3.8% per year.[3]

Another study has indicated a biphasic pattern of AFC decline. It was documented as 4.8% per year before the age of 37 years compared with 11.7% per annum thereafter.[4]

The number of quantity and quality of the follicles in the ovary thus remaining determine the ovarian reserve.[5]

When number of ova drops to less than 1,000, menopause occurs. The age of menopause varies between 40 years and 60 years with an average age of 51 years. But after the age of 42 years, fertility of the female decreases drastically.[6]

Number of ova available:
- At 20 weeks: 6–7 million
- At birth: 2 million
- At puberty: 3–4 hours
- After 30 years: 25,000
- After 40 years: 8,000
- At menopause: <1,000

DEFINITION

The ovarian reserve is the capacity of the ovaries to produce fertilizable ova. This depends on the quality and quantity of ovarian antral and preantral follicles.[5]

OVARIAN RESERVE NEEDS TO BE ASSESSED[7]

- Females of more than 35 years of age.
- Females with unexplained infertility and in females who have had a previous cycle of ovulation induction with gonadotropins and had a poor response.
- In the females who have a history of ovarian surgery in the past.
- Smokers.
- Females who have maternal relations with early menopause. In these females the ovarian reserve assessment needs to be done at an age much earlier than 35 years as they may be genetically predisposed to low ovarian reserve and early ovarian failure. These females need special advise for advancement of fertility treatment.
- But it should be emphasized that decrease in ovarian reserve does not mean inability to conceive.[7]

Though it is important to mention here that at this stage the pattern of reproductive ageing as assessed by hormonal and ultrasonographic ovarian reserve tests does not appear to show an abrupt change at a certain age, but follows a continuously increasing rate of decline in the third decade of life. The changes in serum follicle-stimulating hormone (FSH) levels and ultrasonographic ovarian reserve tests follow a quadratic model in regularly menstruating women.[8]

As no test is perfect to comment on fertility potential and plan of treatment, evaluation by combination of tests may be required for the assessment of ovarian reserve.[8] All the ovarian reserve tests are considered as screening tests and abnormal tests should be confirmed by another tests.[7]

OVARIAN RESERVE TESTS

Ovarian reserve can be assessed by various clinical, biochemical or ultrasound features and these are known as markers of ovarian reserve. These can be divided under three heads.

- Clinical markers
- Endocrinal markers
- Ultrasound markers.

Clinical Markers

- Age
- Menstrual pattern.

Age

It has been already discussed earlier in this chapter that advancing age decreases the ovarian reserve due to apoptosis. This means that age is the most consistent factor that decides the quantity of the ova in the ovary. Moreover the quality of the ova available has also been negatively correlated with the increasing age.

But chronological age and ovarian age are not always correlating. A young woman may have low ovarian reserve and a woman of 40 years may also have several antral follicles in her ovaries. Therefore, other tests of ovarian reserve are required for assessment of ovarian reserve and deciding the line of treatment.

The monthly fecundity rate is about 20% in young couple desiring pregnancy but not undergoing treatment. With increasing age, fecundity decreases and may take longer time to achieve conception. Society of Assisted Reproductive Treatment (SART) and Centers for Disease Control and Prevention (CDC) have constantly demonstrated that age is the single most important factor affecting the probability of success of in vitro fertilization (IVF).

This is because twenty four percent of oocytes in a woman of less than 35 years will be chromosomally abnormal, but this number reaches 52% at the age of 35 years. After 40 years, more than 90% of the oocytes are abnormal.[9] At the age of 30 years, 75% of the women are expected to conceive naturally within a year, while only 66% will do so at the age of 35 years. So age is an important criteria to decide the fertility potential of a woman.[10]

Chronological age is more related to quality of the ova rather than increased FSH. Young women with high FSH may give good ova, but old women with low FSH have a high chance of aneuploidy in the ova. This means that the abnormal tests in younger patients have poor prognosis, but normal tests do not improve the age related poor prognosis in older patients.

Menstrual Pattern

Length of the menstrual cycle depends on the length of the follicular phase. Length of the normal cycle is 21–35 days (28 days—mean) of which the length of the luteal phase is constant (14 days). There will be high FSH and low serum inhibin B level in these patients. This is common as age advances.[11] This may be responsible for faster follicular growth and short cycles but may also be the cause of more aneuploid ova.

Endocrinal Tests

These may be divided under two heads:
- Static tests:
  - Day 2 or 3 S FSH (serum FSH)
  - Day 2 or 3 S E2 (serum estradiol)
  - Day 3 S FSH and S LH (serum luteinizing hormone)
  - Inhibin B
  - Anti-Müllerian hormone (AMH).

- Dynamic tests:
  - Clomiphene citrate challenge test (CCCT)
  - Gonadotropin-releasing hormone analogue stimulation test (GAST)
  - Exogenous FSH ovarian reserve test (EFORT).

Day 2 or 3 Follicle-stimulating Hormone

Follicle-stimulating hormone level in serum when is assessed, it must be combined and correlated with estrogen. This is because there is a negative feedback system between FSH and estrogen. On day 2–3 all follicles in the ovary are small (antral) so the estrogen level is low and FSH levels at this stage are at their baseline levels. Normal FSH with low E2 indicates normal hypothalamo-pituitary-gonadal axis. The level of FSH increases with increasing age due to falling basal estrogen levels and indicates low ovarian reserve. Fluctuations in the serum FSH levels in different cycles also indicate diminished ovarian reserve.[12]

Normal basal FSH is less than 10 mIU/mL (Table 2.1). Levels between 10 mIU/mL and 15 mIU/mL are considered borderline. The ovarian reserve is predicted as very low when the level of FSH is more than 15 mIU/mL. But it has a poor predictive value for nonpregnancy. No single cutoff of S.FSH has been established to predict nonpregnancy. Therefore, cycle cancellation should not be advised only on the ground of high serum FSH levels.

TABLE 2.1: Correlation of follicle-stimulating hormone (FSH) level and response to ovulation induction drugs.

FSH level	Response
<8 mIU/mL	Reassure
8–12 mIU/mL	Average reserve
12–17 mIU/mL	Decreased ovarian reserve
>17 mIU/mL	Extremely poor pregnancy rates

Though a recent study has demonstrated 100% specificity for failure to achieve a live birth at FSH values above 18 mIU/mL.[13]

Follicle-stimulating hormone is released from anterior pituitary in a pulsatile manner and also has circadian variations. Moreover isoforms of FSH are also known and there may be fluctuations in these also. This may lead to variable results when serum FSH levels are assessed at different times in the same patient. Single nucleotide polymorphism in FSH receptive gene may have normal FSH with poor response. Single nucleotide polymorphisms (SNPs) at 307 and 680 are common.[14]

In this case, it is best to consider the highest value of S.FSH (when FSH is assesssed several times in a single female) for the decision making and counseling with the patient for fertility treatment planning. What ever is the ovarian response, pregnancy rates are poor with high serum FSH levels.

Day 2 or 3 Serum Estradiol

Estradiol is secreted from granulosa cells and reflects the follicular activity.

High E2 level on day 2–3 of the menstrual cycle indicates early follicular recruitment. This is reflected on ultrasound as a follicle of 10 mm or larger on day 2–3 of the cycle. This is because of high basal FSH. Cycle cancellation is much higher in IVF cycles when E2 is 80 pg/mL or more or 20 pg/mL or less on day 2-3 of the menstrual cycle.[15] Day 2 FSH and E2 have high predictive value for ovarian reserve, and when both are high indicates poor ovarian reserve.[16] But it must be remembered here that high E2 may mask an abnormal FSH concentration in a patient with diminished ovarian reserve due to negative feed back mechanism.

In patients with polycystic ovarian syndrome (PCOS), E2 level on day 2 is high because of cumulative E2 produced from granulosa cells of multiple small follicles. E2 level alone therefore is never used as a sole marker for ovarian reserve.

Follicle-stimulating Hormone/ Luteinizing Hormone Ratio

High FSH/LH ratio indicates poor ovarian reserve. FSH rises earlier than LH and frequent measurements may diagnose this rise earlier. FSH/LH ratio is an early indicator of ovarian aging and rising FSH/LH ratio could be the first marker of ovarian aging and decreased ovarian reserve.[17]

Inhibin B

It is secreted from small antral follicles and selectively inhibits FSH release. As the number of eggs decreases with advancing age, it will lower inhibin B level which in turn gives higher FSH value because of negative feedback mechanism. Decrease in Inhibin B occurs earlier than rise in FSH with decreasing ovarian reserve, but inhibin B assays are variable, requires validation and there is cycle to cycle variability.[18] This is why it is not used as a routine investigation for evaluation of ovarian reserve.

Though, Inhibin B measurement in early stages of the ovarian stimulation provides useful information in making decision to cancel the cycle or to modulate the doses of gonadotropin. The level more than 45 pg/mL on day 2–3 is indicative of hyper-response to ovulation induction.

Anti-Müllerian Hormone

It is known as anti-mullerian hormone because it prevents development of the Müllerian duct when expressed in males from testis. In females, AMH is produced by granulosa cells of primordial, preantral, and small antral follicles[19] to inhibit the early stages of follicular development. Its expression is maintained till the follicle is 6 mm in diameter, beyond which follicles grow under the effect of FSH. It is not expressed in atretic follicles, dominant follicles or corpus lutea. Therefore AMH is considered to be reflective of FSH independent follicular growth.

Physiology of anti-Müllerian hormone: The function of AMH is to modulate primordial follicle recruitment. It inhibits the action of FSH on the follicular growth and selection of dominance of the follicles. The function of AMH is inhibition of initial recruitment of primordial follicles and inhibits the activity of granulosa cells and decreases if follicular growth starts with FSH stimulation.[20-22] So AMH is a negative regulator of follicular growth and reduces follicular sensitivity to FSH. FSH exerts negative influence on AMH secretion in small follicles.[23] AMH reflects quantitative and qualitative assessment of ovarian reserve. AMH level helps in counseling the woman before chemotherapy as it can predict menopause. Its level becomes negligible, 5 years before actual menopause. It is undetectable before puberty and when the primordial follicle enters the preantral stage, production of AMH starts (follicle size of 2–6 mm). When follicle starts growing AMH decreases and that is because of decrease in the primordial pool. High androgen causes anovulation and anovulatory ovary produces more AMH. Hyperinsulinemia also increases androgen secretion which in turn increases serum AMH and anovulation as is observed in patients with polycystic ovarian syndrome (PCOS). Metformin (insulin sensitizer) decreases AMH concentration.[24] There is inverse correlation between E2 and AMH in follicular fluid of small antral follicle, so AMH and FSH activity are interdependent. More than 3.5 ng/mL level of AMH predicts excessive response in those three studies.[25]

The AMH level is constant throughout the menstrual cycle, except that it has lower thresholds in late luteal phase. In poor reserve patients AMH level varies from 0.5 ng/mL to 1.1 ng/mL (ng/mL × 7.14 = pmol/mL) but low level of AMH alone can not be used as a single parameter to deny fertility treatment for the patient. Higher doses of gonadotropins are not much useful in decreased ovarian response but flare up protocol and addition of LH can improve the results. These protocols will be discussed later in this book. Normal AMH has good prognosis and they are normal responders. High AMH indicates exaggerated response after gonadotropin stimulation. So low dose protocol will be useful in these patients to avoid ovarian hyperstimulation syndrome (OHSS) as well as to improve implantation rates because of lower steroids.

In hypogonadotropic hypogonadism patients, AMH concentration increases in consecutive cycles after human menopausal gonadotropin (HMG) stimulation because of stimulation of FSH dependent follicles. So AMH has a limitation that it only reflects the growing follicular pool, responsive to gonadotropin and may not be reflecting underlying primordial pool.

Actions of AMH are as follows:
- Inhibition of follicular activation and growth
- Inhibition of FSH dependent growth
- Inhibition of granulosa cell growth
- Inhibition of aromatase
- Inhibition of recruitment of primordial follicles in pool of growing follicle
- Decreases follicular sensitivity to gonadotropin stimulation to control follicular growth.

Normal values of AMH and its interpretation (Table 2.2):
- *Extremely low levels:* Less than 1 pmol/L [diagnostic systems laboratory (DSL)] or less than 1.1 pmol/L (Gen II assay). These patients are poor responders and cycle cancellation rates are very high. These patients may be offered ovum donation.

TABLE 2.2: Normal values of anti-Müllerian hormone (AMH) and its interpretation.

Gen II	DSL-AMH in pmol/L	Interpretation
<1.1	<1	Cancel cycle-ovum donation
1.1–6.9	1–5	Poor response
7.0–20	5–15	Adequate response
>20	>15	Chances of hyperstimulation

(DSL: diagnostic systems laboratory)

- *Low levels*: 1–5 pmol/L (DSL) or between 1.1 pmol/L and 6.9 pmol/L in Gen II assay. These patients are poor responders and have decreased ovarian reserve and less number of ova can be retrieved when they are stimulated for IVF. In these cases, high doses of FSH should be used, may be maximum permissible maximum and antagonist protocol should be used.
- *Normal levels*: 5–15 pmol/L (DSL) and it is 7–20 pmol/L by Gen II assay. These are normal responders. In these cases agonist protocol is used and maximum dose of FSH required is 225 IU/day for IVF patients.
- *High level*: AMH is more than 15 pmol/L (DSL) or more than 20 pmol/L (gen II assay). These patients are hyper-responders. According to Faddy et al and Nelson et al. Maximum dose used in these patients is 150 IU daily. But even lower doses and antagonist protocols are preferred.[26,27]

Anti-Müllerian hormone assays: Formerly two companies having different immunoassays were marketing the kits for AMH assessment. One was DSL and other one was IOT (Immunotech branded as Beckman Coulter). IOT had 4–5 times higher values than DSL. This is why there was a confusion and low reliability of the results for AMH assessment

numbers and units. Fortunately the two companies have consolidated now and single new commercially available assay the Gen II enzyme linked immune-absorbent assay is made available and that has replaced DSL and IOT. Now the new assay is reported as ng/mL like IOT.

Anti-Müllerian hormone immunoassays:
- DSL: P mol/mL
- IOT: (ng/mL)
  ng/mL × 7.14 = pmol/mL
- Combination of both Gen II Eliza: (ng/mL).

Though AMH assessment done during ovarian stimulation gives erroneous results therefore it must always be assessed only before ovulation induction is started. With chronic low dose protocol, FSH administration mimics the natural cycle and significant decrease in AMH is observed till the day of follicular dominance.[28] In IVF cycles with multifollicular development, there is decreased AMH because of decrease in number of small follicles.[27] Assessing AMH during ovarian stimulation is not useful. It is also not justified[7] as a routine screening test for decreased ovarian reserve in low risk population.

The AMH is a negative regulator of follicular growth and reduces follicular sensitivity to FSH. FSH exerts negative influence on AMH secretion in small follicles.[23] There is no significant difference between the performance of AMH and AFC in predicting the oocyte yield, however both have a false positive rate of 10–20%.[30]

Clinical uses of anti-Müllerian hormone:
- To confirm presence of testicular tissue in children.
- D/D of patients with intersex disorders.
- In patients with nonpalpable gonads.
- In granulosa cell tumors, it is elevated.
- For diagnosis of PCOS. AMH is increased due to hyperandrogenism and

hyperinsulinemia. But according to the new amendments in the Rotterdam criteria, done in July 2018, AMH can not be used as the only criteria to diagnose PCOS.

- Metformin reduces AMH concentration and so treatment efficacy can be evaluated for insulin sensitizers.
- High AMH in older patients indicate sustained reproductive life span.
    - It helps in deciding stimulation protocol
    - Can be used as a hormone contraception
    - AMH antagonist can be used in PCOS.

Endocrine Dynamic Tests

Clomiphene citrate challenge test: The test is based on the fact that clomiphene citrate, when given for ovulation induction, will stimulate the follicle to produce more inhibin and E2 that will in turn lower FSH on day 10.

Basal level of serum FSH is assessed on day 3 and then is repeated on day 10 after clomiphene citrate challenge (CC) stimulation. Higher value of FSH (more than 10 mIU/mL) either on day 3 or on day 10 indicates diminished ovarian reserve. The total of both values more than 26 IU indicates poor reserve.[29,31] Normally LH rises more than FSH after clomiphene stimulation. But in patients with low reserve FSH rises more than LH. The speculated mechanism is that, smaller follicles produce less inhibin B and less E2, resulting in less negative feedback to FSH that is released due to clomiphene stimulation.[32,33]

This test does not have a high prognostic value as there is no standardized definition of abnormal test. Because of availability of better tests like AFC and AMH, this test is routinely not used.[34]

Normally LH rises more than FSH after clomiphene stimulation. But in patients with low reserve, FSH rises more than LH. The mechanism thought of is that smaller follicles produce less inhibin β and less E2, resulting in less negative feedback inhibition to FSH. Release on clomiphene induced pituitary FSH release.[33,34]

Gonadotropin releasing hormone analog stimulation test: In this test gonadotropin-releasing hormone (GnRh) agonist (leuprolide acetate 1 mg) is given subcutaneously. This causes massive release of FSH and LH from the pituitary which in turn increases the production of E2 from the follicles within 24 hours time frame. This increase in E2 level (twice the baseline level) or flare up of E2 level in response to stimulation indicates early development of follicles, indicating good ovarian reserve.[34,35] But it lacks in standardization in terms of type of the drug, dose and timing, etc. Therefore this test is not used routinely in clinical practice.

Exogenous follicle-stimulating hormone ovarian reserve test: 300 IU of recombinant FSH (rFSH) is given to a patient on day 3 of the cycle. After 24 hours E2 and inhibin levels are assessed. Increase in E2, more than 30 pg/mL is predictive of good response.[26,36]

This test like CCCT and GAST is far from uniform and not used in clinical practice.

This means that no dynamic tests can be used at present in routine practice. These are not better than basal tests and these cannot predict nonpregnancy in any patient.

Ultrasound Markers

- Ovarian volume
- Antral follicle count
- Ovarian blood flow.

Ovarian Volume

Ovarian volume can be measured by B mode or by three-dimensional (3D) ultrasound. To assess it on B mode, the ovary is located first.

The probe is rotated to find the long axis of the ovary. The probe is then spanned across the long axis of the ovary to find the longest section of the ovary. Now the probe is rotated 90° to get a true transverse section of the ovary. On the long axis section measure the largest longitudinal diameter, and AP diameter of the ovary perpendicular as the largest diameter perpendicular to the longitudinal diameter and measure the transverse diameter on the transverse section. The volume is calculated as D1 × D2 × D3 × 0.523.[37,38] Three dimensional ultrasound is recommended for more accurate volume calculation. It has low interobserver and intraobserver variability. 3 cc is taken as a lower cutoff for a normal reserve ovary. Ovarian volume of less than 3 cc was significantly predictive of more than 50% cancellation rates in IVF cycles.[39] But this has poor predictive value for response to ovulation induction and possibility of pregnancy.[40]

Ovarian volume of more than 10cc indicates a possibility of PCOS and may require lower stimulating dose for ovulation induction. But ovarian volume alone is not predictive of ovarian reserve.

Antral Follicle Count

Antral follicle count is defined as the total number of follicles seen in both ovaries, up to 9 mm in diameter, detected by transvaginal ultrasound (TVS) in early follicular phase (day 2–3 of the menstrual cycle). AFC can predict hyperstimulation as well as poor response after gonadotropin stimulation. Low AFC predicts poor response. AFC is also used to predict hyper-response and thus using safe and successful stimulation regimes and to prevent OHSS.[41]

Antral follicle count is found to be as effective as AMH in determining ovarian response.[30,42] Smaller follicles (between 2 mm

and 6 mm) decline in number with age and these indicate real ovarian reserve.[43]

Antral follicle count is a better marker than day 3 FSH, E2, and inhibin.[44] Another study concludes that AFC and AMH both correlate with each other, but have independent significance for estimating follicles larger than 12 mm on the day of ovulation trigger. For ova retrieved on ovum pickup (OPU), in PCOS group both AMH and AFC have similar significance.[45] AFC can be correlated to the quality as well as quantity of the oocytes.[46] AFC has low intercycle as well as interobserver variability. Intercycle variability is more significant in young woman when AFC is higher. Low AFC with ovulatory cycle does not indicate poor reserve. 3D is extremely useful for counting antral follicles. Inversion mode rendering is most convenient when follicles are multiple.

Anti-Müllerian hormone and Antral follicle count: Receiver operating characteristic curves showed high accuracy for AMH and AFC for the prediction of poor ovarian response but limited accuracy for nonpregnancy prediction. These data does not show a better predictive ability than AFC.[42,47,48] For prediction of poor ovarian response a model including AFC + AMH was found to be almost similar to that of (p value 0.001) using AFC alone.[38] Our own study on comparison of AFC and AMH for assessment of ovarian reserve also concluded that AFC alone may suffice as a test for assessing the ovarian reserve.[46]

Antral follicle count has low intercycle as well as interobserver variability. Though, intercycle variability is more significant in young women when AFC is high. Low AFC with ovulatory cycle does not indicate poor reserve. 3D is extremely useful for counting antral follicles and Sono automated volume calculation (AVC) is the most convenient and accurate amongst all. More exact value of AFC was acquired when counted by 3D ultrasound. Number of follicles more than 12 mm on day of oocyte retrieval correlated significantly with AFC counted by 3D ultrasound rather than 2D ultrasound. Inversion mode with Sono AVC is most convenient method for counting antral follicles when they are multiple.[49]

Ovarian Blood Flow

- Ovarian blood flow as a predictor of IVF outcome was assessed by many workers. Though another study shows ovarian stromal peak systolic velocity (PSV) after pituitary suppression is predictive of ovarian responsiveness and outcome of IVF treatment.[50] Kupesic et al. have shown correlation in the ovarian stromal flow index (FI) and number of mature oocytes retrieved in an IVF cycle and pregnancy rates. Stromal FI (<11 low responder, 11–14 good, >15 risk of OHSS).[51] *Total number of antral follicles achieved the best predictive value for favorable IVF outcome, followed by ovarian stromal FI, total ovarian stromal area and total ovarian volume.*[51]

Measurement of ovarian stromal flow in early follicular phase is related to subsequent ovarian response in IVF treatment.[52] *Total ovarian vascularization index (VI), and vascularization flow index (VFI) were significantly lower in women aged more than and equal to 41 years.*[49]

But it was not found to be accurate and it cannot predict future fertility. It can only predict response to IVF treatment.

The ovarian volume, AFC and VI, FI and VFI determined by 3D power Doppler, all have excellent intraobserver and interobserver reproducibility.[53]

Table 2.3 presents finding of our unpublished study.

It is essential to mention here that AFC, ovarian volume, and ovarian 3D power

TABLE 2.3: 3D PD indices in PCOS, normal and poor response ovaries.

Index	PCOS	Normal	Poor responding
VI	5–10	2–5	<2
VFI	2–3	1–2	<0.5

(PCOS: polycystic ovarian syndrome; VFI: vascularization flow index; VI: vascularization index)

Doppler flow indices did not significantly change after a short-term treatment of GnRH agonist for pituitary downregulation[54] and can therefore be reliably used for downregulated as well as nondownregulated cycles for assessment of ovarian response.

CLINICAL APPLICATIONS

Anti-Müllerian hormone and AFC are most widely used tests. These can assess the ovarian reserve quantitatively and qualitatively. No significant difference is observed between the two in terms of accuracy. Both may contribute and act synergistically.[55]

The new ovarian response predictive index (ORPI) has been presented based on age, AMH, and AFC.[56] It is calculated as AMH × AFC/patient's age. This can be positively correlated to number of oocytes retrieved and metaphase II stage (MII) oocytes collected.

We decide the stimulation protocol based on the parameters like AFC, ovarian volume, ovarian stromal resistance index (RI), ovarian stromal PSV, stromal FI, age, and body mass index (BMI). The calculation can be simplified as given in Table 2.4.[57]

To select the correct stimulation protocol, doses are titrated depending on findings present in a particular patient from high-dose table or low-dose table.

INTEGRATED PREDICTORS (TABLE 2.5)

La Marca et al. developed an ORPI. This is based on age, AMH, and AFC. ORPI less than

TABLE 2.4: Calculation of ovarian response predictive index.

	Increase the dose when..	Decrease the dose when..
Age	>35 years	<25 years
BMI	>28 kg/m^2	<20 kg/m^2
AFC	<3 (FNPO)	>12 (FNPO)
Stromal RI	>0.7	<0.5
Stromal PSV	<5 cm/sec	>10 cm/sec
Stromal FI	<11	>15
Ovarian volume	< 3cc	>10 cc

(AFC: antral follicle count; BMI: body mass index; FI: flow index; FNPO: follicle number per ovary; PSV: peak systolic blood flow velocity; RI: resistance index)

TABLE 2.5: Summary of ovarian reserve tests.

Ovarian reserve test	Favorable result	Unfavorable result
Age (in years)	<35	>35
FSH (IU/L)	<10	>10
Day 3 E2 (pg/mL)	<75	>75
Day 10 progesterone	<0.9	>1.1
AMH (p/mol/L)	15.7–48.5	<15.7
Day 3 inhibin B (pg/mL)	>45	<45
AFC	>5	<5
Ovarian vascularity	Lower PI	Higher PI
Ovarian volume (cc)	>3	<3
CCCT (FSH only- IU/L)	<12	>12
GAST	Early E2 flare	Persistent high E2/no response

(AFC: antral follicle count; AMH: anti-Müllerian hormone; CCCT: clomiphene citrate challenge test; E2: estradiol; FSH: follicle-stimulating hormone; GAST: gonadotropin-releasing hormone analogue stimulation test; PI: predictive index)

0.2 has 86% sensitivity and 89% specificity in predicting poor ovarian response (<3 oocytes), with 88% efficacy. ORPI more than 0.9 has same sensitivity, specificity, and 82% efficacy in prediction of high response (>15 follicles).[58]

Another study has recently been published in which a scoring system has been devised based on the ultrasound parameters, ovarian volume, AFC, ovarian stromal RI and ovarian stromal PSV with age and BMI[59] and has shown zero severe ovarian hyperstimulation (OHSS) rate, very low incidence of mild OHSS and acceptable multiple pregnancy rates.

BOLOGNA CRITERIA[60]

European Society of Human Reproduction and Embryology (ESHRE) group has come to the consensus that out of three, two criteria should be present to define poor ovarian reserve for future research.

- Maternal age more than 40 years or other risk factors for poor ovarian reserve (genetic or acquired conditions).
- Previous history of less than 3 oocytes with a conventional stimulation protocol.
- Abnormal ovarian reserve test, i.e. AFC less than 5–7 or AMH less than 0.5–1.1 ng/mL.

Many patients, above 40 years of age, may be infertile, though the menstrual cycles are normal. So the patient with good reserve benefit better with IVF and should be offered IVF if AFC is good.[61]

GENETIC PREDICTORS

Single nucleotide polymorphism in gonadotropins and its receptors is not associated with change in ovarian reserve. But some polymorphism in FSH receptors (FSHR) particularly Ser680 genotype are related with resistance to FSH stimulation. These patients require high doses of FSH in spite of other ovarian reserve markers being normal.[45,62] These observations require further validation by larger studies.

CARRY HOME MESSAGE

- All ovarian reserve tests are considered as screening tests and abnormal test result should be confirmed by another test.
- No test or combined test can predict nonpregnancy.
- Age is the single reliable factor.
- Short follicular phase indicates diminishing ovarian reserve (DOR).
- Day 2–3 FSH more than 12–15 indicates DOR.
- Day 2 E2 more than 80 pg/mL indicates DOR.
- FSH/LH ratio if high indicates DOR.
- Inhibin B > 45 pg/mL indicates good reserve.
- CCCT, GAST, and EFORT are not used in clinical practice.
- AMH is extremely reliable for counseling (5–15 pmol/L indicates good reserve).
- Ovarian volume is as reliable as AMH and AFC more than 5 indicates normal reserve.
- Stromal flow decides the doses required and response to stimulation.
- AMH and AFC both are equally reliable, synergistic, and show no difference between the performances.

REFERENCES

1. Ventura SJ, Mosher WD, Curtin SC, et al. Trends in pregnancy rates for the United States 1976-97: an update. Nat Vital Stat Rep. 2001:49:1-9.
2. Menken J, Trusell J, Larsen U. Age and Infertility. Science. 1986;233(4771):1389-94.
3. Ng EHY, Yeung WSB, Fong DYT, et al. Effects of age on hormonal and ultrasound markers of ovarian reserve in Chinese women with proven fertility. Hum Reprod. 2003;18(10):2169-74.
4. Scheffer GJ, Broekmans FJM, Dorland M, et al. Antral follicle counts by transvaginal ultrasonography are related to age in women with proven natural fertility. Fertil Steril. 1999;72:845-51.
5. Broekmans FJ, Kwee J, Hendriks DJ, et al. A systematic review of tests predicting ovarian reserve and IVF outcome. Hum Reprod Update. 2006;12:685-718.
6. Van Noord-Zaadstra BM, Looman CW, Alsbach H, et al. Delaying childbearing: effect of age on fecundity and outcome of pregnancy. BMJ. 1991;302:1361-5.
7. Practice committee of American Society for Reproductive Medicine. Testing and interpreting measures of ovarian reserve: a committee opinion. Fertil Steril. 2012;98:1407-15.
8. Tufan E, Elter K, Durmusoglu F. Assessment of reproductive ageing patterns by hormonal and ultrasonographic ovarian reserve tests. Hum Reprod. 2004;19(11):2484-9.
9. Alvin ST, Lim BS, Maurine FH, et al. Age related decline in fertility: A link to degenerative oocytes? Fertil Steril. 1997;68:265-71.
10. Leridon H. Can assisted reproduction technology compensate for natural decline in fertility with age? A model assessment. Hum Reprod. 2004;19:1548-53.
11. Van Zonneveld P, Scheffer GJ, Broekmans FJ, et al. Do cycle disturbances explain the age related decline of female fertility? Cycle characteristics of women aged over 40 years compared with a reference population of young women. Hum Reprod. 2003;18(3):495-501.
12. Perloe M, Levy DP, Sills ES. Strategies for ascertaining ovarian reserve among women suspected of subfertility. In J Fertil Womens Med. 2000;45:215-24.
13. Scott RT Jr, Elkind-Hirch KE, Styne Gross A, et al. The predictive value for in vitro fertility delivery rates is greatly impacted by the method used to select the threshold between normal and elevated basal FSH. Fertil Steril. 2008;89:868-78.
14. Oschsenkuhn R, von Schonfeldt V, Simoni M. FSH receptor polymorphisms and ovarian function. Gynécologie Endocrinologie. 2009;11(4):265-70.
15. Frattarelli JL, Bergh PA, Drews MR, et al. Evaluation of basal oestradiol levels in assisted reproductive technology cycles. Fertil Steril. 2000;74(3):518-24.

16. de Carvalho BR, Rosa E, Rosa E, et al. Use of ovarian reserve markers and variables of response to gonadotropic stimulus as predictors of embryo implantation in ICSI cycles. J Brasileiro de Reproducao Assistida. 2009;13(3):26-9.

17. Mukherjee T, Copperman AB, Lapinski R, et al. An elevated day three follicle-stimulating hormone: luteinizing hormone ratio (FSH:LH) in the presence of a normal day 3 FSH predicts a poor response to controlled ovarian hyperstimulation. Fertil Steril. 1996;65:588-93.

18. Al-Azemi M, Killick SR, Duffy S, et al. Multi-marker assessment of ovarian reserve predicts oocyte yield after ovulation induction. Hum Reprod. 2011;26(2):414-22.

19. Visser JA, de Jong FH, Laven JS, et al. Anti-Müllerian hormone: a new marker for ovarian function. Reproduction. 2006;131:1-9.

20. Durlinger AL, Visser JA, Themmen AP. Regulation of ovarian function: the role of anti- Müllerian hormone. Reproduction. 2002;124:601-9.

21. Di Clemente N, Goxe B, Remy JJ, et al. Inhibitory effect of AMH upon aromatase activity and LH receptors of granulosa cells of rat and porcine immature ovaries. Endocrine. 1994;2:553-8.

22. Josso N, di Clemente N, Gouedard L. Anti-Müllerian hormone and its receptors. Mol Cell Endocrinol. 2001;179:25-32.

23. Anderson CY, Byskov AG. Estradiol and regulation of anti-Müllerian hormone, inhibin A and inhibin B secretion: analysis of small antral and preovulatory human follicles' fluid. J Clin Endocrinol Metab. 2006;91:4064-9.

24. Piltonen T, Morin Papunen L, Koivunen R, et al. Serum anti-Müllerian hormone levels remain high until late reproductive age and decrease during metformin therapy in women with polycystic ovary syndrome. Hum Reprod. 2005;20(7):1820-6.

25. La Marca A, Sighinolfi G, Radi D, et al. Anti-Müllerian hormone (AMH) as a predictive marker in assisted reproductive technique (ART). Hum Reprod Update. 2010;16:113-30.

26. Faddy MJ, Gosden RG, Gougeon A, et al. Accelerated disappearance of ovarian follicles in mid-life: implications for forecasting menopause. Hum Reprod. 1992;7(10):1342-6.

27. Nelson SM, Yates RW, Fleming R. Serum anti-Müllerian hormone and FSH: prediction of live birth and extremes of response in stimulated cycles-implications for individualization of therapy. Hum Reprod. 2007;22:2414-21.

28. Catteau-Jonard S, Pigny P, Reyss AC, et al. Changes in serum anti-Müllerian hormone level during low dose recombinant follicle-stimulating hormone therapy for anovulation in polycystic ovary syndrome. J Clin Endocrinol Metab. 2007;92:4138-43.

29. La Marca A, Malmusi S, Giulini S, et al. Anti-Müllerian hormone plasma levels in spontaneous menstrual cycle and during treatment with FSH to induce ovulation. Hum Reprod. 2004;19:2738-41.

30. Broer SL, Dolleman M, Opmeer BC, et al. AMH and AFC as predictors of excessive response in controlled ovarian hyperstimulation: A meta-analysis. Hum Reprod Update. 2011;17:46-54.

31. Maheshwari A, Gibreel A, Bhattacharya S, et al. Dynamic tests of ovarian reserve: a systematic review of diagnostic accuracy. Reprod Bio Med Online. 2009;18(5);717-34.

32. Kwee J, Schats R, McDonnell J, et al. The Clomiphene citrate challenge test versus the exofenous follicle stimulating hormone ovarian reserve test as a single test for identification of low responders and hyperresponders to in vitro fertilization. Fertil Steril. 2006;85(6):1714-22.

33. Hofmann GE, Danforth DR, Seifer DB. Inhibin-B: the physiologic basis of the clomiphene citrate challenge test for ovarian reserve screening. Fertil Steril. 1998;69(3):474-7.

34. Hendricks DJ, Mol BW, Bansci LF, et al. The CCCT for the prediction of poor ovarian response and nonpregnancy in patient-s undergoing IVF. Fertil Steril. 2006;86:807-18.

35. Yong PY, Baird DT, Thong KJ, et al. Prospective analysis of the relationships between the ovarian follicle cohort and basal FSH concentration, the inhibin response to exogenous FSH and ovarian follicle number at different stages of the normal menstrual cycle and after pituitary downregulation. Hum Reprod. 2003;18:35-44.

36. Ravhon A, Lavery S, Micheal S, et al. Dynamic assays of inhibin B and oestradiol following buserelin acetate administration as predictors of ovarian response in IVF. Hum Reprod. 2000;15(11):2297-301.

37. Hendriks DJ, Broekmans FJM, Bancsi LFJMM, et al. Repeated clomiphene citrate challenge testing in the prediction of outcome in IVF: a comparison with basal markers for ovarian reserve. Hum Reprod. 2005;20(1):163-9.

38. Kwee J, Etling MW, Schats R, et al. Comparison of endocrine tests with respect to their predictive value on the outcome of ovarian hyperstimulation in IVF treatment: results of a prospective randomized study. Hum Reprod. 2003;18(7):1422-7.

39. Gibreel A, Maheshwari A, Bhattacharya S, et al. Ultrasound tests of ovarian reserve: a systematic review of accuracy in predicting, fertility outcomes. Hum Fertil. 2009;12(2):95-106.

40. Syrop CH, Dawson JD, Husman KJ, et al. Ovarian volume may predict assisted reproductive outcomes better than follicle stimulating hormone concentration on day 3. Hum Reprod. 1999;14(7):1752-6.

41. Lass A, Skull J, McVeigh E, et al. Measurement of ovarian volume by transvaginal sonography before ovulation induction with human menopausal gonadotropin for in-vitro fertilization can predict poor response. Hum Reprod. 1997;12(2):294-97.

42. Hendriks DJ, Kwee J, Mol BW, et al. Ultrasonography as a tool for the prediction of outcome in IVF patients: a comparative meta-analysis of ovarian volume and antral follicle count. Fertil Steril. 2007;87:764-75.

43. Muttukrishna S, McGarrigle H, Wakim R, et al. Antral follicle count, anti-Müllerian hormone and inhibin B: predictors of ovarian response in assisted reproductive technology? BJOG. 2005;112:1384-90.

44. Nardo LG, Christodoulou D, Gould D, et al. Anti-Müllerian hormone levels and antral follicle count in women enrolled in in vitro fertilization cycles: relationship to life-style factors, chronological age and reproductive history. Gynecol Endocrinol. 2007;3:1-8.

45. Haadsma ML, Bukman A, Greon H, et al. The number of small antral follicles (2-6 mm)

determines the outcome of endocrine ovarian reserve tests in subfertile population. Hum Reprod. 2007;22:1925-31.

46. Klinkert ER, Broekmans FJ, Looman CV, et al. The antral follicle count is a better marker than basal follicle-stimulating hormone for the selection of older patients with acceptable pregnancy prospects after in vitro fertilization. Fertil Steril. 2005;83:811-4.

47. Panchal S, Nagori C. Comparison of anti-Mullerian hormone and antral follicle count for assessment of ovarian reserve. J Hum Reprod Sci. 2012;5(3):274-8.

48. Johnstone EB, Rosen MP, Addauan-Andersen C, et al. Is AFC a marker of oocyte quality? Fertile women have higher AFCs than infertile women. Fertil Steril. 2010;94(4):S63.

49. Gruijters MJ, Visser JA, Durlinger AL, et al. Anti-Mullerian hormone and its role in ovarian function. Mol Cell Endocrinol. 2003;211:85-90.

50. Ng EH, Chan CC, Yeung WS, et al. Effect of age on ovarian stromal flow measured by three-dimensional ultrasound with power Doppler in Chinese women with proven fertility. Hum Reprod. 2004;19:2132-7.

51. Krishnakumar J, Agarwal A, Nambiar D, et al. Comparison of antral follicle count, antimullerian hormone and day 2 follicle stimulating hormone as predictor of ovarian response and clinical pregnancy rate in patient with an abnormal ovarian reserve test. Int J Reprod Contracept Obstet Gynecol. 2016;5(8):2762-7.

52. Engmann L, Sladkevicius P, Agrawal R, et al. Value of ovarian stromal blood flow velocity measurement after pituitary suppression in the prediction of ovarian responsiveness and outcome of in vitro fertilization treatment. Fertil Steril. 1999;71(1):22-9.

53. Kupesic S, Kurjak A. Predictors of in vitro fertilization outcome by three dimensional ultrasound. Hum Reprod. 2002;17(4):950-55.

54. Zaidi J, Barber J, Kyei-Mensah A, et al. Relationship of ovarian stromal blood flow at baseline ultrasound to subsequent follicular response in an in vitro fertilization program. Obstet Gynecol. 1996;88:779-84.

55. Merce LT, Gomez B, Engels V, et al. Intraobserver and interobserver reproducibility ovarian volume, antral follicle count and vascularity indices obtained with transvaginal 3-dimensional ultrasonography, power Doppler angiography and virtual computer aided analysis imaging program. J Ultrasound Med. 2005;24:1279-87.

56. Ng EHY, Chan CCW, Tang OS, et al. Effect of pituitary downregulation on antral follicle count, ovarian volume and stromal blood flow measured by three-dimensional ultrasound with power Doppler prior to ovarian stimulation Hum Reprod. 2004:19(12):2811-5.

57. Oliveira JB, Baruffi RL, Petersen CG, et al. A new ovarian response prediction index (ORPI): implications for individualized controlled ovarian stimulation. Reprod Biol Endocrinol. 2012;10:94.

58. Broer SL, Mol BW, Hendriks D, et al. The role of anti-Mullerian hormone in prediction of outcome after IVF: comparison with the antral follicle count. Fertil Steril. 2009;91:705-14.

59. Panchal S, Nagori CB. Baseline scan and ultrasound diagnosis of PCOS. Donald School J Ultrasound Obstet Gynecol. 2012;6(3):290-9.

60. La Marca A, Grisendi V, Guilini S, et al. Individualization of FSH dose in IVF/ICSI cycles using the antral follicle count. J Ovarian Res. 2013;6:11.

61. Panchal S, Nagori C. Ultrasound-based decision making on stimulation protocol for superovulated intrauterine insemination cycles. Int J Infertil Fetal Med. 2016;7(1):7-13.

62. Ferraretti AP, Gianaroli L. The Bologna criteria for the definition of poor ovarian responders: is there a need for revision? Hum Reprod. 2014;29(9):1842-45.

3

Clomiphene Citrate

Chaitanya Nagori

INTRODUCTION

Clomiphene citrate (CC) is in clinical use since 1967 for dysovulatory infertility. CC is a mixture of two isomers; enclomiphene (trans) 62% and zuclomiphene (cis) 38%. Enclomiphene is more potent antiestrogenic agent and responsible for ovulation inducing actions. Enclomiphene has a shorter duration of action and disappears within few days while zuclomiphene is detected in circulation over a month because of its slow clearance rate. It accumulates cycle after cycle but has no clinical consequences. 85% of the drug is eliminated from the system in 7 days and the rest takes more than a month to be completely excreted from the body systems. That is why the antiestrogenic effect because of CC persists for longer time. Enclomiphene is antiestrogenic centrally and estrogenic peripherally and zuclomiphene is the other way round (estrogenic centrally and antiestrogenic peripherally). The efficacy of the drug varies in clinical practice if the proportion of enclomiphene and zuclomiphene are not maintained.

MECHANISM OF ACTION

CC acts purely as antagonist or antiestrogenic agent. It binds with estrogen receptors at hypothalamus, signaling lack of estrogen to hypothalamus. This in turn releases gonadotropin releasing hormone (GnRH) which causes pituitary to secret more follicle-stimulating hormone (FSH) and luteinizing hormone (LH). This stimulates the ovarian follicular development. As the estrogen level rises after follicular development, it does not decrease FSH and LH because it has no negative effect on hypothalamus as receptors are occupied by CC. As the duration of action of CC is longer, it allows more and more FSH and LH to be secreted and so causes multifollicular development. Clomiphene has direct effect on ovary to stimulate follicular estradiol synthesis. It increases the gonadotropin-releasing hormone (GnRH) pulse frequency in ovulatory patients[1] and pulse amplitude in anovulatory patients like polycystic ovary syndrome (PCOS).[2] Clomiphene does not display progestational, corticotropic, androgenic or antiandrogenic properties.

INDICATIONS OF CLOMIPHENE CITRATE

- *WHO group II patients:* Clomiphene citrate is extremely effective in anovulatory patients in whom hypothalamo-pituitary ovarian axis is normal. Normal thyroid function tests and prolactin should be confirmed before starting the treatment. But it is not effective in hypogonadotropic hypogonadism, i.e. WHO group I as no feedback mechanism of estrogen and FSH, LH is present in these patients CC can not induce ovulation.
- *Luteal phase defect (LPD):* Short luteal phase is associated with low levels of FSH in follicular phase causing LPD. CC will increase FSH and LH in follicular phase, develop the good follicle, and correct the abnormality in luteal phase. So CC is the drug of choice in LPD due to short luteal phase.[3] Progesterone does not help in this group of patients.
- *Unexplained infertility:* The rationale of using CC in unexplained infertility is that it corrects subtle hormonal defects due to deficiency of FSH and LH. It increases the number of follicles available for fertilization and corrects LPD. Cochrane database supports the use of CC in unexplained subfertility. Former belief that CC causes cervical dysmenorrhea and decreases endometrial receptivity in unexplained infertility is not accepted now and instead of contraindication, it is the indication for CC in modern era for unexplained infertility. CC with intrauterine insemination (IUI) is beneficial as compared to expectant management.[4] Though there are some studies in which CC has not been found to increase pregnancy rates in ovulatory patients.[5]

CONTRAINDICATIONS OF CLOMIPHENE CITRATE

- Large ovarian cyst more than 5 cm in diameter. The cycle can be started when size of the cyst is less than 5 cm on day 5 of the cycle.
- Liver disease.
- Hypogonadotropic hypogonadism—as the hypothalamic-pituitary-ovarian axis is highly dysfunctional.
- Hypergonadotropic hypogonadism.

PREREQUISITES BEFORE STARTING CLOMIPHENE CITRATE

- Thyroid function tests should be normal.
- Serum prolactin should be normal.
- Male partner should be evaluated and treated if required.
- Progesterone withdrawal bleeding should be present in otherwise amenorrheic patients.
- Adrenal function should be normal.
- Tubal factor should be normal.

TREATMENT REGIMES

- Clomiphene citrate is given as 50 mg dose daily starting between day 2 and day 5 (both inclusive) for 5 days after spontaneous or induced bleeding. Ovulation, conception, and pregnancy rates are same, independent of the day when CC is started.[6] But day 5 is the most accepted day for starting the treatment. On day 5 of the cycle there is a physiological decrease in serum FSH concentration that provides the means for selection of the dominant follicle.[6] Most women (up to 74%)[7] respond to clomiphene with maximum 100 mg daily dose. Higher doses have very poor pregnancy rate.

Several workers have recommended only one dose to start with and maximum, 100 mg daily. The advantage of using this dose is that it can diagnose clomiphene resistant cases earlier and will cut down superfluous cycles of treatment till ovulation occurs. Doses more than 100 mg is not approved by United States Food and Drug Administration (USFDA) and adds only a little to pregnancy rates. Higher doses do not increase the ovulation rate or follicular recruitment.[8] Even though clomiphene is not deposited in adipose tissue, the dose required for obese patient is higher. This is due to high androgen level that inhibits ovulation in obese patients.

- Royal College of Obstetricians and Gynaecologists (RCOG) guidelines with American College of Obstetricians and Gynecologists (ACOG) recommendations is that CC can be used maximum for 6 months continuously and maximum for 12 months in lifetime. Therefore monitoring for evidence of ovulation is must when patient is on CC.
- Patients who do not respond to 150 mg of CC for 5 days, are termed as CC resistant cases (Table 3.1).[9]

Monitoring

Monitoring during CC treatment is must because it can be used only for 3–6 months.

- Serum progesterone in midluteal phase if is more than 3 ng/mL, it is an evidence of ovulation.

TABLE 3.1: Doses of CC and ovulation rates.[10,11]

Dose	Ovulation rate
50 mg	52%
100 mg	22%
150 mg	12%
200 mg	7%
250 mg	5%

- Luteinizing hormone detection kit may help to detect the LH surge. Normally LH surge occurs after 7 days of the last dose of CC.
- Serial sonography just for documenting ovulation is not justified. It does not help to change the line of treatment. It is very inconvenient for the patient as compared to serum progesterone levels being assessed a week before expected date of menstruation.
- If LH may be done on day 8–9 and if it is more than 10 IU/mL success rate is very low because of poor quality ova and embryo.[12-14] This is very common in PCOS patients. So with the first month of CC treatment, assess LH level on day 8–10. If it is more than 10 IU, CC should not be repeated in second month and needs another protocol for ovulation induction.
- Endometrial biopsy (EB) should not be done to know the proliferative or secretory phase as being the invasive test.

Results

- Clomiphene citrate will induce ovulation in approximately 75–80% of cases.
- Up to 70–75% of cumulative pregnancy rate can be achieved in 6–9 months.[7]
- In many series only up to 40% pregnancy rates have been achieved because of antiestrogenic effect on cervical mucous, endometrium, ova, and embryo causing thick cervical mucous, thin endometrium, and is toxic to ova and embryo also.[15]
- 75% of conceptions occur in the first 3 months.[10] So in clinical practice many consultants use it only for 3 months. After 6 months of therapy, only few pregnancies are recorded in literature. This observation is consistent with recommendation of US manufacturer's package inserts for CC. "If pregnancy has not been achieved

after three ovulatory responses, further treatment is generally not recommended".

- So, if the patient has not conceived within 3–6 months with CC, reevaluation of the patient and switching over to further management is required.

High ovulation rate and low pregnancy rate with CC is because of:[16]

- Its antiestrogenic effect on cervix
- Its antiestrogenic effect on endometrium
- High LH, that deteriorates the ovum quality
- Decreased uterine blood flow and decreased PP14, that are required for implantation
- Direct effect on oocytes
- Effect on tubal transport
- Subclinical pregnancy loss.

Side Effects

- Serious side effects are extremely rare.
- Transient hot flushes, mood swings, premenstrual syndrome (PMS) like symptoms, breast tenderness, nausea, and pelvic pain may occur.
- Visual disturbances may occur that are reversible after cessation of treatment. Alternative methods are tried if patient complains of visual disturbances.
- These side effects are due to accumulation of zuclomiphene.

ANTIESTROGENIC EFFECTS OF CLOMIPHENE CITRATE

Antiestrogenic effects on cervix, endometrium, ovary, ovum, and embryo have been described but there is no objective evidence that these effects occur or have clinical consequences. Enclomiphene is a more potent antiestrogenic isomer and has a half life of few days.[17] Endometrial thickness is within normal range in majority of cases. This is because

clomiphene is a selective estrogen receptor modulator and has a negative effect only on few patients. Very rarely endometrium suppression is observed with its thickness is less than 6 mm in spite of a good mature follicle. CC is not given, instead patient is to be shifted over to other therapy because usually same endometrial suppression is repeated in subsequent cycles. This is because zuclomiphene component of CC has a very long half life and its accumulation from cycle-to-cycle leads to depletion of estrogen receptors, so much so that it may also cause hot flushes, postmenopausal syndrome like symptoms, visual scotomata, and also cervical dysmucorrhea.[18] CC can be stored in body fat and accumulate in the body around crucial times of implantation, organogenesis, and embryogeme.[19] Cervical dysmenorrhea can be overcome by IUI. In these patients having antiestrogenic effect, even though ovulation rate is 80%, conception rate is only 40%. Exogenous estrogen supplementation has no effect. Exogenous estrogen should not be used to correct cervical dysmenorrhea or increase endometrial thickness as receptors are already occupied by CC. Tamoxifen and letrozole can be used to overcome these side effects. No significant difference in ovulation rates was found with raloxifene and CC.[20]

It has been found that the endometrium continues to grow till the size of the follicle reaches 24 mm. It is therefore recommended to wait for the endometrium to grow till that size of the follicle if at 18–19 mm size of follicle the endometrium is thin. This means that when the follicle actually attains functional maturity, produces sufficient estrogen, that is when the endometrium grows. This can also be confirmed by Doppler studies. In CC cycles therefore a late trigger may be beneficial. The LH surge that occurs prematurely due to rising estrogen may be prevented in these cases because of blocked estrogen receptors by CC.

The argument against delaying trigger is that even though the endometrium is 6 mm, it continues to grow and implantation will occur 7 days after the trigger, by which time the endometrium might attain the required thickness. Moreover it has also been argued that if the trigger is delayed the estrogen will keep on rising which might be detrimental to implantation.

RISKS OF CLOMIPHENE CITRATE

- *Multiple pregnancy (5–8%)*: Most are twins or triplets—higher order pregnancies are rare (0.08–1.1%).[21]
- *Miscarriage*: It does not increase spontaneous miscarriage rate.[22]
- *Congenital anomalies*: There is no substantial evidence that CC causes any particular birth defects or increases the incidence of birth defects.[23] Neural tube defects and hypospadias are the ones most often found in babies of CC treated mothers. Defects that were found to be associated with CC were Dandy-Walker malformation, muscular ventricular septal defect (VSD), cloacal exstrophy, anencephaly, all septal heart defects combined, coarctation of aorta, esophageal atresia, craniosynostosis, and omphalocele according to this study. Another study though shows that CC cannot be associated with increased incidence of craniosynostosis.[24] The malformations may be due to zuclomiphene, that remains in circulation for a longer time.
- *Ovarian hyperstimulation syndrome (OHSS)*: Mild OHSS may occur in a few cases of PCOS, which requires only conservative management. Severe OHSS is rare and I have not seen any in my practice of 30 years.
- *Breast and ovarian cancer*: Previous studies suggested that if CC is used for more than 12 months. It can increase the occurrence of ovarian malignancy. But subsequent studies have proved that fertility drugs are not associated with any invasive cancers. CC does not increase the risk of breast cancer.

Women on clomiphene therapy must be counseled that no causal relationship has been established between ovulation inducing drugs and breast or ovarian cancer. However, prolonged treatment with CC is futile and should be avoided because it has little success.

Clomiphene resistant cases can be treated with:
- Extended CC regime
- Glucocorticoids
- Estrogen
- Bromocriptine
- Human chorionic gonadotropin
- Gonadotropins
- Gonadotropin-releasing hormone agonist
- Gonadotropin-releasing hormone antagonist
- Insulin sensitizers
- Ovarian drilling.

TREATMENT ALTERNATIVES

Extended Clomiphene Treatment

1. Clomiphene citrate is given for 7–10 days.
2. 150 mg of CC is given for 8 days.
3. 50 mg/day is given for 5 days and increment of 50 mg/day is done every 5 days to reach 250 mg/day.
4. *Stair step protocol*: When there is no follicle development after 14 days of 5 days course of CC, higher dose is given without withdrawal bleed. This reduces the duration of total treatment. But the efficacy of this protocol is controversial.

No factors have been identified that can predict which patient will respond to extended regime. Such extended regimes have extremely poor pregnancy rates and are not much helpful in clinical practice. After CC administration of more than 5 days, FSH first increases but then it decreases and LH goes on rising and remains high, so pregnancy rates are very poor.[25,26]

Clomiphene Citrate + Glucocorticoids

This combination is very useful in chronic anovulatory patients. It is also given to those patients who have high dehydroepiandrosterone sulfate (DHEA-S) and hirsutism. It can be given to all the patients who show increase in adrenal androgen production. It has given good results even with normal DHEA-S and unselected population having clomiphene resistance due to increased androgen. Two large trials evaluated CC-resistant anovulatory patients with normal DHEA-S levels. Those treated with dexamethasone on cycle days 3–12 and CC, showed 75–88% ovulation rates and 40% conception rates as compared to 15–20% and 5% respectively, without dexamethasone.[27] Those patients who are resistant to 100–150 mg of CC, start ovulating when glucocorticoids are added. Glucocorticoids are given in the form of dexamethasone 0.5 mg daily or prednisolone 5 mg daily continuously for 30 days at bed time. When given at night, it reduces the night peak of adrenocorticotropic hormone (ACTH) and reduces the level of androgens.[28] It can be given continuously for 3–6 months. No serious side effects are seen, though water logging and weight gain have been documented. The dose can be reduced to 0.25 mg/day or can be stopped in second phase of the cycle. As the drug is very cheap and effective and does not have any major disadvantage it should be tried in chronic anovulatory patients. Glucocorticoids improve response of follicles to stimulation and the health of their developing oocytes.[29] The Cochrane review 2009 shows that sequential use of dexamethasone in resistant PCOS patients increases the pregnancy rate to five times more.[30]

Clomiphene Citrate + Estrogen

Estrogen was tried to improve cervical mucous and endometrial thickness. But these effects on cervical mucous and endometrium are not dependent on dosage and duration of treatment of CC. It is idiosyncratic response in subgroup of CC treated patients which may reduce conception rate. So combination with estrogen is not of any help as receptors are occupied by CC and should not be used in clinical practice. Empirical treatment with estrogen has no role.

Clomiphene Citrate + Bromocriptine

Bromocriptine is given to the patients of hyperprolactinemia, but there are two definite indications even with normal prolactin level:
1. Galactorrhea with normal prolactin level. In these cases galactorrhea must be confirmed by presence of fat globules under the microscope in the secretions expressed from the breast. It must be differentiated from simple mucoid discharge that does not have fat globules.[31]
2. There are patients who are known as spikers. These patients show nocturnal spikes of prolactin in the first half of the cycle when CC is used for ovulation induction. These patients are given bromocriptine in first half of the cycle. It is not to be continued in second half of the cycle as normal level of prolactin is required for maintenance of corpus luteum. Clinically, these patients show poor endometrium even though there is no local cause and follicle is good and meet all parameters on B mode and

color Doppler for optimum maturity. Bromocriptine can be tried in these patients and if endometrium improves, it can be continued for 3–6 months.

Clomiphene Citrate + Human Chorionic Gonadotropin

Routine use of hCG for rupture of the follicle is not justified. If the follicle is mature it will reflect as serum estradiol level of more than 150 pg/mL. This will initiate the LH surge which in turn will cause rupture of the follicle and exogenous hCG is not required. But if the follicle is not mature and if hCG is given as a trigger for ovulation, it will lead to premature luteinization or atresia. Therefore, hCG must not be given just to cause a follicular rupture,[32,33] when no intervention is planned.

Human chorionic gonadotropin must be combined with clomiphene when IUI is to be done. hCG in these cases is given to time IUI as follicle ruptures at 34–36 hours after hCG injection. A meta-analysis of 7 studies comparing triggering ovulation with hCG (1,461 patients) with urinary LH testing to identify endogenous LH surge (1,162 patients) for timing IUI for women with unexplained infertility treated with CC, reported lower odds of pregnancy when an hCG trigger was used as compared to endogenous LH surge.[34] hCG can also be given in patients proved to have absent, inadequate or delayed LH surge. This is a common occurrence in endometriosis. hCG, therefore must be used for timed intercourse, to time IUI and in cases of delayed LH surge.

Clomiphene Citrate + Gonadotropin

Gonadotropins are often combined with clomiphene with the idea that it would decrease the requirement of gonadotropins. CC by its direct effect on ovary, increases the sensitivity of ovary to gonadotropins. This combination has risks of ovarian hyperstimulation and multiple pregnancies. Increased LH secretion induced by CC, which does not occur with FSH administration, may also reduce the likelihood of conception.[35] Pregnancy rate with CC + human menopausal gonadotropin (HMG) are same as for CC alone.[36] The author is not convinced by this combination and would never use it. It does not increase the pregnancy rate. The argument is that CC increases FSH and LH both. The poor pregnancy rate with CC is because of high LH which will remain in spite of adding gonadotropins. The effect of high LH will decrease the implantation and pregnancy rate. So even though we get a follicle after adding gonadotropins, in many of these patients, the follicular quality is not good and pregnancy rates are only comparable to CC alone and much less than gonadotropins alone. Instead letrozole is a better drug to be combined with gonadotropins. This will be discussed elsewhere.

Low dose FSH protocol is recommended by Professor Roy Homburg as a first line of treatment for ovulation induction instead of CC. The study has shown to double the pregnancy rates, with reduced treatment pregnancy interval and more singleton pregnancies.[37]

Gonadotropin-releasing Hormone Agonist

Gonadotropin-releasing hormone agonists are not used routinely in IUI cycles and are reserved only for in vitro fertilization (IVF) cycles. Agonists are used for downregulation and this in IUI cycles only increases the requirement of gonadotropins, without increasing the pregnancy rate.

Clomiphene Citrate + Antagonist

This makes a good combination in thin lean PCOS patients where LH is tonically raised. It improves the quality of ovum and also the conception rates. For patients on clomiphene therapy, serum LH levels are checked on day 8–9 of the cycle. If it is more than 10 IU/mL, it is an indicator of poor pregnancy rates. These are the ideal patients to start antagonist. Regular use of antagonist is not justified because it sharply decreases LH and it causes regression of follicle as well as LPD. Here antagonist is started when the size of the lead follicle reaches 14 mm and is continued till the day of trigger.

CLOMIPHENE CITRATE + METFORMIN

Several workers have shown that metformin is inferior to CC for ovulation induction and metformin alone should not be used for ovulation induction.[38] But in CC resistant cases of PCOS when metformin is combined with CC, it improves ovulation 4–9 times more than clomiphene alone. But metformin is a very useful drug when patient does not want to conceive immediately. If metformin is taken for 6 months, it will normalize hormonal milieu. It will decrease LH and androgen. So if CC is given when patient wants to conceive, ovulation will occur and will decrease the incidence of multiple pregnancies also. Pretreatment with metformin for patients to be treated with CC has shown to improve ovulation rates[39] and conception rates[40] in several studies. Though another study has clearly shown that metformin pretreatment does not improve the pregnancy rates or extended metformin therapy does not reduce the required dose of CC.[41,42] Though a meta-analysis of 17 randomized control trials (RCTs) in PCOS women has shown both

increased ovulation and pregnancy rates when metformin was added to CC. This effect was found to be statistically significant in obese women with PCOS, where as it failed to reach significance in nonobese women with this condition. It is therefore logical to routinely use metformin with CC in obese women with PCOS and glucocorticoid as the first adjunct of choice for nonobese PCOS women failing to respond to CC.[43] Large randomized study has shown that CC + metformin has no significant advantage over CC for ovulation induction.[44,45]

Clomiphene Citrate + Drilling

It is done in CC resistant cases. Drilling is also done before switching over to gonadotropins. After drilling the medical ovulation induction becomes easier and this is further discussed on the chapter dedicated to ovulation induction in PCOS.

Clomiphene + Low Dose Aspirin

Aspirin may be used to increase the blood flow by vasodilatation which may counter the effect of stress in reducing pelvic blood flow.[46] Though in a meta-analysis this benefit has not been established.[47]

PRIOR TREATMENTS

- *Clomiphene after prior treatment with OC pills (oral contraceptive pills)*: The mechanism of action of OC pills is to decrease the LH. High LH will cause high androgen, which in turn will cause anovulation. So OC pills when given for 2–3 months will decrease the LH and in turn androgen and improves sensitivity to CC with the same dose. Therefore in PCOS patients prior treatment with OC pills was given routinely in CC resistant cases and did show good results.

- *Micronized progesterone*: If it is given for 5 days, it modulates LH pulsatility, reducing LH concentration and induces more favorable environment for CC.[48]

CARRY HOME MESSAGE

- Clomiphene citrate should be used for 3–6 months, 100 mg/day starting from day 5, provided day 8 LH is less than 10 IU.
- Clomiphene citrate + estrogen has no role.
- Clomiphene citrate + dexamethasone is useful in chronic anovulatory patient and DHEA-S is high in resistant PCOS and nonobese PCOS.
- Clomiphene citrate + bromocriptine is used in patients with normal prolactin levels with galactorrhea and spikers when prolactin is high in first half of the cycle.
- Routine use of hCG is not justified just for rupture of the follicle.
- Clomiphene citrate + GnRh agonist for downregulation has no role in IUI cycles.
- Clomiphene citrate + antagonist must be used in thin lean PCOS patients when LH is tonically high.
- Clomiphene citrate + gonadotropins do not improve pregnancy rates.
- Clomiphene citrate + metformin can be used in CC resistant PCOS patients.
- Metformin, OC pills, and progesterone are useful prior to CC.
- Clomiphene citrate without IUI does not increase the fecundity rates in patients with unexplained infertility but does definitely increases the fecundity rates with IUI.[49]
- Ovarian drilling is offered to CC resistant PCOS.

REFERENCES

1. Kerin JF, Liu JH, Phillipou G, et al. Evidence for a hypothalamic site of action of clomiphene citrate in women. J Clin Endocrinol Metab. 1985;61:265-8.
2. Kettel LM, Roseff SJ, Berga SL, et al. Hypothalamic-pituitary-ovarian response to clomiphene citrate in women with polycystic ovary syndrome. Fertil Steril. 1993;59:532-8.
3. The Practice Committee of American Society for Reproductive Medicine. The clinical relevance of luteal phase deficiency. Fertil Steril. 2012;98:112-7.
4. Deaton JL, Gibson M, Blackmer KM, et al. A randomised controlled trial of clomiphene citrate and intrauterine insemination in couples with explained infertility or surgically corrected endometriosis. Fertil Steril. 1190;54:1083-8.
5. Guzick DS, Carson SA, Coutifaris C, et al. Efficacy of superovulation and intrauterine insemination in the treatment of infertility. N Engl J Med. 1999;340(3):177-83.
6. Wu CH, Winkel CA. The effect of therapy initiation on clomiphene citrate therapy. Fertil Steril. 1989;52:564-8.
7. The Thessaloniki ESHRE/ASRM-sponsored PCOS consensus workshop group. Consensus on infertility treatment related to polycystic ovary syndrome. Fertil Steril. 2008;89:505-22.
8. Dickey RP, Taylor SN, Curole DN, et al. Relationship of clomiphene dose and patient weight to successful treatment. Hum Reprod. 1997;12:449-53.
9. National Collaborating Centre for Women's and Children's Health/National Institute for Clinical Excellence. Fertility: assessment and treatment for people with fertility problems. RCOG Press. 2004;11:57-8.
10. Gysler M, March CM, Mishell DR Jr, et al. A decade's experience with an individualized clomiphene treatment regimen including its effect on postcoital test. Fertil Steril. 1982;37:161-7.
11. Gorlitsky GA, Kase NG, Speroff L. Ovulation and pregnancy rates with clomiphene citrate. Obstet Gynecol. 1978;51:265.
12. Shoham Z, Borenstein R, Lunenfeld B, et al. Hormonal profiles following clomiphene citrate therapy in conception and non-

conception cycles. Clin Endocrinol. 1990;33:271-8.

13. Venn A, Lumley J. Clomiphene citrate and pregnancy outcome. Aust N Z J Obstet Gynaecol. 1994;34:56-66.

14. Vandenberg G, Ten SS. Effect of anti-oestrogenic action of clomiphene during the menstrual cycle: evidence for a change in feedback snesitivity. J Clin Endocrinol Metab. 1973;37:356-65.

15. Homburg R. Clomiphene citrate-end of an era? Hum Reprod. 2005;20:2043-51.

16. Out HJ, Coelingh Bennink HJ. Clomiphene citrate or gonadotropins for induction of ovulation? Hum Reprod. 1998;13:2358-61.

17. Young SL, Opsahl MS, Fritz A. Serum concentration of enclomiphene and zuclomiphene across consecutive cycles of clomiphene citrate therapy in anovulatory infertile women. Fetil Steril. 1999;71:639-44.

18. Ghobadi C, Mirhosseini N, Shiran MR, et al. Single dose pharmacokinetic study of clomiphene citrate isomers in anovular patients with polycystic ovary disease. J Clin Pharacol. 2009;49:147-54.

19. Mikkelson TJ, Kroboth PD, Cameron WJ, et al. Single dose pharmacokinetics of clomiphene citrate in normal volunteers. Fertil Steril. 1986;46:392-96.

20. de Paula Guedes Neto E, Savaris RF, von Eye Corleta H, et al. Prospective, randomised comparison between raloxifene and clomiphene citrate for ovulation induction in polycystic ovary syndrome. Fertil Steril. 2011;96(3):769-73.

21. Reefhuis J, Honein MA, Schieve LA, et al. National birth defects prevention study. Use of clomiphene citrate and birth defects. National birth defects prevention study, 1997-2005. Hum Reprod. 2011;26:451-7.

22. Badawy A, Shokeir T, Allam AF, et al. Pregnancy outcome after ovulation induction with aromatase inhibitors or clomiphene citrate in unexplained infertility. Acta Obstet gynecol. 2009;88:187-91.

23. Correy JF, Marsden De, Schokman F. The outcome of pregnancy resulting from clomiphene induced ovulation. Aust N Z J Obstet Gynecol. 1982;22:18-21.

24. Reefhuis J, Honein MA, Show GM, et al. Fertility treatments and craniosynostosis: California, Georgia and Iowa, 1993-1997. Pediatrics. 2003;111:1163-6.

25. Adashi EY. Clomiphene citrate: mechanism(s) and site(s) of action: A hypothesis revisited. Fertil Steril. 1984;42:331-44.

26. Messinis IE, Milingos SD. Future use of clomiphene in ovarian stimulation. Clomiphene in the 21st century. Hum Reprod. 1998;13:2362-5.

27. Elnashar A, Abdelageed E, Fayed M, et al. Clomiphene citrate and dexamethasone in treatment of clomiphene citrate resistant polycystic ovary syndrome: a prospective placebo-controlled study. Hum Reprod. 2006;21:1805-8.

28. Keay SD, Jenkins JM. Adjunctive use of dexamethasone in Clomid resistant patients. Fertil Steril. 2003;80:230.

29. Thurston LM, Norgate DP, Jonas KC, et al. Ovarian modulators of type 1 11 beta-hydroxysteroid dehydrogenase (11 beta HSD) activity and intra-follicular cortisol: cortisone ratios correlate with the clinical outcome of IVF. Hum Reprod. 2003;18:1603-12.

30. Parsanezhad ME, Alborzi S, Motazedian S, et al. Use of dexamethasone and clomiphene citrate in the treatment of clomiphene citrate resistant patient with polycystic ovarian syndrome and normal dehydroepiandrosterone sulfate levels: a prospective double blind, placebo-controlled trial. Fertil Steril. 2002;78:1001-4.

31. Padilla SL, Person GK, McDonough PG, et al. The efficacy of bromocriptine in patients with ovulatory dysfunction and normoprolactinemic galactorrhoea. Fertil Steril. 1985;44:695-8.

32. Agrawal SK, Buyalos RP. Corpus luteum function and pregnancy rates with clomiphene citrate therapy: comparison of human chorionic gonadotropin induced versus spontaneous ovulation. Hum Reprod. 1995;10:328-31.

33. Flukar MR, Wang IY, Rowe TC. An extended 10-day course of clomiphene citrate in women with CC resistant ovulatory disorder. Fertil Steril. 1996;66:761-4.

34. George K, Nair R, Tharyan P. Ovulation triggers in anovulatory women undergoing ovulation induction. Cochrane database Syst Rev. 2008;3:CD006900.
35. Hamilton-Fairley D, Franks S. Common problems in induction of ovulation. Baillieres Clin Obstet Gynaecol. 1990;4:609-25.
36. Vargyas JM, Moernte C, Shangold G, et al. The effect of different methods of ovarian stimulation for human in vitro fertilization and embryo replacement. Fertil Steril. 1984;42:745-9.
37. Homburg R, Hendriks L, Konig TE, et al. Clomiphene citrate or low-dose FSH for the first line treatment of infertile women with anovulation associated with polycystic ovary syndrome: a prospective randomized multinational study. Hum Reprod. 2012;27(2):468-73.
38. De Leo V, la Marco A, Ditto A, et al. Effects of metformin on gonadotropin induced ovulation in women with polycystic ovary syndrome. Fertil Steril. 1999;72:282-3.
39. Kocak M, Caliskan E, Simsir C, et al. Metformin therapy improves ovulation rates, cervical scores and pregnancy rates in clomiphene citrate resistant women with polycystic ovary syndrome. Fertil Steril. 2002;77:101-6.
40. Khorram O, Helliwell JP, Katz S, et al. Two weeks of metformin improves clomiphene citrate induced ovulation and metabolic profiles in women with polycystic ovary syndrome. Fertil Steril. 2006;85:1448-51.
41. Silbert TI, Kruger TF, Lombard C. Evaluating the equivalence of clomiphene citrate with and without metformin in ovulation induction in PCOS patients. J Assist Reprod Genet. 2009;26:165-71.
42. Cataldo NA, Barnhart HX, Legro RS, et al. Extended-release metformin does not reduce the clomiphene citrate dose required to induce ovulation in polycystic ovary syndrome. J Clin Endocrinol Metab. 2008;93:3124-7.
43. Creanga AA, Bradley HM, McCormick C, et al. Use of metformin in polycystic ovary syndrome: a meta-analysis. Obstet Gynecol. 2008;111:959-68.
44. Tahng T, Lord JM, Norman RJ, et al. Insulin sensitizing drugs (metformin, Rosiglitazone, pioglitazone, D-chiro-inositol) for women with polycystic ovarian syndrome, oligo-amenorrhoea and subfertility. Cochrane Database Syst Rev. 2012;16(5):CD003053.
45. Palomba S, Pasquali R, Orio Jr F, et al. Clomiphene citrate, metformin or both as first step approach in treating anovulatory infertility in patients with polycystic ovarian syndrome (PCOS): a systematic review of head-to-head randomised controlled studies and meta-analysis. Clin Endocrinol (Oxf). 2009;70:311-21.
46. Ebbesn SM, Zaachariae R, Mehlsen MY, et al. Stressful life events are associated with poor in-vitro fertilization (IVF) outcome: a prospective study. Hum Reprod. 2009;24:2173-82.
47. Khairy M, Banerjee K, El-Toukhy T, et al. Aspirin in women undergoing in-vitro fertilization treatment: a systematic review and meta-analysis. Fertil Steril. 2007;88:822-31.
48. Homburg R, Weissglass L, Goldman J. Improved treatment for anovulation in polycystic ovary syndrome on the inappropriate gonadotropin release and clomiphene response. Hum Reprod. 1988;3:285-8.
49. The practice committee of American Society of reproductive medicine. Use of clomiphene citrate in infertile women: a committee opinion. Fertil Steril. 2013;100(2):341-8.

4

Letrozole: An Aromatase Inhibitor

Chaitanya Nagori

INTRODUCTION

Letrozole is an aromatase inhibitor used for ovulation induction. It is the third generation of aromatase inhibitor (Fig. 4.1). First and second generations of aromatase inhibitors are not used in clinical practice. The main advantage of the drug is that it is a reversible enzyme inhibitor. It was for the first time used by Mitwally et al. in 2001 for ovulation induction.[1]

MECHANISM OF INDUCTION OF OVULATION

- *Central*: At brain level
- *Peripheral*: On uterus and ovaries.

Central Mechanism

Estrogen withdrawal centrally causes increase in activins produced from pituitary and several other tissues.[2] This stimulates synthesis of follicle-stimulating hormone (FSH) by a direct action on gonadotropes.[3] This causes increase in FSH and luteinizing hormone (LH) from pituitary.

Peripheral Mechanism

Androgens have a stimulatory role in early follicular growth[4] mediated directly through testosterone augmentation of follicular FSH receptor expression[5,6] and directly through androgen stimulation of insulin-like growth factor 1 (IGF-1), which may synergize with FSH to promote folliculogenesis.[7,8] High androgen sensitizes follicle to lower doses of FSH.

Aromatase, a cytochrome P450 dependent enzyme acts as ultimate step in synthesis of estrogen, catalyzing the conversion of androgen to estrogen (Fig. 4.1). This conversion also occurs at peripheral sites such as muscle, fat and liver. Letrozole inhibits aromatase enzyme by completely binding to the heme of cyto 450 subunits of enzyme, so that androgen

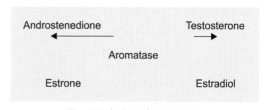

Fig. 4.1: Action of aromatase.

is not converted to estrogen. Androstenedione is not converted into estrone and testosterone is not converted into estradiol (E2) as the aromatase is inhibited. This leads to increased androgen with letrozole.

The end result is low estrogen causing negative feedback at hypothalamus and releasing FSH and LH releasing factors resulting in high FSH and LH causing folliculogenesis. As androgen is not converted into estrogen, there is slightly higher level of androgen which also causes folliculogenesis by sensitizing follicles to FSH. Letrozole has no effect on estrogen receptors (ERs) and acts on hypothalamus. So, it has no deleterious effect on LH surge, cervical mucous, and endometrium.

As FSH and LH stimulate folliculogenesis, estrogen will rise and will cause negative feedback on FSH release and so FSH level will decrease. This decrease in FSH is responsible for monofollicular development as other follicles will not grow. This is not the case with clomiphene citrate (CC), that binds to the Estrogen receptors (ERs) and FSH will go on rising in spite of high estrogen, leading to multifollicular development with CC. Another important advantage is that along with FSH, LH will also decrease as the estrogen rises because of follicular growth and estrogen and will have negative effect on FSH and LH, and so quality of an ovum is not disturbed and does not affect implantation. This is another advantage over CC, which causes persistent high LH along with FSH.

- No antiestrogenic effect
- Decreases the dose of gonadotropins
- Monofollicular development
- Low abortion and congenital malformation rate
- Improves endometrial receptivity.

BOX 4.1: Indications of letrozole.

- Clomiphene citrate (CC) resistant cases
- Day 10 luteinizing hormone (LH) > 10 IU in CC cycle
- In polycystic ovary syndrome (PCOS) patients as baseline estradiol (E2) is high
- Antiestrogenic effect of CC on cervix and endometrium
- Poor responders, refuse lower doses of gonadotropins
- Endometriosis
- Elderly women
- In breast cancer patients, for ovum preservation
- Can replace CC
- It can be combined with gonadotropins.

INDICATIONS OF LETROZOLE (BOX 4.1)

- *Clomiphene citrate resistant cases*: When 100–150 mg of CC fails to induce ovulation, letrozole should be tried.[9]
- *Polycystic ovary syndrome (PCOS):* Here baseline E2 is elevated which blocks hypothalamus causing anovulation. Letrozole will reduce estrogen and stimulate hypothalamus to release LH-releasing hormone (LHRH) to secrete more FSH and induce folliculogenesis.
- It is useful in cases where CC induces cervical dysmenorrhea and poor endometrium. Letrozole is devoid of antiestrogenic effect as it does not bind to ERs.
- When LH is elevated on day 8 or day 9 after CC, letrozole should be tried.
- It is useful in poor responders as it improves response to gonadotropins.[10]

CHARACTERISTICS OF LETROZOLE

Letrozole causes total suppression of estrogen (up to 97–99%) with doses up to 5 mg/day. Maximum suppression occurs between 48 hours and 72 hours. After day 7, estrogen level will rise due to folliculogenesis because of increasing FSH after negative feedback of estrogen due to letrozole. This rise of estrogen will continue for 5–7 days. This E2 peak because of positive feedback mechanism will cause LH surge for ovulation. So, LH surge occurs after 12 days unlike CC when it occurs early. Estrogen rise after 7 days will decrease FSH, which is responsible for monofollicular development. Half-life of letrozole is 48 hours which allows once daily dosage. Temporary rise of androgen improves the sensitivity of follicle to gonadotropin. It therefore requires lower dose of gonadotropins when it is combined with letrozole.

It has no antiestrogenic effect on cervical mucus or endometrium as it does not deplete ERs. Total E2 production is lower with letrozole and prevents supraphysiological levels of E2 which alters endometrial receptivity. Moreover, recovery of endometrium is complete before implantation, due to its short half-life.[11,12]

ADVANTAGES OF LETROZOLE

For Ovulation

- It is almost free from side effects and is well tolerated.
- Monofollicular development, as hypo-thalamic-pituitary-ovarian (HPO) axis is intact.
- Low multiple pregnancy rate due to monofollicular development.
- Higher androgen stimulates and sensitizes follicle to FSH and so lower doses of gonadotropins are required. There is a transient accumulation of androgens in the ovary when letrozole is given for ovulation induction. This creates an androgenic microenvironment in the maturing follicle that enhances the follicular sensitivity to FSH for a short duration (half-life of letrozole is approximately 45 hours). This action is of help in poor responders in

whom ovarian aging has already reduced ovarian androgens.
- It is useful in patients with high body mass index (BMI).[13]

For Implantation: Letrozole and Endometrial Receptivity

- No antiestrogenic effect leads to higher pregnancy rates. Low E2 because of letrozole does not allow rapid degradation of its own receptors and so there is upregulation of ERs. This improves response of endometrium to rising E2 and improves blood flow giving positive effect for implantation.[14] Letrozole positively influences a number of markers of endometrial receptivity compared with CC. This is because of change in endometrial gene expression, leukemia inhibitory factor (LIF) and vascular endothelial growth factor (VEGF), and GGF-22. Letrozole increases LIF protein expression that helps in implantation. This LIF expression is not increased with CC.[15] It improves the level of marker of endometrial receptivity better than CC.[15] Aromatase inhibition may potentially improve endometrial receptivity especially in patients with endometriosis.[16] Endometrium of PCOS females is dysfunctional.[17] ERs in the endometrium, which should normally reduce in the midsecretory phase[18] are not reduced, with altered status of other receptors also. This functional derangement leads to progesterone resistance. This is why antiestrogenic agents for ovulation induction may be beneficial in PCOS patients. Moreover, these agents would also improve endometrial receptivity by suppressing the action of ERα and also has a positive impact on endometrial expression of αvβ3.[19] Concomitant use of aromatase inhibitors with gonadotropins reduces the doses of gonadotropins required[20] and improve the response of gonadotropins in poor responders.[10] It also reduces the supraphysiological levels of estrogen seen with development of multiple ovarian follicles and improves treatment outcome.[21] Low estrogen levels decrease ubiquitination to allow upregulation of ERs and increasing sensitivity to subsequent estrogen rise.[22] This in turn leads to improved endometrial blood flow and faster proliferation of the endometrium, which might have a positive impact on implantation.[14]

- Low abortion rate because of thick and vascular endometrium. It also increases integrin expression that reduces miscarriage rate.

For Fetal Outcome

Letrozole stimulus reduces the risk of miscarriage by increasing integrin expression, with no increase in risk of major congenital fetal malformation or adverse pregnancy or neonatal outcome compared to natural cycle in women undergoing assisted reproductive technology (ART). So, it is safe for mild ovarian stimulation.[23]

The incidence of cardiac anomalies in the letrozole group was slightly lower than the 1 in 400 rate quoted in general population[24] whereas the CC cardiac anomaly rate was about seven times higher.

MATERNAL COMPLICATIONS

Letrozole also leads to reduction in secretion of estrogen from granulosa cells leading to less circulating estrogens, therefore less chances of thrombosis in hyperestrogenic states during controlled ovarian hyperstimulation (COH) and also an additional safety for women with hormone-dependent cancers undergoing fertility therapy.[16]

DOSES

- Recommended dose is 2.5 mg from day 3–7.
- Some workers suggest 5 mg daily dose. The disadvantage of 5 mg dose as a routine is not justified as 2.5 mg can suppress 97–99% of estrogen. 5 mg may suppress more estrogen causing more FSH to be secreted. So, it may not cause monofollicular development. As it is a chemotherapeutic agent, it may be toxic to ovum and embryo. Higher dose has no advantage in terms of pregnancy rates.[25]
- 20 mg on day 3: It has advantage of having short half-life and reduces embryotoxic effect. But symptoms of hyperestrinism may develop.
- It is superior to anastrozole 1 mg from days 3 to 7 or anastrozole 5 mg single dose as anastrozole is weak and less-effective for follicular growth.[26]

SIDE EFFECTS (DRAW BACKS)

- It increases intrafollicular androgen, which may arrest the growth of follicle. But optimum level of androgen is not yet decided.
- As it is chemotherapeutic agent for carcinoma breast, it may be teratogenic to ovum and embryo. But it is not proved.
- In a multicentric study of 911 newborns conceived after CC[27] and letrozole and also one another recent study[28] have shown that there was no increase in congenital malformations following use of letrozole. In recent randomized control study of letrozole for ovulation induction in 900 patients of unexplained infertility, found no increase in congenital malformations than CC or gonadotropins.[29]

FUTURE USES

Infertility

- It stimulates follicles for in vitro maturation (IVM) in PCOS. Letrozole may be used to reduce the risk of ovarian hyperstimulation syndrome (OHSS) and thrombosis due to hyperestrinism-when given in luteal phase, after human chorionic gonadotropin (hCG) trigger in an in vitro fertilization (IVF) patient, it reduces estrogen levels and thus reduces the risk of OHSS[30] without any effect on progesterone and LH.
- Improves implantation in IVF. Some women have high levels of aromatase P450 in endometrium and are related to poor IVF results. Letrozole can be useful to them. Decreased supraphysiological estrogen and decreased aromatase will improve implantation. Use of letrozole in patients undergoing frozen embryo transfer (FET) is associated with higher chance of clinical pregnancy and lower rate of miscarriage.
- Letrozole challenge test may be used for predicting the ovarian response to gonadotropin stimulation. This test is done by evaluating FSH on day 3 and day 7 of a letrozole cycle. Ratio of day 7: day 3 FSH more than 1.5 predicts poor response to gonadotropins.[31]

For Endometriosis

- Letrozole may reduce the chronic pelvic pain of endometriosis.[9]
- Letrozole can be used to treat endometriosis as it decreases local estrogen production and prevents progression of endometriosis.[32]

For Male Infertility

Aromatase inhibitors are also used to treat male subfertility. Anastrozole 1 mg/day or letrozole 2.5 mg/day is the recommended dose for patients with high aromatase activity and increased testosterone to estrogen ratio in nonobstructive azoospermic patients. Therefore, in patients with low testosterone levels, use of aromatase inhibitors is justified.[33]

AUTHOR'S VIEW

Should Letrozole Replace Clomiphene Citrate?

The author strongly believes that letrozole should be used as the first-line of drug. The argument is that it has comparable pregnancy rate with CC and it does not increase congenital malformations. The main advantage is that, it has no antiestrogenic effect on cervical mucus and endometrium and so it will cut down superfluous cycles of treatment. No antiestrogenic effect is the single most important benefit with letrozole that prevents the use of CC.

Efficacy wise, letrozole gives better ovulation and pregnancy rate compared to CC.[34] Results of the trial by Amer et al. are consistent with the recent Cochrane review indicating letrozole is better as primary ovulating agent in PCOS with 40% increase in pregnancy rates and with shorter time to pregnancy.[35]

Letrozole + Gonadotropins

We have found letrozole + recombinant FSH (rFSH) as a very useful combination for giving equivalent pregnancy rates like gonadotropins with advantage that lower number of ampoules are required. Apart from this, it gives lower rate of multiple births. It sensitizes ovary by rise in androgen level, is an added advantage as reduces number of gonadotropin ampoules. We have used this combination routinely in superovulation with intrauterine insemination (IUI).[36]

So letrozole is superior in PCOS and poor responders than CC. Anastrozole has been tried for ovulation induction. It appears from clinical studies that anastrozole is less effective than letrozole for ovulation induction.[37,38] Our personal experience is that in elderly patients (around 40 years), letrozole combined with gonadotropins with IUI gives good pregnancy rates.[39]

CARRY HOME MESSAGE

- Letrozole causes monofollicular development.
- It has no antiestrogenic effect.
- It is a drug of choice in PCOS and poor responders.
- Letrozole + gonadotropins is an excellent combination.
- Letrozole may replace CC as first-line of treatment in future.
- Letrozole does not increase the incidence of congenital malformations in fetus.
- It improves endometrial receptivity.

REFERENCES

1. Mitwally MF, Casper RF. Use of aromotase inhibitor for ovulation induction in patients with an inadequate response to clomiphene citrate. Fertil Steril. 2001;75:2-8.
2. Roberts V, Meunier H, Vaughan J, et al. Production and regulation of inhibin subunits in pituitary gonadotropes. Endocrinology. 1989;124:552-4.
3. Weil SJ, Vendola K, Zhou J, et al. Androgen receptor gene expression in the primate ovary: cellular localization, regulation and functional correlations. J Clin Endocrinol Metab. 1989;837:2479-85.
4. Mason AJ, Berkemeier LM, Schmelzer CH, et al. Activin B: precursor sequences, genomic structure and in vitro activities. Mol Endocrinol. 1989;3:1352-58.
5. Weil S, Vendola K, Zhou J, et al. Androgen and follicle-stimulating hormone interactions in primate ovarian follicle development. J Clin Endocrinol Metab. 1999;84:2951-56.
6. Vendola KA, Zhou J, Adesanya OO, et al. Androgens stimulate early stages of follicular growth in the primate ovary. J Clin Invest. 1998;101:2622-9.
7. Vendola K, Zhou J, Wang J, et al. Androgens promote oocyte insulin-like growth factor I expression and initiation of follicle development in the primate ovary. Biol Reprod. 1999;61:353-7.
8. Giudice LC. Insulin like growth factors and ovarian follicular development. Endocr Rev. 1992;13:641-69.
9. Pavone ME, Bulun SE. Aromatase inhibitors for the treatment of endometriosis: A review. Fertil Steril. 2012;98(6):1370-79.
10. Mitwally MF, Casper RF. Aromatase inhibition improves ovarian response of follicle stimulating hormone in poor responders. Fertil Steril. 2002;77:776-80.
11. Lamb HM, Adkins JC. Letrozole. A review of its use in postmenopausal women with advanced breast cancer. Drugs. 1998;56:1125-40.
12. Healey S, Tan SL, Tulandi T, et al. Effects of letrozole on superovulation with gonadotropins in women undergoing intrauterine insemination. Fertil Steril. 2003;80:1325-29.
13. McKnight KK, Nodler JL, Cooper JA, et al. Body mass index-associated differences in response to ovulation induction with letrozole. Fertil Steril. 2011;96(5):1206-8.
14. Nirmala PB, Thampan RV. Ubiquitination of the rat uterine oestrogen receptor: dependence on oestradiol. Biochem Bio Phys Res Commun. 1995;213:24-31.
15. Wallace KL, Johnson V, Sopelak V, et al. Clomiphene citrate versus Letrozole: molecular analysis of endometrium in women with PCOS. Fertil Steril. 2011;96:1651-6.
16. Garcia-Valesco JA. The use of aromatase inhibitors in in vitro fertilization. Fertil Steril. 2012;98(6):1356-58.
17. Giudice LC. Endometrium in PCOS: implantation and predisposition to endocrine CA. Best Pract Res Clin Endocrinol Metab. 2006;20:235-44.
18. Lessey BA, Killam AP, Metzger DA, et al. Immunohistochemical analysis of human

uterine oestrogen and progesterone receptors throughout the menstrual cycle. J Clin Endocrinol Metab. 1988;67:334-40.

19. Lessey BA, Palomino WA, Apparao KB, et al. Estrogen receptor alpha and defects in uterine receptivity in women. Repro Biol Endocrinol. 2006;(Suppl 1):59.

20. Mitwally MF, Casper RF. Aromatase inhibition reduces the dose of gonadotropin required for controlled ovarian hyperstimulation. J Soc Gynecol Invest. 2004;11:406-15.

21. Fatemi H, Popovic-Todorovic B, Donoso P, et al. Luteal phase oestradiol suppression by letrozole: a Pilot study in oocyte donors. Reprod Biomed Online. 2008;17:307-11.

22. Mitwally MF, Witchel SF, Casper Rf. Troglitazone: a possible modulator of ovarian steroidogenesis. J Soc Gynecol Invest. 2002;9:163-7.

23. Tatsumi AT, Jwa SC, Kuwahara A, et al. No increased risk of major congenital anomalies or adverse pregnancy or neonatal outcomes following letrozole used in ART. Hum Reprod. 2017;32:125-32.

24. Hoffman JI. Incidence of congenital heart disease: I. Postnatal incidence. Pediatr Cardiol. 1995;16:103-13.

25. Badawy A, Metwally M, Fawzy M. Randomised controlled trial of three doses of letrozole for ovulation induction in patients with unexplained infertility. Reprod Biomed Online. 2007;14:559-62.

26. Griesinger G, von OS, Schultze-Mosgau A, et al. Follicular and endocrine response to anastrozole versus clomiphene citrate administered in follicular phase to normo-ovulatory women: a randomised comparison. Fertil Steril. 2009;91:1831-6.

27. Franks S, Adams J, Mason H, et al. Ovulatory disorders in women with polycystic ovarain syndrome. Clin Obstet Gynecol. 1985;12:605-32.

28. Hull MGR. The causes of infertility and relative effectiveness of treatment. In: Templeton AA, Drife JO (Eds). Infertility. London: Springer-Verlag; 1992. pp. 33-62.

29. Legro DM, Raivero CC, Robinson R, et al. Letrozole, clomiphene or gonadotropin for unexplained infertility. N Engl J Med. 2015;373:1230-40.

30. Fatemi H, Popovic-Todorovic B, Donoso P, et al. Luteal phase oestradiol suppression by letrozole: a pilot study in oocyte donors. Reprod Biomed Online. 2008;17:307-11.

31. Bentov Y, Burstein E, Esfandiari N, et al. Use of letozole challenge test t adjust gonadotropin dose in non down regulated cycles. Fertil Steril. 2011;95(8):2492-3.

32. Vignali M, Infantino M, Matrone R, et al. Endometriosis: Novel etiopathogenetic concepts and clinical perspectives. Fertil Steril. 2002;78:665-78.

33. Schlegel PN. Aromatase inhibitors for male infertility. Fertil Steril. 2012;98(6)1359-62.

34. Begum RM, Ferdous J, Begum A, et al. Comparison of efficacy of aromatase inhibitor and clomiphene citrate in induction of ovulation in PCOS. Fertil Steril. 2009;92:853-7.

35. Amer SA, Smith J, Mahran A, et al. Double blind randomised controlled trial of letrozole versus clomiphene citrate in subfertile women with PCOS. Hum Reprod. 2017;32:1631-8.

36. Ibrahim MI, Moustafa RA, Abdel-Azeem AA. Letrozole versus clomiphene citrate for superovulation in Egyptian women with unexplained infertility: a randomised controlled trial. Arch Gynecol Obstet. 2012;286:1581-87.

37. Tredway D, Schettz JC, Bock D, et al. Anastrozole vs clomiphene citrate in infertile women with ovulatory dysfunction: a phase II randomised, dose-finding study. Fertil Steril. 2011;95:1720-24.

38. Tredway D, Schettz JC, Bock D, et al. Anastrozole single dose protocol in women with oligo or anovulatory infertility: results of a randomised, phase II dose-response study. Fertil Steril. 2011;95:1724-8.

39. Bedaiwy MA, Shorky M, Mousa N, et al. Letrozole co-treatment in infertile women 40 years old and older receiveing controlled ovarian stimulation and intrauterine insemination. Fertil Steril. 2009;91:2501-7.

Gonadotropins

Chaitanya Nagori

INTRODUCTION

Gonadotropins are direct stimulation to ovaries in contrast to clomiphene citrate and letrozole, which stimulate hypothalamus and indirectly increases follicle-stimulating hormone (FSH) and luteinizing hormone (LH) simultaneously. Professor Bruno Lunenfeld first reported the use of human menopausal gonadotropin (HMG) followed by pregnancy in 1963. Now purified preparations of gonadotropins are also available. The availability of recombinant FSH (rFSH) has changed the picture for demand of gonadotropins.

PHYSIOLOGY

- Primordial follicles are independent of gonadotropin stimulation and they take 10 weeks to develop into antral follicles.
- Antral follicles can respond to gonadotropin stimulation.
- Under the influence of FSH and LH, antral follicle grows, matures, and ovulates in two weeks.

- Follicle-stimulating hormone rise in the late luteal phase of previous cycle decides the dominant follicle.
- For follicular cohort minimum level of FSH is required and this is called FSH threshold.
- Follicle-stimulating hormone window means number of days the FSH levels are above threshold.
- As the sensitivity of follicle to FSH increases with development, lower amount of FSH is required for further growth of the follicle.
- As the amount of FSH decreases, it stops growth of other follicles except the dominant follicle. The process of selection of follicle is completed in seven days. But when gonadotropins are given from outside, we do not decrease the dose of FSH and so there will be larger number of follicles to grow and ovulate in controlled ovarian stimulation (COS).
- All oocytes are arrested in prophase stage in meiosis in preantral follicles. This inhibition is removed by LH surge and first meiotic division will be complete with extrusion of first polar body. Oocytes

should be fertilized within 48–72 hours and second meiotic division occur otherwise oocyte dies.

FOLLICLE-STIMULATING HORMONE PREPARATIONS AVAILABLE

- *Human menopausal gonadotropin*: 75 IU of FSH and 75 IU of LH activity with human chorionic gonadotropin (hCG) which acts as LH surrogate.
- *Human menopausal gonadotropin-HP (highly purified)*: 75 IU of FSH and 75 IU of LH with less than 5% of urinary proteins.
- *Urinary FSH (uFSH)*: 75 IU of FSH and 1 IU of LH.
- *Follicle-stimulating hormone-HP*: 75 IU of FSH with less than 0.1 IU of LH and more than 5% of urinary proteins.
- *Recombinant FSH*: 75 IU of FSH and no LH activity.
- Recombinant FSH + rLH combination.

PRINCIPLES OF GONADOTROPIN THERAPY

The basic principles were suggested by Insler and Lunenfeld in 1974.[1]
- *Effective dose*: Ovarian response is seen when certain dose of FSH is given. Below this dose, the ovaries do not respond.
- *Latent phase*: This phase lasts for 3–7 days. It starts with onset of stimulation, but there is no estrogen rise or ultrasound demonstrable follicular growth during this phase.
- *Active phase*: This phase starts with ultrasound demonstrable follicle growth to ovulation and it lasts for 4–6 days.

PHYSIOLOGY OF OVULATION

- Follicle-stimulating hormone stimulates the follicle to grow. But continuous stimulation is required for follicle to grow.
- Follicle secretes estrogen, that has negative feedback on hypothalamus to secrete less FSH and LH.
- When follicle is mature and estrogen secretion is at its peak, pituitary receives a positive feedback for LH surge by the short loop.
- Luteinizing hormone surge causes ovulation to occur.
- Mature follicle is 16–18 mm and estrogen secretion from such a follicle is 150 pg/mL/follicle.

DIFFERENT REGIMES OF GONADOTROPIN THERAPY

- Step-up protocol
- Step-down protocol
- Chronic low-dose protocol.

When to use which protocol depends on the baseline scan and has been discussed in the chapter on baseline scan.

Indications of Gonadotropins Therapy

- Hypogonadotropic hypogonadism (substitutional therapy)
- Hypothalamo-pituitary dysfunction:
  - Clomiphene resistant patients
  - Clomiphene failure patients
  - Superovulation combined with intra-uterine insemination (IUI)
  - Gonadotropin as first line of treatment
  - Controlled ovarian hyperstimulation (COH) in assisted reproductive technique (ART) cycles.

Step-up Protocol

Baseline scan guides to decide the stimulating dose. Conventionally in normal responding ovary, 1 amp i.e. 75 IU of FSH is started from day 5 for 5 days. Ultrasound scan is done on day 6 of stimulation. If this scan shows a follicle of 10–12 mm and/or there is 2–3 mm increase in endometrial thickness, the same dose is continued till follicle and endometrium become mature. If there is no increase in the size of the follicle or not much change in the endometrial thickness, the dose is doubled and scan is repeated after 3 days. If the follicle or endometrium grows, the same dose is continued till follicle and endometrium are mature; otherwise dose is further increased by 75 IU/day. But this is rarely the case now as each patient is assessed on day 2–3 of period (baseline scan), and if this scan diagnose poorly responding ovaries, in these patients stimulation is to be started with higher doses.

This protocol has been blamed for higher rates of multiple pregnancies and ovarian hyperstimulation syndrome (OHSS).[2] But I personally do not agree with the statement of higher risk of OHSS as step-up protocol is never used in polycystic ovary syndrome (PCOS) patients. Conventional protocol gives excellent pregnancy rates in normal responding ovary (Fig. 5.1). We never do estradiol (E2) level before increasing the dose though some centers do. Good ultrasound monitoring can replace hormonal estimations.

Step-down Protocol (Fig. 5.2)

This protocol is very useful for the poor responding ovaries or low reserve ovaries. According to this protocol, stimulation is started with higher dose, i.e. 150–225 IU FSH from day 5 for 5 days. Once the follicle grows to 10–12 mm, the dose is reduced to 75–150 IU FSH, once the follicle size reaches 14 mm, the dose is further reduced, if it was 150 IU, or is continued with 75 IU FSH till follicle and endometrium mature.

Chronic Low-dose Protocol (Fig. 5.3)

This protocol is very useful in PCOS patients. PCO contains almost twice the number of available FSH sensitive antral follicles in

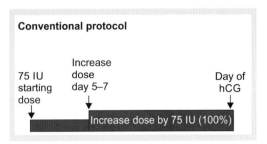

Fig. 5.1: Conventional protocol. (hCG: human chorionic gonadotropin)

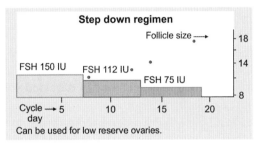

Fig. 5.2: Step-down protocol. (FSH: follicle-stimulating hormone)

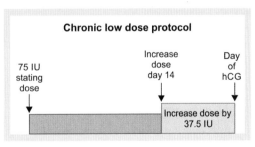

Fig. 5.3: Chronic low-dose protocol. (hCG: human chorionic gonadotropin)

cohort as compared to normal ovaries. This protocol gives good pregnancy rates with very little risk of OHSS or multiple pregnancies. But it is essential that PCOS is confirmed on baseline ultrasound scan. In this protocol, stimulation is started with 75 IU of FSH and same dose is continued for 14 days. If follicle or endometrium grows, the same dose is continued till mature follicle and endometrium are achieved otherwise the dose is increased by 37.5 IU for other 7 days. Almost all the patients

TABLE 5.1: Scoring system depending on the initial score of the patient on the baseline scan.[5]

Score	1	2	3	4	5
Age	>40	35–40	30–35	25–30	<25
BMI	>30	30–28	28–25	25–22	<22
AFC	<5	5–10	10–15	15–20	>20
Ovarian volume	<3	3–5	5–7	7–10	>10
Stromal RI	>0.75	0.75–0.65	0.65–0.55	0.55–0.45	<0.45
Stromal PSV	<3	3–5	5–7	7–10	>10

(AFC: antral follicle count; BMI: body mass index; RI: resistance index; PSV: peak systolic velocity)

develop good follicle and endometrium and incidence of multiple pregnancy and OHSS is extremely low.[3] Majority of the patients develop good follicle within 14 days and we should strongly resist ourselves to increase the dose till then. There may be spotting or some bleeding during this period, which should be ignored. With chronic low-dose protocol, there is monofollicular development in 70% of cycles, OHSS can be almost totally eliminated and multiple pregnancy rate less than 6% with same pregnancy rate as conventional protocol.[4]

Though the stimulation protocols can be tailor made for individual patients, depending on the antral follicle count (AFC), ovarian volume, ovarian stromal resistance index (RI), and peak systolic velocity (PSV). This reduces the risk of OHSS to less than 1%. According to this study, depending on the above-described ultrasound parameters, age and body mass index (BMI), the scoring system is devised and depending on the initial score of the patient on the baseline scan the starting dose of rFSH can be decided (Table 5.1).[5,6]

For IUI:

Score of ≥ 25	25 IU
20–24	37.5 IU
15–20	75 IU
10–15	112.5 IU
6–10	150 IU

For in vitro fertilization (IVF):

Score of ≥ 23	75 IU
20–22	150 IU
16–20	225 IU
11–15	300 IU
6–10	375 IU

RECOMBINANT FOLLICLE-STIMULATING HORMONE

The invent of rFSH has changed the management of infertile patients. In 1990, 6 lacs urine donors were required for 120 million liters of urine for urinary gonadotropin production. This was becoming extremely difficult as with developing techniques in ART, the need for gonadotropins were further increasing. Therefore, there was an urgent need for FSH production by alternate route. The first rFSH was introduced in 1995. But it was in 1992 that Professor Paul Devroey and Germond reported the clinical utility of rFSH.

How is Recombinant Follicle-stimulating Hormone Produced?

The objective of recombinant deoxyribonucleic acid (rDNA) technology is to insert genes in the cell to produce desired proteins. The gene that is coded for desired protein is isolated enzymatically from DNA chain. The isolated gene is put in vector (a large segment of DNA).

TABLE 5.2: Product with their specific bioactivity.

Product	Specific bioactivity
HMG (1950)	8 IU/mg protein
uFSH (1980)	100–150 IU/mg protein
uHMG-HP	2,000 IU/mg protein
uFSH-HP (1990)	9,000 IU/mg protein
rFSH (1995)	10,000 IU/mg protein

(HP: highly purified; HMG: human menopausal gonadotropin; rFSH: recombinant follicle-stimulating hormone; uFSH: urinary follicle-stimulating hormone)

TABLE 5.3: Comparison of recombinant follicle-stimulating hormone (rFSH) with urinary FSH (uFSH).

	rFSH	uFSH
Higher number of oocytes	10.8	8.9
Lower dose of FSH	2,138 IU	2385 IU
Shorter period	10.7	11.3
High quality embryos	3.1	2.6
Pregnancy rate with cryopreservation	25.5%	20.4%

This is known as rDNA in host cell. This rDNA produces desired proteins—rFSH. Therefore, human DNA genes into a mammalian cell line produces rFSH, which is 99.9% pure without LH activity. rFSH has bioactivity of 10,000 IU/mg of protein (Table 5.2).

Preparation

Follitropin alpha is produced by transfecting Chinese hamster ovary cells with genes for the α and β subunits of human FSH.

The secretory products of these cells undergo six-step purification process to get a final preparation, which is highly pure biochemically (>99% FSH).

Properties

- It has highest bioactivity
- It has no LH or hCG like activity
- It has no protein
- It has high batch to batch consistency
- It does not produce FSH antibodies in patients
- It has low level of oxidation and/or degradation, i.e. 10% compared to 40% with uFSH
- Bioactivity mimics the preovulation FSH in normal cycles.

Comparison of rFSH with uFSH

The study conducted by Hedan B clearly indicates superiority of rFSH (Table 5.3).[7]

The meta-analysis conducted by Salim Daya and Gunby of 12 randomized controlled trials has proved that rFSH is 20% more likely to achieve pregnancy than uFSH. The amount of FSH used was 400 IU less.[8]

The meta-analysis data was summarized by the author as "The overall conclusion from this meta-analysis is that rFSH is more effective than uFSH because of the higher rates of clinical pregnancy per cycle started and is more efficient because the total dose of gonadotropin required was lower",[8] i.e. 400 IU less.

Prospective meta-analysis has proved that clinical pregnancy rate is 5% higher in rFSH and if cryopreserved embryos are taken into account, pregnancy rate is 6.4% higher.[9]

Though a recently published Cochrane review has shown no difference in pregnancy outcomes with fresh embryo transfers when rFSH and uFSH were compared. It was concluded that "all available gonadotropins in clinical practice are equally effective and safe" and the choice is based on availability, convenience, and cost.[10]

Comparison of rFSH with uFSH-HP

Recombinant follicle-stimulating hormone is more effective than highly purified FSH in multiple follicular development (Table 5.4).[11]

Frydman and associates also published the data that rFSH gives more number of

TABLE 5.4: Comparison of recombinant follicle-stimulating hormone (rFSH) with highly purified urinary FSH (uFSH-HP).[11]

	rFSH	uFSH	P value
Number of ampoules	21.9 ± 5.1	31.9 ± 13.4	<0.0001
FSH days	11 ± 1.6	13.5 ± 3.7	<0.001
Oocytes retrieved	12.2 ± 5.5	7.6 ± 4.4	<0.0001
Embryos transferred	2 ± 0.19	1.9 ± 0.4	NS
Pregnancy rates	53/119 (45%)	42/114 (37%)	NS
Implantation	32	31	NS

oocytes, more embryos with lesser number of injections.[12]

Gearon and Abdalla from Lister hospital, London in an unpublished study have reported for the first time improvement in quality of oocytes in older women treated with rFSH instead of uFSH-HP. Another randomized single blind, multicentric multinational study by Schats et al. also confirmed the same findings.

Recombinant follicle-stimulating hormone gives more embryos with lesser ampoules. More than four embryos in culture have higher chance of achieving pregnancy.[13] The chances of blastocyst transfer is increased if more than four oocytes are retrieved.[14] But some randomized trials have failed to show the difference in terms of pregnancy rate or miscarriage rate in normal as well as PCOS.[15,16]

Recombinant follicle-stimulating hormone was associated with higher per cycle pregnancy rate than uFSH-HP, when used at the same dose, whereas the pregnancy rates were similar when the dose of rFSH was 50% lower.[17]

Recombinant Follicle-stimulating Hormone versus Human Menopausal Gonadotropin

Meta-analysis of eight randomized controlled trials comparing rFSH with HMG has shown that rFSH has 50% higher pregnancy rates.[18]

The FIVNAT (French National Register on in vitro fertilization) report 1999 showed that the pregnancy rates were higher with rFSH than HMG.

Prospective analysis of 24,000 ART cycles from Germany also showed higher birth rate and lower dosage with rFSh than HMG.[19] In patients where LH and FSH ratio is high in PCOS, only FSH rather than HMG will improve the results.[20] There is a subgroup of patients like poor responders and elderly patients when HMG-HP is given. It has given higher pregnancy rates, so either rLH or HMG-HP is useful in a sub-group of patients.[21,22]

Meta-analysis including 400,000 IVF cycles showed that compared to rFSH, HMG resulted in fewer oocytes and higher doses.[23]

Facts about Highly Purified Human Menopausal Gonadotropin

- The process is partially successful with specific activity of 2,000 IU/mg of protein.
- In many cases, LH activity has to be added using hCG which has longer half-life.
- Presence of variable amount of hCG may further increase variation between different batches of product and result in follicular atresia.[24]
- The HMG-HP contains 30% extraneous proteins including leukocyte elastase inhibitor protein C inhibitor and Zn-α2 glycoprotein apart from hCG.

Different Types of Recombinant Follicle-stimulating Hormone

- Follitropin α; 1995.
- Follitropin β; 1996.
- Immunopotency, biopotency, and internal carbohydrate complexity are same for both but follitropin α contains higher proportion of acidic glycoforms.
- Follitropin α has a specific activity of 13,645 IU/mg whereas that for follitropin β is 9,396 IU/mg.

There is a difference in tolerability between rFSH preparations favoring follitropin alpha over beta.[25] Though follitropin alpha has a higher incidence of OHSS as compared to follitropin beta (4.1% as compared to 2.7%).[26]

Fill by mass Concept

Dose of gonadotropin is expressed in international units (IU). But recent fill by mass (FbM) technique reflects a constant relationship between mass and bioactivity and guarantees consistency of dose from batch to batch. So, drawbacks of vivo bioassay can be avoided. Bioassay of FSH preparation is 50 years old. Steelman-Pohley bioassay, which is cumbersome, requires large number of animals and variation can be 10–20%. But FbM is by liquid chromatography supported by glycine mapping isoelectric focusing that demonstrates physicochemical consistency of the product.

Duration of stimulation was significantly shorter in FbM group and embryo quality and implantation rates were significantly higher (28.6% in FbM vs 18.6% in FbIU).[27,28]

Clinical Benefits of Recombinant Follicle-stimulating Hormone[29]

- Improved logistics of pharmaceutical process
- Controlled manufacturing
- Reduced batch to batch variability
- Potentially unlimited supply—no shortage
- Not reliant on the urine supply
- No risk of infection
- No risk of contamination with drugs or metabolites
- No seroconversion to antigonadotropin antibodies
- Effective, safe, and less traumatic subcutaneous administration
- Greater purity and specific activity
- Smaller doses required
- More predictable response
- Cost benefit.

There are reports also that there is no difference in pregnancy rate when rFSH was compared with uFSH or urinary gonadotropins[30] and there is no difference in OHSS also.

PROTOCOLS FOR ASSISTED REPRODUCTIVE TECHNIQUE

Gonadotropins in Assisted Reproductive Technique

In ART cycles also, stimulation protocol is decided by baseline scan.

Long Agonist Protocol

Downregulation from 21st day of previous cycle as nasal spray or subcutaneous injections of GnRH agonist (leuprolide acetate 0.5 mg or decapeptyl 0.1 mg) and is continued till periods. The dose is halved from the day of period. Depot preparations of agonist can be used instead of daily agonist injections on day 21 of the previous cycle. The most common starting dose for COS with rFSH is 150–225/day. Increasing the dosage in elderly women does not result in increased oocyte yield.[31] It has been found that 150 IU of rFSH is equivalent to 225 IU of uFSH for follicular growth. The dose of 150 IU is optimum,[32] rather than 100 IU that has been mentioned in a comparative study for IVF patients.

Short Protocol

This protocol exploits the flare-up effect of agonist during the ovarian stimulation. Agonist is started with the beginning of the menstrual cycle and flare up provides the surge of gonadotropins secretion. A few days later, exogenous gonadotropins are administrated to supplement the flare. Both agonist and gonadotropins are continued till the day of trigger. This protocol is preferred for poor responders.

Ultrashort Protocol

Agonist is given on day 2, 3, and 4 of the stimulation cycle in the dose of 500-1,000 μg per day and then gonadotropins are given subsequently till day of hCG.

Antagonist Protocol

High resistance, low velocity stromal flow, fewer antral follicles, smaller ovarian volume, high BMI, and age more than 35 years are the parameters which decide higher doses for stimulation with antagonist protocol where as low resistance, high velocity stromal flow, polycystic ovaries, low BMI, and age less than 24 years are the parameters which would be in favor of lower doses with antagonist protocol. Antagonist is started from day 6 and continued till the day of trigger. In these patients, GnRh agonist can be used for ovulation trigger, instead of hCG. This protocol reduces the incidence of OHSS significantly. This is known as fixed antagonist protocol. Antagonist can also be used as flexible protocol, when antagonist is started when at least one follicle is 14 mm in diameter.[33] Antagonist protocol has high cumulative pregnancy rate in both groups, high anti-Müllerian hormone (AMH) (40.1–63.6%) and low AMH (11.1–18.7%).[34] A meta-analysis of 45 randomized controlled trials involving 7,511 women comparing GnRH antagonist protocol and long agonist protocol for COS in ART has found no significant differences in live birth or ongoing pregnancy rates, but marked decrease in OHSS with antagonist protocols.[35] Another meta-analysis comparing agonist and antagonist protocols for poor responders has shown advantage in terms of FSH stimulation, but no statistically significant difference in terms of oocytes retrieved or clinical pregnancy rates.[36]

Antagonist-agonist Protocol

This protocol is especially used for PCOS patients. It is known as OHSS free protocol. Fixed antagonist protocol is used for downregulation and then agonist is used for ovulation trigger.

Antagonist-agonist Protocol with Human Chorionic Gonadotropin as Luteal Support

The above-mentioned protocol is very likely to lead to luteal phase defect. It is therefore recommended to supplement the luteal phase with 1,500 IU of hCG on day 3-7-10 of ovum pick-up.[37]

PREDICTORS OF OVARIAN RESPONSE

Predictors of ovarian response are as follows:
- Age
- Body mass index
- Baseline FSH
- Anti-Müllerian hormone (AMH) (not mentioned in Collin-Howles study)
- Antral follicle count.

A nomogram can be prepared using these predictors. *Howles and colleagues have prepared a manuscript on the same.*[38] The cost effectivity has been mentioned in the results presented in Table 5.5. These are the results of computer modeling study.

Individualized dose calculation for COS[34] is presented in Table 5.6.

TABLE 5.5: Cost-effectivity of predictors of ovarian response.

	rFSH	uFSH
UK	5,906£	6,060£
USA (social)	40,688$	47,096$
(insurance)	28,481$	32,967$
Spain (public insurance)	12,791€	13,007€
Spain (private)	19,739€	20,467€
Germany	21,686€	22,189€

(rFSH: recombinant follicle-stimulating hormone; uFSH: urinary follicle-stimulating hormone)

Newer Developments

- *Long-acting FSH:* Long-acting FSH is corifollitropin alpha. It keeps the FSH above the threshold level for multifollicular growth. It is convenient for the patients for having less number of injections. There is no difference in live births and OHSS rate.[39]
- Sustained release rFSH.
- Oral FSH.

LUTEINIZING HORMONE SUPPLEMENTATION: FOR WHOM, WHEN, AND WHY?

Two-cell–two-gonadotropins Theory

- Both FSH and LH are required for E2 synthesis. LH binds to theca cells to induce androgen synthesis. Androgen diffuses into granulosa cells, where FSH-stimulated aromatization leads to estrogen synthesis.[40]
- Luteinizing hormone in follicular phase helps conversion of progesterone to androgen to reduce follicular phase progesterone, that is detrimental to endometrial receptivity.[41] A combination of rFSH and rLH in a ratio of 2:1 is indicated for women with severe gonadotropin deficiency— hypogonadotropic hypogonadism.[42]

Luteinizing Hormone Threshold

Luteinizing hormone is required for terminal stages of follicular maturation, for meiosis, and ovulation.

Luteinizing Hormone Ceiling Effect

- High LH causes follicular atresia, premature luteinization and oocyte quality may be compromised.[43]
- In patients over responding to FSH, adding 30 mg rLH, leads to monofollicular development.[44] This indicates LH ceiling effect.

Current Opinion

- Current opinion is that there is no absolute requirement for LH supplementation in unselected patient population.[45]
- However, LH may have benefit in women aged more than 35 years and

TABLE 5.6: Individualized dose calculation for COS.

AMH level	Predicted response to COS	Treatment strategies
15 pmol/L	High responders (150 IU)	GnRH antagonist protocol Normal oocyte yield, very low excess response, low embryo cryopreservation, high/maintained fresh CPR
5–15 pmol/L	Normal responders (225–300 IU)	GnRH agonist protocol: very low cancellation of oocyte pick-up and OHSS
<5 pmol/L	Poor responders (375 IU)	High dose FSH: long stimulation, high cancellation Antagonist strategy: short stimulation, moderate cancellation

(AMH: anti-Müllerian hormone; COS: controlled ovarian stimulation; CPR: clinical pregnancy rate; OHSS: ovarian hyperstimulation syndrome)

those who are poor responders to COS.[46] Though Cochrane review[37] and studies subsequently published have shown that LH supplementation, including for women with advanced age, has no benefit on ongoing pregnancy, with an adjusted odds ratio (OR) of 0.99 [confidence interval (CI) 0.76–1.29].[45]

- Luteinizing hormone supplementation may improve outcomes in patients with suboptimal response to FSH stimulation.[47]
- No LH cutoff value is known to identify a female requiring LH supplementation and LH assessment is therefore of no use.[48]
- In antagonist cycle, LH supplementation is controversial. Though some studies have shown that it improves results in selected groups.
- Luteinizing hormone estimation may not be a reliable guide to decide for LH supplementation because of variable bioactivity and polymorphism.

Summary

Adding LH increases the number of developmentally competent oocytes in woman with endogenous LH suppressed below 1 IU/L at the start of stimulation. However, with LH more than 1 IU/L, adding LH is associated with significant lower embryo quality and implantation rate compared with rFSH alone.[49] Recombinant human LH (r-hLH) alone can trigger follicular growth arrest in a significant number of patients supporting the existence of LH ceiling during late follicular maturation.[50] rFSH with r-hLH 150 IU from day 6 might be beneficial in subgroup women in older reproductive age, having LH polymorphism and less sensitivity to LH.

The results of analysis by age showed a trend towards higher implantation rate with rFSH alone in patients aged less than 35 years. In contrast, the group aged more than 35 years

had numerically higher implantation rate in the rFSH plus r-hLH group.[51,52]

Recombinant human LH supplementation on day 8 in patients having E2 less than 180 pg/mL and no follicles more than 10 mm, significantly increases the number of oocytes retrieved and requirement of rFSH was also decreased.[53]

In Summary

Recombinant human LH supplementation when:
- Age more than 35 years
- Poor initial response to rFSH.
  Stimulation protocol at Bourn Hall Clinic, London:
- *Preprocedure investigations*:
  - Serum FSH
  - Serum LH
  - Serum estradiol
  - Serum prolactin.
- Review response to previous stimulation
- Gonadotropin-releasing hormone antagonist (GnRHa) 500 µg (buserelin) from day 21
- Dose of GnRHa is reduced to 200 µg in first few days of menstruation when:
  - Estradiol less than 50 pg/mL
  - Luteinizing hormone less than 5 IU/L
  - Progesterone less than 2 pg/mL.

Dose in first IVF cycle:
- *Age less than 35 years*: 150 IU rFSH daily
- *Age 35–39 years*: 225 IU of rFSh daily
- *Age more than 40 years*: 300 IU of rFSH daily.

After 5-7 days, dose is adjusted according the response.

Recombinant luteinizing hormone is added when:
- Age more than 38 years
- Serum LH less than 1.5 IU
- H/O poor response
- Serum estradiol is low

- Poor response in current cycle
- Gonadotropin-releasing hormone antagonists are used.

Recombinant human chorionic gonadotropin (rhCG) is given when:

- Two follicles are 18 mm
- Estradiol more than 100 pg/follicle of 12–14 mm size
- 34–36 hours prior to pickup.

Luteal support:

- Only progesterone 400 mg bd vaginally from day of ovum pick-up (OPU)
- Progesterone gel can be used
- Human chorionic gonadotropin is never used
- Beta hCG on 15th day after OPU
- Ultrasound on day 35 after OPU.

CARRY HOME MESSAGE

- Gonadotropins give better pregnancy rates than clomiphene citrate.
- Step-up protocol is used for normal responding ovaries.
- Chronic low dose protocol is best for PCOS.
- Recombinant FSH requires lower dosage with better efficacy.
- Recombinant FSH is better than all urinary preparation.
- Recombinant LH is used in poor responders and patients of age more than 35 years.

REFERENCES

1. Lunenfeld B, Insler V, Rabau E. The principles of gonadotrophin therapy. Acta Endocrinol Suppl (Copenh). 1970;148:52-101.
2. Westergard LG, Erb K, Laursen SB, et al. HMG versus rFSH in normogonadotrophic women down regulated with gonadotrophic releasing hormone agonist who were undergoing IVF and ICSI, a prospective randomised study. Fertil Steril. 2001;76(3):543-49.
3. Homburg R, Levy T, Ben-Rafael Z. A comparative prospective study of conventional regimen with chronic low dos administration of follicle stimulating hormone for anovulation associated with polycystic ovary syndrome. Fertil Steril. 1995;63(4):729-33.
4. Driebergen R, Baer G. Quantification of follicle stimulating hormone (follitropin alpha): is in vivo bioassay still relevant in recombinant age? Curr Med Res Opin. 2003;19:41-6.
5. Panchal S, Nagori C. Ultrasound based decision making on stimulation protocol for superovulated intrauterine insemination cycles. Int J Infertil Fetal Med. 2016;7(1):7-13.
6. Panchal S, Nagori CB. Ultrasound based decision making on stimulation protocol in IVF. Donald School J Ultrasound Obstet Gynecol. 2016;10(3):330-7.
7. Hedon B, Out HJ, Hugues JN, et al. Efficacy and safety of recombinant follicle stimulating hormone (Puregon) in infertile women pituitary suppressed with triptorelin undergoing in-vitro fertilization: a prospective randomized, assessor-blind, multicentre trial. Hum Reprod. 1995;10:3102-6.
8. Daya S. Updated meta-analysis of recombinant follicle-stimulating hormone (FSH) versus urinary FSH for ovarian stimulation in assisted reproduction. Fertil Steril. 2002;77(4):711-14.
9. Out HJ, Driessen SG, Mannaerts BM, et al. Recombinant follicle-stimulating hormone (follitropin beta, Puregon) yields higher pregnancy rates in in vitro fertilization than urinary gonadotropins. Fertil Steril. 1997;68:138-42.
10. van Wely M, Kwan I, Burt AL, et al. Recombinant versus urinary gonadotrophin for ovarian stimulation in assisted reproductive technology cycles. Cochrane Database Syst Rev. 2011;(2):CD005354.
11. Bergh C, Howles CM, Borg K, et al. Recombinant follicle stimulating hormone (r-h-FSH; Gonal-F) versus highly purified urinary FSH (Metrodin HP): results of a randomized comparative study in women undergoing assisted reproductive techniques. Hum Reprod. 1997;12:2133-39.
12. Frydman R, Haverell C, Camier B. A double blind randomized study comparing the efficacy of recombinant human (FSH:

Gonal-F) versus highly purified urinary FSH (Metrodin-HP) in inducing superovulation in women undergoing assisted reproductive techniques. Hum Reprod. 1998;13:180-5.

13. XV FIGO World Congress of Gynecology and Obstetrics. Copenhagen, Denmark, 3-8 August 1997. Abstracts. Part 1. Acta Obstet Gynecol Scand Suppl. 1997;167 Pt 1:1-119.

14. Scholtes MC, Zeilmaker GH. Blastocyst transfer in day-5 embryo transfer depends primarily on the number of oocytes retrieved and not on age. Fertil Steril. 1998;69:78-83.

15. Yaralli H, Bukulmez O, Gurgan T. Urinary follicle stimulating hormone (FSH) versus recombinant FSH in clomiphene citrate resistant, normogonadotrophic, chronic anovulation: a prospective randomized study. Fertil Steril. 1999;72:276-81.

16. Bayram N, van Wely M, van der Veen F. Recombinant FSH versus urinary gonado-trophins or recombinant FSH for ovulation induction in subfertility associated with polycystic ovary syndrome. Cochrane database Syst Rev. 2002;(1):CD002121.

17. Matorras R, Osuna C, Exposito A, et al. Recombinant FSH versus highly purified FSH in intrauterine insemination: systematic review and meta-analysis. Fertil Steril. 2011;95:1937-42.

18. Daya S, Gunby J, Hughes EG, et al. Follicle stimulating hormone versus human menopausal gonadotrophins for in-vitro fertilization cycles: a meta-analysis. Fertil Steril. 1995;27:347-54.

19. Ludwig M, Rabe T, Buhler K, et al. Wirksamkeit von recombinanten humane FSH in Vergleich zu urinarem hMG nach Downregulation im langen Protokoll–eine Analyse von 24.764 ART-Zyklen in Deutschland. J Reprod Med Endocrinol. 1994;4:284-8.

20. Hughes E, Collins J, Vandekerckhove P. Ovulation induction with urinary follicle stimulating hormone versus human menopausal gonadotropin for clomiphene-resistant polycystic ovary syndrome. Cochrane Database Syst Rev. 2000;(2):CD000087.

21. Coomarasamy A, Afnan M, Cheema D, et al. Urinary HMG versus recombinant FSH for controlled ovarian hyperstimulation following an agonist long down-regulation protocol in IVF or ICSI treatment: a systematic review and meta-analysis. Hum Reprod. 2008;23:310-5.

22. Al-Inany HG, Abou-Setta AM, Aboulghar MA, et al. Efficacy and safety of human menopausal gonadotrophins versus recombinant FSH: a meta-analysis. Reprod Biomed Online. 2008;16:81-8.

23. Lehert P, Schertz JC, Ezcurra D. Recombinant human follicle stimulating hormone produces more oocytes with low total dose per cycle in assisted reproductive technologies compared with highly purified HMG: a meta-analysis. Reprod Biol Endocrinol. 2010;8:112.

24. Filicori M. Cognigni GE, Taraborrelli S, et al. Luteinizing hormone activity in menotropins optimizes folliculogenesis and treatment in controlled ovarian stimulation. J Clin Endocrinol Metab. 2001;86(1):337-43.

25. Brinsden P, Akagbosu F, Gibbons LM, et al. A comparison of the efficacy and tolerability of two recombinant human follicle-stimulating hormone preparations in patients undergoing in vitro fertilization-embryo transfer. Fertil Steril. 2003;73:114-6.

26. Devroey P, Boostanfar R, Koper NP, et al. A double blind non-inferiority RCT comparing corifollitropin alpha and rFSH during first seven days of ovarian stimulation using GnRH antagonist protocol. Hum Reprod. 2009;24(12):3063-72.

27. Balasch J, Fabergues F, Penarrubia J, et al. Outcome from consecutive assisted reproduction cycles in patients treated with recombinant follitropin alfa filled-by-bioassay and those treated with recombinant follitropin alfa filled-by-mass. Reprod Biomed Online. 2004;8:408-13.

28. Hugues JN, Barlow DH, Rosenwaks Z, et al. Improvement in consistency of response to ovarian stimulation with recombinant human follicle stimulating hormone resulting from a new method for calibrating the therapeutic preparation. Reprod Biomed Online. 2003;6:185-90.

29. Ludwig M, Diedrich K. Evaluation of an optimal luteal phase support protocol in IVF. Obstet Gynecol Scand. 2001;80:452-66.

30. van Wely M, Kwan I, van der Veen F, et al. Recombinant FSH versus urinary gonadotrophins for ovarian hyperstimulation in IVF and ICSI cycles. A systematic review and meta-analysis. Hum Reprod. 2009;24:S1-34.

31. Out HJ, Braat DD, Linsten BM, et al. Increasing the daily dose of recombinant follicle stimulating hormone (Puregon) does not compensate for the age-related decline in retrievable oocytes after ovarian stimulation. Hum Reprod. 2000;15:29-35.

32. Hughes JN, Barlow DH, Rosenwaks Z, et al. Improvement in consistency of response to ovarian stimulation with recombinant human follicle stimulating hormone resulting from a new method for calibrating the therapeutic preparation. Reprod Biomed Online. 2003;6:185-90.

33. Ludwig M, Katalinic A, Banz C, et al. Tailoring the GnRH antagonist ceterorelix acetate to individual patients' needs in ovarian stimulation for IVF: results of a prospective, randomized study. Hum Reprod. 2002;17(11):2842-5.

34. Nelson SM, Yates RW, Lyall H, et al. Anti-Müllerian hormone based approach to controlled ovarian stimulation for assisted conception. Hum Reprod. 2009;24:867-75.

35. Al-Inany HG, Youssef MA, Aboulghar M, et al. Gonadotropin-releasing hormone antagonists for assisted reproductive technology. Cochrane Database Syst Rev. 2011;5:CD001750.

36. Pu D, Wu J, Liu J. Comparison of GnRH antagonist versus GnRH agonist protocol in poor ovarian responders undergoing IVF. Hum Reprod. 2011;26(10):2742-9.

37. Humadian P, Ejdrup BH, Westergaard LG, et al. 1,500 IU human chorionic gonadotrophins administered at oocyte retrieval rescues the luteal phase when gonadotrophins-releasing hormone agonist is used for ovulation induction: a prospective randomised controlled study. Fertil Steril. 2010;93:847-54.

38. Howles CM. Predictive factors of ovarian reserve. Reprod Biomed Online. 2008;16(S2):pS-5.

39. Pouwer AW, Farquhar C, Kremer JA. Long acting FSH versus daily FSH for women undergoing assisted reproduction. Cochrane Database Syst Rev. 2012;6:CD009577.

40. Kobayashi M, Nakano R, Ooshima A. Immunohistochemical localization of pituitary gonadotrophins and gonadal steroids confirms the 'two cell two gonadotrophins hypothesis of steroidogenesis in the human ovary. J Endocrinol. 1990;126(3):483-88.

41. Fanchin R, Righini C, Olivennes F, et al. Computerized assessment of endometrial echogenicity: clues to the endometrial effects of premature progesterone elevation. Fertil Steril. 1999;71(1):173-81.

42. Bosch E. Recombinant human FSH and recombinant human LH in a 2:1 ratio combination: a new tool for ovulation induction. Exp Rev Obstet Gynecol. 2009;4(5):491-8.

43. Hillier SG. Current concepts of the roles of follicle stimulating hormone and luteinizing hormone in folliculogenesis. Hum Reprod. 1994;9:188-91.

44. Hughes JN, Soussis J, Calderon I, et al. Recombinant LH study group 2005. Does the addition of recombinant LH in WHO group II anovulatory women over-responding to FSH treatment reduce the number of developing follicles? A dose-finding study. Hum Reprod. 2005;20:629-35.

45. Mochtar MH, Van der Veen F, Zeich M, et al. Recombinant luteinizing hormone (rLH) for controlled ovarian hyperstimulation in assisted reproductive cycles. Cochrane Database Syst Rev. 2007;2:CD005070.

46. Howles CM. Luteinizing hormone supplementation in ART. In: Kovacs G (Ed). How to Improve Your ART Success Rates. Cambridge, UK: Cambridge University Press; 2011. pp. 99-104.

47. Lisi F, Rinaldi L, Fischel S, et al. Use of recombinant FSH and recombinant LH in multiple follicular stimulation for IVF: a preliminary study. Reprod Biomed online. 2001;3(3):190-4.

48. Loumaye E, Engrand P, Howles CM, et al. Assessment of the role of serum luteinizing hormone an estradiol response to follicle stimulating hormone on in vitro fertilization treatment outcome. Fertil Steril. 1997;67:889-99.

49. Tesarik J, Mendoza C, et al. Effects of exogenous LH administration during ovarian stimulation of pituitary down regulated young oocyte donors on oocyte yield and developmental competence. Hum Reprod. 2002;17:3129-37.

50. Loumaye E, Engrand P, Shoham Z, et al. Clinical evidence for an LH 'ceiling' effect induced by administration of recombinant human LH during the late follicular phase of stimulated cycles in World Health Organization type I and type II anovulation. Hum Reprod. 2003;18:314-22.

51. Marrs RP, Meldrum DR, Muasher SJ, et al. Randomized trial to compare the effect of recombinant human FSH (follitropin alfa) with or without recombinant human LH in women undergoing assisted reproduction treatment. Reprod Biomed Online. 2004;8:175-82.

52. Humadian P, Bungum M, Bungum L, et al. Effects of recombinant LH supplementation in women undergoing assisted reproduction with GnRh agonist down-regulation and stimulation with recombinant FSH: an opening study. Reprod Biomed online. 2004;8:635-43.

53. De Placido, Alviggi C, Mollo A, et al. Effects of recombinant LH (rLH) supplementation during controlled ovarian stimulation(COH) in normogonadotrophic women with an initial inadequate response to recombinant FSH (rFSH) after pituitary downregulation. Clin Endocrinol. 2004;60:637-43.

6

Ultrasound Monitoring of ART Cycle

Sonal Panchal

INTRODUCTION

Ultrasound has been long considered now to be the modality of choice for monitoring of the patients on treatment for infertility, may it be intrauterine insemination (IUI) cycles or in vitro fertilization (IVF) cycles. The reason for this is that it is patient friendly, easy to use repeatedly and is also financially viable. Moreover, when used with Doppler it gives precise idea not only about the morphological changes but also about the hormonal changes occurring during the entire cycle. It is important to mention here that ultrasound is the modality that gives idea about the instantaneous endocrinological status, unlike the hormonal assessment reports, that take a few hours to give the results.

The discussion about of the role of ultrasound during the entire treatment cycle will be divided into three parts:
1. Baseline scan and deciding the stimulation protocol
2. Preovulatory scan and decision on trigger
3. Luteal phase scan.

BASELINE SCAN AND DECIDING THE STIMULATION PROTOCOL

This scan is done when hormonal levels are at baseline on day 2–3 of the menstrual cycle. The ovaries are silent, and have no active follicle or corpus luteum at this stage. Route of scan has to be transvaginal always to allow better resolution and more anatomical details of ovary and endometrium. All the scans are done using B-mode ultrasound with color Doppler, pulse Doppler, three-dimensional (3D) ultrasound, and 3D power Doppler. Using color Doppler in this assessment is mandatory because a large number of biochemical or hormonal changes occur during the menstrual cycle, which reflect as vascular and morphological changes in the ovaries and uterus and vascular changes can be assessed by Doppler.

One of the earliest studies, by Ravhon et al.[1] has used dynamic assessment of inhibin B and estradiol after buserelin acetate as predictors of ovarian response and have found these to be highly correlating with the ovarian response in IVF patients. The two major drawbacks of this study are that this required several blood tests at different times and the study sample was pretty small (n = 37).

In 2002, Kupesic et al.[2] used 3D ultrasound for assessment of ovarian response in IVF cycles. The antral follicle count (AFC) and ovarian stromal flow parameters on the baseline scan were shown to be most predictive of the ovarian response after pituitary down regulation in this study, followed by total ovarian volume, ovarian stromal area, and age. This study could predict favorable IVF outcome in 50% (11/22) of patients and poor outcome in 85% (29/34) of patients. Though the study results were fairly convincing the sample volume was only 56 patients. Popovic-Todorovic et al.[3] in 2003, combined age, body mass index (BMI), cycle length, and smoking status and ultrasound features of the ovaries also to design a dosage nomogram of recombinant follicle-stimulating hormone (rFSH) for IVF/intracytoplasmic sperm injection (ICSI) patients. This was a prospective study and also had a larger sample volume than the previous two studies (n = 145). According to this study, total number of antral follicles and ovarian stromal blood flow were the two most significant predictors of ovarian response and ovarian volume was highly significant predictor of number of follicles and oocytes retrieved. Using this nomogram for dose calculation was evaluated by the same group in another study. The results of this study were in absolute favor of individualizing dose according to the dosage nomogram proving the reliability of ultrasound parameters and age and BMI for decision on stimulation doses. Whereas, a study by Ng EH et al.[4] showed basal FSH to be the most reliable parameter for assessment of ovarian response followed by AFC and BMI. Where AFC was predictive of number of follicles (serum estradiol level) on the day of human chorionic gonadotropin (hCG) and BMI was predictive of gonadotropins dosage.

Another landmark study by oliveness and Howles et al.[5]—The CONSORT study, used basal FSH, BMI, age, and AFC for individualizing FSH dose for ovarian stimulation.

A dose calculator was developed using these factors as predictors and was evaluated in a prospective clinical trial.

An ultrasound based study on prediction of ovarian response in 2007 by Merce et al.[6] evaluated ovarian volume, AFC, and 3D power Doppler indices vascularization index (VI), flow index (FI), and vascularity flow index (VFI) for their reliability to calculate the number of follicles grown, oocyte retrieved embryos transferred.

This study clearly showed the relevance of ovarian volume and AFC to the number of follicles matured and oocytes retrieved. It also mentioned that 3D power Doppler indices made the assessment of ovarian response to stimulation protocols easier.

The only study that worked on the dose calculations for IUI patients was by Freiesleben NL et al.[7] in 2008 with 159 patients. They evaluated age, spontaneous cycle length, body weight, BMI, smoking status, total ovarian volume, AFC, total Doppler score of ovarian stromal blood flow, baseline FSH, and estradiol as possible predictive factors of ovarian response. This study concluded that body weight and AFC may be used to achieve appropriate ovarian response for IUI in ovulatory patients. Study by the same investigators for IVF and ICSI patients concluded that AFC and age could predict the low response better where as to predict hyper response AFC and cycle length were better parameters.

The parameters that we have used to calculate the dose of gonadotropins for stimulation protocol for IUI cycles in our study are age, BMI, AFC, ovarian volume stromal RI, and peak systolic velocity (PSV).

Antral follicle count showed the best correlation with women's age and declines linearly at a rate of 3.8% per year according to Ng et al.[8]

Antral follicle count declines at a rate of 4.8% per year before the age of 37 years and declines at rate of 11.7% after 37 years according to another study.[9]

Anti-Müllerian hormone (AMH) and AFC both have reflections of primordial follicles and both are stable between cycles.[10]

Linear correlation is seen between AFC and AMH and both help to predict the extremes of response. Therefore, we have included AFC as one of the parameters for ovarian reserve and omitted AMH. Age is known to be one of the most important factors that reduce not only the ovarian reserve but also the oocyte quality. It has been shown in several studies, above mentioned, that BMI may be an important determinant of the ovarian response. This is because flow in the ovarian stroma is less in obese patients as compared to controls.[10]

A study indicates that AFC is the most useful marker in predicting the ovarian response. Doing AFC assessment alone would be more cost-effective for predicting the ovarian response in patients undergoing controlled ovarian stimulation with gonadotropin-releasing hormone (GnRH) antagonist. AFC had the highest accuracy for predicting ovarian response in patients with abnormal ovarian reserve test and was statistically significant (number of oocyte aspirated p value <0.001) than AMH (p value 0.06) and FSH (p value 0.212) in predicting ovarian response. For prediction of poor ovarian response a model including AFC + AMH was found to be almost similar to that of (p value 0.001) using AFC alone.[11]

Precise calculation of AFC therefore can help in predicting the ovarian response. This can be done on 2D ultrasound or by 3D with inversion mode rendering and sonography-based automated volume count (SonoAVC) a specialized 3D ultrasound software for calculation of antral follicle number and volumes. This method is more precise as there is least chance of follicles being missed or being counted twice because of color coding. But postprocessing is required for accurate calculations. It takes longer to perform, because of the need for postprocessing, and obtains values that are lower than those obtained by the 2D and 3D-manual multiplanar view (MPV) techniques (Fig. 6.1).[12,13]

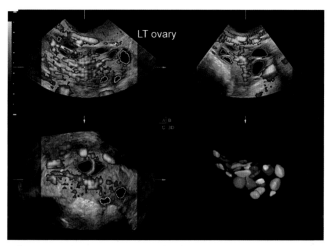

Fig. 6.1: Three-dimensional ultrasound image of the ovary with sonography-based automated volume count (SonoAVC) for calculating antral follicle counts.

Ovarian volume less than 3 cc was significantly predictive of higher IVF cancellation rates more than 50%[14] (Fig. 6.2) and ovarian volume was also used in decision-making for stimulation protocol for ovarian induction. AFC and ovarian volume provide direct measurements of ovarian reserve.[15]

Inclusion of stromal blood flows (Fig. 6.3) as one of the decision-making parameters is also considered. It has been shown that measurement of ovarian stromal flow in early follicular phase is related to subsequent ovarian response in IVF treatment.[16]

Ovarian stromal PSV after pituitary suppression is predictive of ovarian responsiveness and outcome of IVF treatment.[17] Kupesic has shown correlation between the ovarian stromal flow index and number of mature oocytes retrieved in IVF cycles and pregnancy rates (Fig. 6.4).[2] It is shown in this study that stromal FI [<11, low responder; 11–14, good; >15, risk of ovarian hyperstimulation

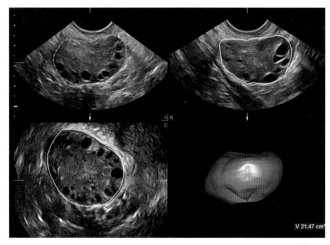

Fig. 6.2: Three-dimensional ultrasound calculated ovarian volume by a soft ware called VOCAL (virtual organ computer-aided analysis).

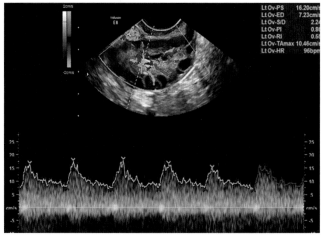

Fig. 6.3: Ovarian stromal flow as seen on color Doppler and pulse Doppler.

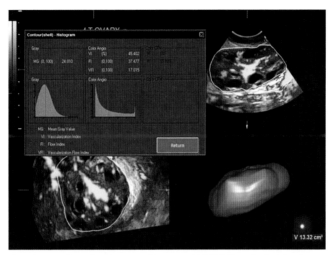

Fig. 6.4: Three-dimensional power Doppler ultrasound image with VOCAL calculated volume with volume histogram (blue box) showing VI, FI, and VFI parameters. (FI: flow index; VFI: vascularity flow index; VI: vascularization index; VOCAL: virtual organ computer-aided analysis)

syndrome (OHSS)] can be correlated to ovarian response in ovulation induction.

The ovarian stromal blood flow was found to be negatively correlated with age. Ovarian blood flow predicts ovarian responsiveness and hence provides a noninvasive and cost-effective prognostic factor of IVF outcome.[18]

Based on all these facts and findings, it is understood that ovaries that have high resistance, low velocity flow require higher doses of gonadotropins for stimulation. Whereas those with low resistance, high velocity flow require lower doses of gonadotropins for stimulation.

The final dose calculation can be based on factors certain factors and we would prefer to simplify it as mentioned in Table 6.1.

A scoring system was developed based on clinical and ultrasound findings (Table 6.2).

The ovulation induction in all patients was done by rFSH and the stimulation doses were based on the scores of individual patient based on Table 6.2. The doses according to the patient's score were decided as follows:

≥25	25 IU
20–24	37.5 IU
15–20	75 IU

TABLE 6.1: Final dose calculation.

	Increase the dose when..	Decrease the dose when..
Age	>35 years	<25 years
BMI	>28 kg/m²	<20 kg/m²
AFC	<3 (FNPO)	>12 (FNPO)
Stromal RI	>0.7	<0.5
Stromal PSV	<5 cm/sec	>10 cm/sec
Stromal FI	<11	>15
Ovarian Volume	<3 cc	>10 cc

(AFC: antral follicle count; BMI: body mass index; FI: flow index; FNPO: follicle number per ovary; PSV: peak systolic velocity; RI: resistance index)

10–15	112.5 IU
6–10	150 IU

The doses for stimulation for IVF cycle according to the patient's score was decided as follows:

Score of

>23	75 IU
20–22	150 IU
16–20	225 IU
11–15	300 IU
6–10	375 IU
1–5	450 IU

TABLE 6.2: Scoring system based on clinical and ultrasound findings.

Score	1	2	3	4	5
Age	>40	35–40	30–35	25–30	<25
BMI	>30	30–28	28–25	25–22	<22
AFC	<5	5–10	10–15	15–20	>20
Ovarian volume	<3	3–5	5–7	7–10	>10
Stromal RI	>0.75	0.75–0.65	0.65–0.55	0.55–0.45	<0.45
Stromal PSV	<3	3–5	5–7	7–10	>10

(AFC: antral follicle count; BMI: body mass index; PSV: peak systolic velocity; RI: resistance index)

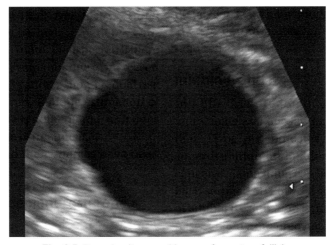

Fig. 6.5: B-mode ultrasound image of a mature follicle.

As per the results of our study, we believe that the scoring system devised in this study for deciding the stimulation protocol is highly reliable for safe planning of stimulation protocols in assisted reproductive technology (ART) cycles as the OHSS rates and cycle cancellation rates due to poor response are negligible. Multiple pregnancy rates are also acceptable. This study, we believe, may prove to be an important guide for safe use of gonadotropins for ovulation induction in ART cycles.[19,20]

A follicle that is of more than 10 mm in diameter, grows at a rate of 2–3 mm per day has no internal echogenicity and has thin (pencil line like) walls is not only more likely to become the leading follicle but will also give mature healthy ovum.

B-MODE FEATURES OF A MATURE FOLLICLE

The follicular diameter is measured when the follicle is seen as a rounded structure or at least three measurements must be taken perpendicular to each other and take a mean measurement as follicular diameter. A mature follicle is 16–18 mm (Fig. 6.5), has thin walls, regular round shape, and no echogenicity in the lumen and shows a thin hypoechoic rim surrounding the follicle and sometimes (about 35–40%) cumulus-like shadow may be seen. This

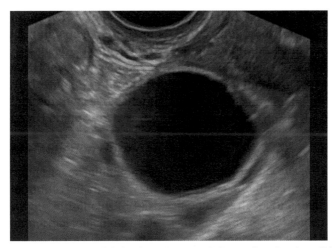

Fig. 6.6: B-mode ultrasound image of a follicle of which rupture is impending showing mild separation of inner wall at 2 o'clock and 6 o'clock positions.

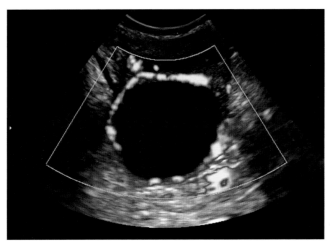

Fig. 6.7: Perifollicular vascularity seen on color Doppler.

thin hypoechoic rim and cumulus-like shadow develops approximately 36 hours before rupture. A flimsy irregular line or low level scany echoes are seen inside the follicle parallel to the wall about 6–10 hours before rupture (Fig. 6.6).

DOPPLER FEATURES OF A GOOD PRE-HUMAN CHORIONIC GONADOTROPIN FOLLICLE

Increase in perifollicular vascularity of dominant follicle in theca layer starts developing as early as 8th day of the cycle. Fall in perifollicular resistance index (RI) starts 2 days before ovulation, reaches nadir at ovulation, remains low for 4 days, and then with gradual rise reaches 0.5 in midluteal phase.[21]

When functionally mature, on color Doppler, the follicle shows blood vessels covering at least 3/4th of the follicular circumference (Fig. 6.7). Chui et al. graded the follicular flow on the day of oocyte collection as grade 1–4 when in a single cross area slice the flow covered less than 25%, 25–50%, 50–75%,

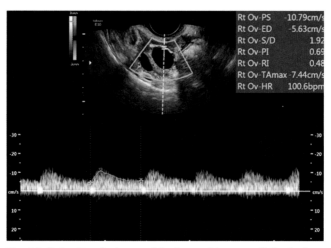

Fig. 6.8: Pulse Doppler image of the low resistance perifollicular flow.

and more than 75% of follicular circumference. The conception was related to grade 3–4 vascularity.[22]

On pulse Doppler, these blood vessels show RI of 0.4–0.48[22] and PSV of more than 10 cm/sec (Fig. 6.8).

The pulse repetition frequency (PRF) settings for color Doppler are set at 0.3 and wall filter at the lowest. The perifollicular vessels are only those that obliterate the follicular wall with color. If the follicular wall is seen and the vessel is seen just besides it, it is not a perifollicular vessel. Ovarian flow correlates well with oocyte recovery rates and hence may be useful in determining the most appropriate time to administer hCG to optimize oocyte recovery rate. It has been quoted in a study by Nargund et al.[22,23] that embryos produced by fertilization of the ova obtained from the follicles which had a perifollicular PSV of less than 10 cm/sec, are less likely to result in grade I embryos and also have higher chance of chromosomal malformations. In the same study, it has been shown that the probability of developing a grade 1 or 2 embryo is 75% if PSV was more than 10 cm/sec, 40% if PSV was less than 10 cm/sec, and 24% if there was

no perifollicular flow. There is yet another study that supports this finding. Oocytes from severely hypoxic follicles are associated with high frequency of abnormalities of organization of chromosomes on metaphase spindle and may lead to segregation disorders and catastrophic mosaics in embryo.[24]

On 3D ultrasound, the follicular volume of 3–7.5 cc has been found to be optimum in our study.[25] This agrees with the study by Wittmack et al.[26] which says that: In IVF-embryo transfer (ET) cycles, follicles with mean follicular diameter of 12–24 mm are associated with optimal rates of oocyte recovery, fertilization, and cleavage.[26] This corresponds to the follicular volumes of between 3 mL and 7 mL. The accuracy of 3D ultrasound measurement of follicular volume compared to the standard 2D techniques by comparing the volume of individual follicles estimated by both methods with the corresponding follicular aspirates using the formula of ellipse the limits of agreement between aspirates and calculated volume was + 3.47 to –2.42 as compared to +0.96 to –0.43 when calculated by 3D ultrasound using virtual organ computer-aided analysis (VOCAL) (Fig. 6.9).[27]

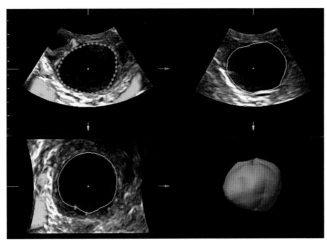

Fig. 6.9: Three-dimensional ultrasound acquired virtual organ computer-aided analysis (VOCAL) calculated volume of follicle.

It has been shown that follicular fluid concentrations of leptin, a follicular angiogenesis related factors are inversely related to the stromal blood flow index.[28]

It has also been suggested that the follicles containing oocytes capable to produce a pregnancy have a perifollicular vascular network more uniform and distinctive.[29]

In our study,[25] we have found perifollicular VI of between 6 and 20 and perifollicular FI more than 35 as most optimum.

About 68.4% of patients conceived when the VI was between 6 and 18 and 50% when it was between 18 and 20. However, the pregnancy rates were less than 25% when VI was less than 6 and only 7.4% when VI was more than 20. It was only 7.4% of patients with FI less than 27 who conceived whereas beyond 27, the conception rates rose consistently. It was 50% with FI between 27 and 35, 70% when FI was between 35 and 43, and almost all patients had conceived when FI was more than 43. Although it is possible to assess the follicular flow as expressed by the PSV and perifollicular color map,[30] it is the 3D power Doppler that gives the most precise information about the vascularization and follicular blood flow.[31]

The hCG plays a major role in inducing influx of blood within follicles. At the luteinizing hormone (LH) surge the perifollicular PSV is 10 cm/sec. This means that if the follicle is said to be functionally mature when PSV is 10 cm/sec, that is the time when the LH surge starts and under the effect of that LH, the perifollicular PSV keeps on rising constantly.[32]

This derives that a rising PSV with steady low RI suggests that the follicle is close to rupture.

Implantation has been the weakest link in the success of infertility treatment. Endometrium is a receptor organ for majority of the hormones involved in fertility and therefore study of its morphology and vascularity is thought to explain the mysteries of implantation failure. Therefore, like follicle, endometrium is also assessed by transvaginal 2D ultrasound and color Doppler before planning for hCG during any ART.

B-MODE FEATURES OF ENDOMETRIUM WITH GOOD RECEPTIVITY

On transvaginal ultrasonography (TVS), an endometrial thickness of minimum 6 mm

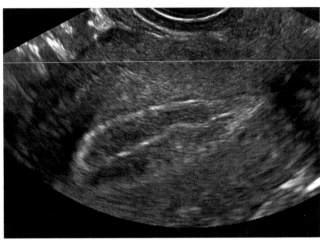

Fig. 6.10: B-mode ultrasound image of grade A endometrium with intact endometrio-myometrial junction.

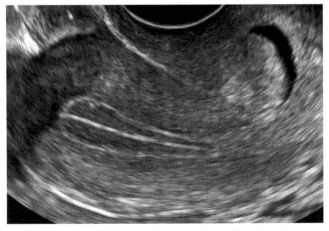

Fig. 6.11: B-mode ultrasound image of grade B endometrium.

is required on the day of ovulation trigger but 8–10 mm is optimum. Endometrial thickness has more negative predictive value for implantation. Morphology of the endometrium is as important as thickness of the endometrium. In all the healthy endometria, the endometrio-myometrial interface is always seen as a clear hypoechoic halo surrounding the whole endometrium (Fig. 6.10). Breach or irregularity of endometrio-myometrial junction is an indication of unhealthy endometrium and therefore poor receptivity.

Popularly multilayered endometrium is considered as a desired endometrial pattern. Morphologically the endometrium is graded as the best grade A, when it is a triple line endometrium with the intervening area is as echogenic as the anterior myometrium. The echogenicity is attributed to the development of multiple vessels penetrating in the endometrium producing multiple

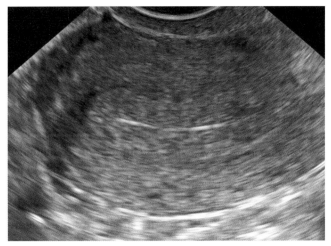

Fig. 6.12: B-mode ultrasound image of grade C endometrium.

tissue interfaces and therefore causing the echogenicity, due to stromal edema and due to glycogen storage in the endometrial columnar epithelium (Fig. 6.11). The endometrium is graded as intermediate or grade B when it is multilayered or triple line with hypoechoic intervening area. Grade C (Fig. 6.12) or the most unfavorable endometrium would be a homogeneous isoechoic endometrium.[33] Though some studies have shown no significant difference in pregnancy rates among different morphological patterns.

DOPPLER FEATURES OF ENDOMETRIUM WITH GOOD RECEPTIVITY

There are several reports by different groups[34] that agree on the fact that implantation rates can be more correlated to the vascularity of the endometrium rather than the thickness and morphology of the endometrium.

Segmental uterine artery perfusion demonstrates significant correlation with hormonal and histological markers of uterine receptivity, reaching the highest sensitivity for subendometrial blood flow. On color Doppler the endometrium which is mature shows vascularity in zone 3 and 4 or may be called subendometrial and endometrial layers (Fig. 6.13).

The zones of vascularity are defined according to Applebaum[34] as: Zone 1 when the vascularity on power Doppler is seen only at endometrio-myometrial junction, zone 2 when vessels penetrate through the hyperechogenic endometrial edge, zone 3 when it reaches intervening hypoechogenic zone, and zone 4 when they reach the endometrial cavity (central line). The pregnancy rates related to the zones of vascular penetration: 26.7% for zone 1, 36.4% for zone 2, and 37.9% for zone 3.

One more comparison of two studies have also shown similar pregnancy rates:[20]

- Zone 1   3.5–7.5%   5.2%
- Zone 2   15.8–29.7%   28.7%
- Zone 3   24.2–47.8%   52%
- Zone 4   67.3%   74%

Another study also compares the conception rates and miscarriage rates with the endometrial vascularity in different zones.[35]

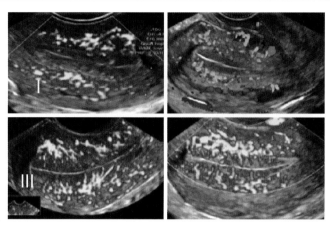

Fig. 6.13: Power Doppler images of the grade 1–4 endometrium.

ENDOMETRIAL VASCULARITY: ITS RELATION TO IMPLANTATION AND MISCARRIAGE RATES[35]

	Zone 1	Zone 2	Zone 3	Zone 4
• Vascularity in				
• % of patients	6.69%	20.73%	58%	14.47%
• + βhCG	19%	21.87%	39.77%	70.14%
• Gestational sac	9.6%	14.58%	36.8%	68.65%
• Miscarriage rate	50%	23.8%	5.6%	1.5%

Zaidi et al. found that absence of flow in the endometrial and subendometrial zones on day of hCG indicate total failure of implantation.[36]

The vessels that reach the endometrium are the spiral arteries. The pulse Doppler of these arteries should have an RI of up to 0.6 for the endometrium to be called mature for implantation.

Moreover, the pulse Doppler analysis of the uterine artery waveform is done and its RI should not be more than 0.9 and PI should be less than 3.2 (Fig. 6.14).

Several authors have shown that the optimum uterine receptivity was obtained when average PI of the uterine artery was between 2 and 3 on the day of transfer or on the day of hCG.[37,38]

Coulam et al. have also shown that no pregnancy was achieved after ET when uterine artery PI was above 3.3 in an IVF program.[39]

Cacciatore et al. suggest that implantation is unlikely when PI is more than 3.3 and RI more than 0.95 or when no velocities are seen at the end of the diastole.[40]

In such cases therefore in IUI cycles, hCG is withheld or postponed and in IVF cycles, embryos are frozen for transfer in subsequent cycles.

Endometrial volume by 3D ultrasound volume calculation of the endometrium may help to correlate the cycle outcome with quantitative parameter rather than endometrial thickness.[26]

A study by Raga et al.[41] shows pregnancy and implantation rates were significantly lower when endometrial volume less than 2 mL, while no pregnancy was achieved when endometrial volume was less than 1 mL. Study by Kupesic et al. also shows no pregnancy when endometrial volume was less than 2 mL, or when exceeded 8 mL.[42]

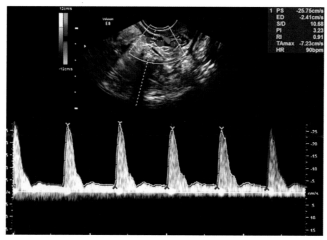

Fig. 6.14: Pulse Doppler image showing high resistance uterine artery flow waveform.

TABLE 6.3: Optimum pretrigger parameters of follicle and endometrium.

	Follicle	Endometrium
Size/thickness	16–18 mm	8–10 mm
Morphology	Thin wall, no internal echoes, halo	Grade A/B
Vascularity	3/4th circumference	Zone 3–4
RI	0.4–0.48	<0.5
PSV	>10 cm/sec	–
Uterine artery PI	–	<3.2
Volume	3–7 cc	3–7 cc
3D morphology	Cumulus	Intact endo-myo junction
3D power Doppler	More symmetrical the better	Higher the better

(PI: pulsatility index; PSV: peak systolic velocity; RI: resistance index; 3D: three-dimensional)

The optimum parameters for follicle and endometrium before the trigger are mentioned in Table 6.3.

SECRETORY PHASE ASSESSMENT

Rupture of the follicle leads to formation of corpus luteum. Corpus luteum is responsible for progesterone production. The functional efficacy of the corpus luteum can be assessed by Doppler by assessing the pericorpus luteal vascularity.

Segmental uterine and ovarian artery perfusion demonstrates a significant correlation with histological and hormonal markers of uterine receptivity and may aid assessment of luteal phase defect.[43] A clear correlation between RI of corpus luteum and plasma progesterone levels has been seen in natural cycle. RI of the corpus luteum can therefore be used as an adjunct to plasma progesterone assay as an index of luteal function.[44]

A corpus luteum that is functionally normal and produces adequate amount of progesterone shows corpus luteal flow: RI (0.35–0.50) and PSV (10–15) (Figs. 6.15A and B).

The receptor organ for progesterone also (like estrogen) is endometrium and its vascular studies can be a reliable clue to adequate progesterone production. Endometrium also becomes hyperechoic as a result of progesterone exposure. Soon after rupture of the follicle, the outer margin of the endometrium starts becoming fluffy and blurred. With adequate progesterone levels, that are achieved in the midluteal phase,

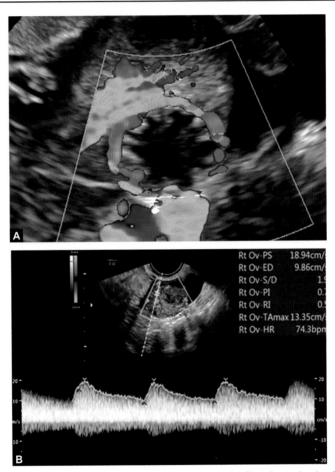

Figs. 6.15A and B: Normal corpus luteal flow seen on color Doppler and pulse Doppler.

the spiral arteries show RI of 0.48–0.52 (low resistance flow) and uterine artery shows PI of 2.0–2.5. This PI is lower than in the preovulatory phase because of smooth muscle relaxing effect of progesterone. Inadequate progesterone production and therefore corpus luteal inadequacy is suggested by high resistance flow in corpus luteal vessels.[44]

Whereas, high spiral artery resistance would suggest inadequate response of endometrium to progesterone. This is because of inadequate progesterone receptors in the endometrium or because of local endometrial cause, like endometrial injury or chronic endometritis.

In luteal phase defect because of low progesterone levels, the resistance in the pericorpus luteal vessels is high. Because of low progesterone levels there is inadequate relaxation of the muscularis of the uterine artery and therefore the uterine artery resistance is high along with higher resistance in its branches—the spiral vessels.

Corpus luteal flow and spiral artery flow in normal cycle and luteal phase defect are shown in Tables 6.4A and B.[43]

TABLE 6.4A: Corpus luteal flow and spiral artery flow in normal cycle and luteal phase defect.

	Normal	LPD
Perifollicular	0.56 ± 0.06	0.58 ± 0.04
LH peak day	0.44 ± 0.04	0.58 ± 0.04
Midluteal phase	0.42 ± 0.06	0.58 ± 0.04
Late luteal phase	0.50 ± 0.04	0.58 ± 0.04

(LH: luteinizing hormone; LPD: luteal phase defect)

TABLE 6.4B: Corpus luteal flow and spiral artery flow in normal cycle and luteal phase defect.

Phase	Control RI	LPD RI
Periovulatory	0.53 ± 0.04	0.70 ± 0.06
Midluteal	0.50 ± 0.02	0.72 ± 0.06
Late luteal	0.51 ± 0.04	0.72 ± 0.04

(LPD: luteal phase defect; RI: resistance index)

CORRELATION OF PROGESTERONE TO ULTRASOUND FINDINGS

Blurring of outer margin of multilayered endometrium suggests initiation of progesterone secretion (Fig. 6.16).

Blurring of Outer Margins of Multilayered Endometrium

Low resistance flow in corpus luteum, with echogenic endometrium (Figs. 6.17A and B) and low resistance endometrial vascularity in midluteal phase suggests normal luteal phase.

High resistance corpus luteal flow suggests corpus luteal inadequacy. High resistance endometrial flow in midluteal phase suggests either inadequate progesterone levels or inadequate progesterone receptors in endometrium.

CONCLUSION

Ultrasound is an excellent tool for assessment of the menstrual cycle. Hormonal changes occurring day to day during the menstrual cycle reflects as morphological and vascular changes in the ovary and the uterus. Assessing these changes by transvaginal ultrasound and Doppler and correctly interpreting can explain the hormonal basis of these changes. Ultrasound with Doppler can thus be used as the only modality for cycle assessment in

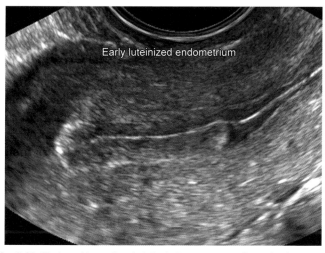

Fig. 6.16: Endometrium of early luteal phase seen on B-mode ultrasound.

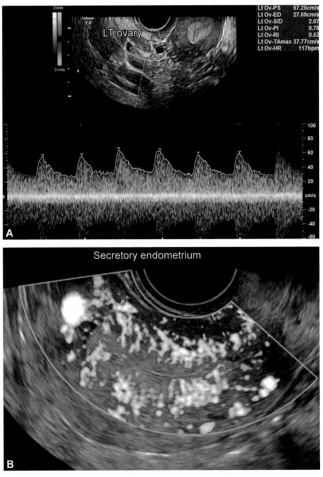

Figs. 6.17A and B: (A) Low resistance blood flow of the corpus luteum demonstrated on pulse Doppler; (B) High-definition power Doppler showing blood flow in the secretory endometrium.

patients undergoing assisted reproduction technology and may be of help to reduce the cost of the cycle by avoiding certain hormonal assessments and still maintaining close and accurate watch on the hormonal changes occurring during treatment cycle.

REFERENCES

1. Ravhon A, Lavery S, Michael S, et al. Dynamic assays of inhibin B and oestradiol following Buserelin acetate administration as predictors of ovarian response in IVF. Hum Reprod. 2000;15(11):2297-301.

2. Kupesic S, Kurjak A. Predictors of IVF outcome by three-dimensional ultrasound. Hum Reprod. 2002;17(4):950-5.

3. Popovic-Todorovic B, Loft A, Lindhard A, et al. A prospective study of predictive factors of ovarian response in 'standard' IVF/ICSI patients treated with recombinant FSH. A suggestion for recombinant FSH dosage normogram. Hum Reprod. 2003;18(4):781-7.

4. Ng EH, Tang OS, Chan CC, et al. Ovarian stromal blood flow in the prediction of ovarian response during in vitro fertilization treatment. Hum Reprod. 2005;20(11):31147-51.

5. Oliveness F, Howles CM, Borini A, et al. Individualizing FSH dose for assisted

reproduction using a novel algorithm: the CONSORT study. Reprod Biomed Online. 2009;18(2):195-204.

6. Merce LT, Barco MJ, Bau S, et al. Prediction of ovarian response and IVF/ICSI outcome by three dimensional ultrasonography and power Doppler angiography. Eur J Obstet Gynecol Reprod Biol. 2007;132(1):93-100.

7. Freiesleben NL, Lossl K, Bogstad J, et al. Predictors of ovarian response in intrauterine insemination patients and development of a dosage nomogram. Reprod Biomed Online. 2008;17(5):632-41.

8. Yu Ng EH, Yeung WS, Tak Fong DY, et al. Effects of age on hormonal and ultrasound markers of ovarian reserve in Chinese women with proven fertility. Hum Reprod. 2003;18(10):2169-74.

9. Scheffer GJ, Broekmans FJ, Dorland M, et al. Antral follicle counts by TVS are related to age in women with proven natural fertility. Fertil Steril. 1999;72:845-51.

10. Lam PM, Johnson IR, Rainne-Fenning NJ. Three dimensional ultrasound features of the polycystic ovary and the effect of different phenotypic expressions on these parameters. Hum Reprod. 2007;22(12):3116-23.

11. Krishnakumar J, Agarwal A, Nambiar D, et al. Comparison of antral follicle count, antimullerian hormone and day 2 follicle stimulating hormone as predictor of ovarian response and clinical pregnancy rate in patient with an abnormal ovarian reserve test. Int J Reprod Contracept Obstet Gynecol. 2016;5(8):2762-7.

12. Rainne-Fenning NJ. What is in a number? The polycystic ovary revisited. Hum Reprod. 2011;26(11):3118-22.

13. Deb S, Jayaprakasan K, Campbell BK, et al. Intraobserver and interobserver reliability of automated antral follicle counts made using three-dimensional ultrasound and SonoAVC. Ultrasound Obstet Gynecol. 2009;33(4):477-83.

14. Lass A, Skull J, McVeigh E, et al. Measurement of ovarian volume by transvaginal sonography before ovulation induction with human menopausal gonadotrophin for in vitro fertilization can predict poor response. Hum Reprod. 1992;12(2):294-7.

15. te Velde ER. Advances in fertility studies and reproductive medicine [thesis]. Durban: IFFS; 2007. p. 306.

16. Zaidi J, Barber J, Kyei-Mensah A, et al. Relationship of ovarian stromal blood flow at baseline ultrasound to subsequent follicular response in an in vitro fertilization program. Obstet Gynecol. 1996;88:779-84.

17. Engmann L, Saldkevicius P, Agrawal R, et al. Value of ovarian stromal blood flow velocity measurement after pituitary suppression in the prediction of ovarian responsiveness and outcome of in vitro fertilization treatment. Fertil Steril. 1999;71(1):22-9.

18. Arora A, Gainder S, Dhaliwal L, et al. Clinical significance of ovarian stromal blood flow in assessment of ovarian response in stimulated cycle for in vitro fertilization. Int J Reprod Contracept Obstet Gynecol. 2015;4(5):1380-3.

19. Panchal S, Nagori C. Ultrasound-based decision making on stimulation protocol for superovulated intrauterine insemination cycles. Int J Infertil Fetal Med. 2016;7(1):7-13.

20. Panchal S, Nagori C. Ultrasound Based decision making on stimulation protocol in IVF. Donald School J Ultrasound Obstet Gynecol. 2016;10(3):330-7.

21. Jokubkeine L, Sladkevicius P, Rovas L, et al. Assessment of changes in volume and vascularity of ovaries during the normal menstrual cycle using three dimensional power Doppler ultrasound. Hum Reprod. 2006;21(10):2661-8.

22. Nargund G, Doyle PE, Bourne TH, et al. Ultrasound derived indices of follicular blood flow before HCG administration and prediction of oocyte recovery and preimplantation embryo quality. Hum Reprod. 1996;11:2512-17.

23. Nargund G, Bourne TH, Doyle PE, et al. Association between ultrasound indices of follicular blood flow, oocyte recovery and preimplantation embryo quality. Hum Reprod. 1996;11:109-13.

24. Blerkom V, Antezak M, Schrader R. The developmental potential of human oocyte is related to the dissolved oxygen content of follicular fluid: association with vascular

endothelial growth factor levels and perifollicular blood flow characteristics. Hum Reprod. 1997;12(5):1047-55.

25. Panchal S, Nagori C. Can 3D PD be a better tool for assessing the pre HCG follicle and endometrium? A randomized study of 500 cases. Presented at 16th World Congress on Ultrasound in Obstetrics and Gynecology, 2006, London. J Ultrasound Obstet Gynecol. 2006;28(4):504.

26. Wittmack FM, Kreger DO, Blasco L, et al. Effect of follicular size on oocyte retrieval, fertilization, cleavage and embryo quality in in vitro fertilization cycles: a 6 year data collection. Fertil Steril. 1994;62:1205-10.

27. Kyei-Mensah A, Zaidi J, Pittrof R, et al. Transvaginal three dimensional ultrasound reproducibility of ovarian and endometrial volume measurements. Fertil Steril. 1996;66:718-22.

28. Wu MH, Tsai SJ, Pan HA, et al. Three dimensional power Doppler imaging of ovarian stromal blood flow in women with endometriosis undergoing in vitro fertilization. Ultrasound Obstet Gynecol. 2003;21:480-5.

29. Vlaisavljevic V, Reljic M, Gavric Lovrec V, et al. Measurement of perifollicular blood flow of the dominant preovulatory follicle using three dimensional power Doppler. Ultrasound Obstet Gynecol. 2003;22:520-6.

30. Merce LT. Ultrasound markers of implantation. Ultrasound Rev Obstet Gynecol. 2002;2:110-23.

31. Merce LT, Barco MJ, Kupesic S, et al. 2D and 3D power Doppler ultrasound from ovulation to implantation. In: Kurjak A, Chervenak F (Eds). Textbook of Perinatal Medicine. London: Parthenon Publishing; 2005.

32. Bourne TH, Jurkovic D, Waterstone J, et al. Intrafollicular blood flow during human ovulation. Ultrasound Obstet Gynecol. 1991;1:53-9.

33. Smith B, Porter R, Ahuja K, et al. Ultrasonic assessment of endometrial changes in stimulated cycles in an in vitro fertilization and embryo transfer program. J In Vitro Fert Embryo Transf. 1984;1(4):233-38.

34. Applebaum M. The 'steel' or 'teflon' endometrium ultrasound visualization of endometrial vascularity in IVF patients and outcome. Presented at The third World Congress of Ultrasound in Obstetrics and Gynecology. Ultrasound Obstet Gynecol. 1993;3(Suppl 2):10.

35. Nagori C, Panchal S. Endometrial vascularity: its relation to implantation rates. Int J Infertil Fetal Med. 2012;3(2):48-50.

36. Zaidi J, Campbell S, Pittrof R, et al. Endometrial thickness, morphology, vascular penetration and velocimetry in predicting implantation in an in vitro fertilization program. Ultrasound Obstet Gynecol. 1995;6:191-8.

37. Steer CV, Campbell S, Tan SL, et al. The use of transvaginal color flow imaging after in vitro fertilization to identify optimum uterine conditions before embryo transfer. Fertil Steril. 1992;57:372-6.

38. Zaidi J, Pittrof R, Shaker A, et al. Assessment of uterine artery blood flow on the day of human chorionic gonadotropin administration by transvaginal color Doppler ultrasound in an in vitro fertilization program. Fertil Steril. 1996;65:377-81.

39. Coulam CB, Stern JJ, Soenksen DM, et al. Comparison of pulsatility indexes on the day of oocyte retrieval and embryo transfer. Hum Reprod. 1995;10:82-4.

40. Cacciatore B, Simberg N, Fusaro P, et al. Transvaginal Doppler study of uterine artery blood flow in in vitro fertilization embryo transfer cycles. Fertil Steril. 1996;66:130-4.

41. Raga F, Bonilla-Musoles F, Casan EM, et al. Assessment of endometrial volume by three dimensional ultrasound prior to embryo transfer: clues to endometrial receptivity. Hum Reprod. 1999;14:2851-4.

42. Kupesic S, Bekavac I, Bjelos D, et al. Assessment of endometrial receptivity by transvaginal colour doppler and three dimensional power Doppler ultrasonography in patients undergoing in vitro fertilization procedures. J Ultrasound Med. 2001;20:125-34.

43. Kupesić S, Kurjak A, Vujisić S, et al. Luteal phase defect: comparison between Doppler velocimetry, histological and hormonal markers. Ultrasound Obstet Gynecol. 1997;9(2):105-12.

44. Glock JL, Brumsted JR. Color flow pulsed Doppler ultrasound in diagnosing luteal phase defect. Fertil Steril. 1995;64:500-4.

Gonadotropin-releasing Hormone Analogs

Chaitanya Nagori

GONADOTROPIN-RELEASING HORMONE AGONISTS

INTRODUCTION

Premature luteinizing hormone (LH) surge was the common problem in assisted reproductive technology (ART) leading to cancellation of cycles and decreased pregnancy rate in initial phase of ART era. Premature LH surge is because of positive feedback mechanism due to high estrogen level because of multiple follicular development. So agonist was tried on the patient to resolve the problem.[1] Gonadotropin-releasing hormone agonist (GnRHa) decreases the follicle-stimulating hormone (FSH) and LH secretion from the pituitary and prevents the LH surge. It also abolishes FSH secretion, so follicle develops through only exogenous FSH which allows development of optimum number of follicles by adjusting the dose of FSH.

MECHANISM OF ACTION (TABLE 7.1)

Gonadotropin-releasing hormone agonist causes flare-up effect initially followed by downregulation. This flare-up effect causes increased secretion of FSH and LH initially followed by decrease in their secretion if analog is continued. Within 12 hours of administration it liberates high amount of FSH (5-folds increase) and LH (10-folds increase).[2] Flare-up effect can be used for short protocol and ovulation trigger.

The decrease in FSH and LH secretion is because of internalization of receptor-agonist complex and there is reduction in number of receptors causing reduction in FSH and LH content and release.[3]

TABLE 7.1: Mechanism of action of GnRHa.

GnRHa	Dose	Route
Decapeptyl	100–500 mg/day	SC
Triptorelin	3.75 mg depot	IM
Naperelin	400 mg bd	Nasal
Goserelin	3.6 mg/month	SC/implant
Buserelin	300–400 mg	Intranasal
	200–500 mg	SC
Leuprolide	0.5–1 mg daily	SC
	3.75 ng/month	IM

(GnRHa: gonadotropin-releasing hormone agonist; IM: intramuscular; SC: subcutaneous)

Gonadotropin-releasing hormone agonist, as mentioned in the Table 7.1, can be given subcutaneously, intranasally, as depot preparation, as intramuscular (IM) injection or as implants. Intranasal is better than daily subcutaneous (SC) injections but in rhinitis and allergy, absorption varies from patient to patient. The depot preparation as well as daily preparation achieved same estradiol (E2) level, oocyte quality, fertilization, and pregnancy rates. But depot preparation causes prolonged desensitization, so dose of gonadotropin and days needed are more for stimulation.[4] The effect of depot preparation may last for 8 weeks after the injection[5] and this is the reason for giving low implantation and pregnancy rate. The depot preparation might interfere with luteal phase and embryo development. In recent meta-analysis, it has been found that pregnancy rates are same, but it required longer days of stimulation and more number of gonadotropins and therefore not advocated in terms of cost-effectiveness.[4]

Lahat et al. reported a high incidence of attention deficit hyperactivity disorder in long-term follow-up of children exposed to GnRHa early in pregnancy.[6]

GONADOTROPIN-RELEASING HORMONE AGONIST PROTOCOLS FOR ASSISTED REPRODUCTIVE TECHNOLOGY

- Long protocol
- Short protocol
- Ultrashort protocol
- Microdose protocol.

Long Protocol

Gonadotropin-releasing hormone agonist is started from midluteal phase, i.e. day 21 of the cycle. Leuprolide acetate 1 mg daily can be given to the patient or depot preparation of 3.75 mg can be given. This 1 mg dose is continued till the patient gets periods. Normally patient gets period after 7–10 days. Period comes when there is adequate downregulation. At this stage, E2 level will be between 30 pg/mL and 50 pg/mL. LH less than 2.5 IU/L and endometrium will be single line (<4 mm). Gonadotropins are started from day 2 of menstruation. The dose is decided based on ultrasound parameters in our practice, but other workers may decide the dose of gonadotropins based on anti-Müllerian hormone (AMH) levels or age and AMH together. As the pituitary is already downregulated, the dose of GnRHa can be reduced to half in the daily dose protocol (0.25–0.5 mg daily). This dose is given till the day of ovulation trigger. According to Nelson et al.,[7] long protocol is best used for normal responding patients having AMH levels of between 5 pmol/L and 15 pmol/L.

The advantage of long protocol is that it almost abolishes unwanted LH surge, prevents cancellation of cycles and improves pregnancy rates that was about 20–30%.[8] With this long protocol follicles develop depending on exogenous FSH dosage so there is complete elimination of endogenous control of sequences of follicular recruitment and selection. This leads to synchronization of the cohort of follicles and time for pick up can be adjusted. Majority of the studies have proved that long protocol gives better results than short or ultrashort protocols.[9] The disadvantage of this protocol is that it requires more total doses of gonadotropins and longer duration of treatment. As there is initial flare-up for about 3 days because of increase in FSH and LH, there may be cyst formation. High E2 and LH due to this may rescue corpus luteum giving high progesterone levels on the starting day of gonadotropin stimulation. In these cases, stimulation may have to be delayed till the cyst and corpus luteum resolve. Corpus luteum can lead to luteinization of small follicles and in some cases may also cause ovulation. Pretreatment with oral contraceptive (OC) pills for 14 days prior to starting GnRHa can reduce the cyst formation without negative effect on pregnancy rates.[10] But recent studies have shown that prior treatment with OC pills can reduce the pregnancy rates.

Downregulation can be confirmed by:

- Estradiol less than 30 pg/mL
- Luteinizing hormone less than 2.5 IU/L
- Progesterone less than 2 ng/mL
- Endometrial thickness less than 4 mm.

Short Protocol

In short protocol 1 mg of leuprolide acetate is given daily from day 1 or 2 of the menstrual cycle. Gonadotropins are started from day 2 or day 3, i.e. 1 day after the agonist is started. Agonist is continued till the day of trigger with gonadotropins. This protocol is used for poor responders and the advantage is the initial flare-up effect can be used for development of the follicle. It is less expensive and has a lower incidence of ovarian hyperstimulation syndrome (OHSS), but does not give big homogeneous cohort of follicles. The other disadvantage is that it can also rescue the corpus luteum of the previous cycle. It can cause luteinization of small follicles because of high levels of progesterone due to high FSH and LH, and can also lead to ovulation from bigger mature follicles. Prolonged downregulation for more than 28 days may improve the endometrial receptivity and may increase pregnancy rate. Quiet endometrium in postmenopausal patients also increases the pregnancy rate. Therefore, OC pills or progesterone should be given before starting short protocol.[11]

Ultrashort Protocol

In this protocol, GnRHa is started from day 1–2 of the menstruation in a dose of 0.5–1 mg/day. It is given for 3 days only. Gonadotropins are started from day 2 or day 3, that is 1 day after GnRHa is started. In this protocol, advantage of the flare-up effect is taken for stimulation of the follicles. It decreases the dose of agonist as well as gonadotropins and thus decreases the cost and risk of OHSS. But the disadvantage is the higher chance of a premature LH surge as the agonist is not continued. This also gives poor pregnancy rates.

Microdose Flare Protocol

This is the short protocol in which the dose of agonist is reduced to quarter of the short protocol. Instead of 200 microgram of daily dose, only 50 microgram is given daily.[12] Moreover, GnRHa can be stopped when gonadotropin is started. Suppression lasts up to gonadotropin introduction, but more studies are required for this protocol.[13,14]

CLINICAL APPLICATION OF GONADOTROPIN-RELEASING HORMONE AGONIST

Long protocol has a better pregnancy rate than short or ultrashort protocol.[15,16] Pregnancy rates are equivalent to antagonist protocols.[17] It has low cycle cancellation and high oocyte recovery rates. But it is associated with high gonadotropin consumption, increased cost due to increased days of stimulation, increased incidence of OHSS and cyst formation. Ultrashort protocols are used for poor responders, but have poor pregnancy rates because of premature LH surge.

All GnRHa protocols cause luteal phase defect and judicious luteal support should be given. This is discussed in the chapter of luteal phase support. GnRHa can be used as ovulation trigger. This is also discussed in detail in the chapter on ovulation trigger.

When long protocol is used, there is profound suppression of LH. When recombinant FSH (rFSH) is used for stimulation of follicles, in subgroup of patients, supplementation of LH can improve the pregnancy rate. Comparison of short protocol or microdose protocol for poor responders versus antagonist protocol, there is no difference in pregnancy outcome.

There is no clear cut advantage of GnRHa + gonadotropins than gonadotropins alone.[18] Advantages of agonist therapy are as follows:

- Multiple follicles, more embryos
- Prevents LH surge due to high E2
- No spontaneous ovulation
- Less cycle cancellation
- Flexibility of time to start stimulation and ovum pick-up.

There is no advantage of discontinuing GnRHa earlier. It may have deleterious effect.[19,20] Continuous-long protocol in luteal phase has given higher pregnancy rates.[21] But the short protocol increases the ovarian response. Though early release of androgen declines oocyte quality giving lower pregnancy rates.[22]

Delaying human chorionic gonadotropin (hCG) triggers for more than 2 days after more than three follicles of more than 17 mm diameter are seen by ultrasound, is associated with poor pregnancy rates.[23]

Other uses of GnRHa are as follows:

- *Endometriosis*: For 3 months before in vitro fertilization (IVF)
- *Fibroid*: Not used as primary treatment
- *Precocious puberty*: Depot preparation are used
- Gonadal protection during chemotherapy[24]
- Metabolic prostatic cancer
- Breast cancer
- Hirsutism.

CARRY HOME MESSAGE

- Long protocol abolishes the LH surge.
- Initial flare-up is utilized in short and ultrashort protocols.
- Pregnancy rates are highest in long protocol than short or ultrashort protocol.
- Long protocol can cause cyst formation, rescue corpus luteum with high progesterone and requires more gonadotropins for stimulation.
- Daily doses are better than depot preparation in long protocol.
- Ovarian hyperstimulation syndrome incidence is high in long protocol.
- Judicious luteal support is required in agonist trigger.
- Because of low LH, subgroup is benefitted by adding LH.

GONADOTROPIN-RELEASING HORMONE ANTAGONIST

INTRODUCTION

Premature LH surge was common in up to 20–50% of cases of IVF with gonadotropin stimulation. With the advent of GnRHa in early 1980s,[25] it was the breakthrough in prevention of LH surge and allowed consultants for more flexible oocyte retrievals.[26] GnRH antagonist was available at that time, but did not get much popularity due to allergic reaction due to its histamine release property.[27] The use of GnRHa became universal in 1980s, 1990s, and 2000s. But the development of third generation antagonist has completely changed the line of treatment in ART.

MECHANISM OF ACTION

There are two different antagonists available commercially since 1999: (1) Cetrorelix (cetrotide from Merck) and (2) ganirelix

(Orgalutran from Organon). It acts as complete blocker for GnRH receptors and so blocks native GnRH that ultimately stops the release of FSH and LH from pituitary. It immediately blocks gonadotropin release and its action is reversible. LH falls by 70% and FSH by 30% within 6 hours of antagonist administration. Complete reversal of action occurs in 24–72 hours. The incidence of LH surge is extremely rare if the dose is not missed. Any imminent LH surge is blocked within 6–8 hours of administration.

ENDOCRINE CHANGES IN ANTAGONIST CYCLE

Progesterone level may be high (5% cases) on the day of stimulation in a spontaneous ovulatory cycle. Even if we postpone the stimulation for 1 or 2 days, progesterone level will normalize but pregnancy rates are low compared with normal levels.[28] Same is true if E2 level is high because of follicular cyst on day 2. In both these situations, postponing of IVF cycle is advisable.

DOSAGE OF ANTAGONIST

- Daily dose scheme
- Single dose scheme.

In a daily dose scheme, 0.25 mg of cetrorelix or ganirelix is given daily. In single dose scheme, cetrorelix is given as 3 mg dose that inhibits LH surge for 4 days. Both daily dose and single dose scheme gives equivalent pregnancy rate.[29] The fixed protocol is also known as French protocol. It is given on day 7. It lasts for 4 days. If there are no mature follicles to give trigger, single dose of 0.25 mg cetrorelix is given till the day of trigger.[30] In fixed protocol, antagonist is started from day 6, 0.25 mg cetrorelix. The disadvantage of the fixed day is in polycystic ovary syndrome (PCOS) patients and poor responders. Here if follicular development is late unnecessary more antagonists are used and may also increase the consumption of gonadotropins.

TIMING OF ANTAGONIST

Gonadotropin-releasing hormone antagonist can be given as a fixed protocol or flexible protocol. The argument for fixed protocol is the knowledge that after certain days of stimulation with gonadotropins, LH starts rising in majority of the patients and so it should be started on fixed days routinely. Formerly it was considered as 6th day of stimulation.[31] But now recent studies have shown that it should be started from day 5 of stimulation.[32] Fixed protocol is simpler and requires less monitoring (also known as Ludwig's protocol). The flexible antagonist protocol depends on endocrine and ultrasound criteria, which indicate the rise of LH. Antagonist is given when the size of the follicle is more than or equal to 14 mm.[33] The advantage of flexible criteria is that it can avoid unnecessary administration of GnRH antagonist and gonadotropin from day 5 when LH surge is not going to occur as the follicle development was inadequate. There is no significant difference in clinical pregnancy rate in flexible as well as the fixed protocol.[34,35] Flexible protocol should not start after day 8. In patients with PCOS, LH level is high even before antagonist is added in fixed or flexible protocol. This early rise of LH may be detrimental and decrease the pregnancy rates so antagonist is started earlier, i.e. day 2 has an advantage in these patients.

Breakthrough LH surge can occur in spite of GnRH antagonist in patients with diminished ovarian reserve, but the dose of antagonist can be doubled in the subsequent cycle. LH level when is less than 300 pg/mL or more than 1,100 pg/mL on the day of start of antagonist, it gives poor results.

ADVANTAGES OF ANTAGONIST

- It is patient friendly and has a high efficacy.
- There is no estrogen deprivation or cyst formation.
- The action of antagonist is immediate.
- Incidence of OHSS is decreased with antagonist. It is decreased to more than 50%.[36] When antagonist is used for downregulation, agonist can be used as trigger and this reduces the risk of OHSS to almost zero.[37] Here freeze all eggs or judicious luteal support is given.
- Coasting is very effective in antagonist protocol with equivalent pregnancy rates.[38]
- It can avoid oocyte retrievals on weekends and avoid initiation of many cycles and the load for the center. Stimulation can be started on day 3 instead of day 2 and can give trigger also a day later.
- It has no teratogenic or other adverse effect on implantation or embryonic development.[39]
- Duration of treatment is short and the dose of gonadotropin is also reduced, thus reduces the cost of treatment.

DISADVANTAGES OF ANTAGONIST

- Delay of hCG for more than 2 days after three follicles of 17 mm on ultrasound is associated with a significantly decreased probability of pregnancy.[23]
- Pretreatment with OC pills are not to be used in antagonist cycles as there is decreased probability of pregnancy when OC pills are used and it also increases the duration of stimulation required and cost to the patient.[40] Apart from pregnancy rate, it results in higher pregnancy loss and so OC pills pretreatment is not recommended.[41]

- The lower pregnancy rate in antagonist cycle reported earlier in some studies was because clinicians were less trained in using antagonist and learning curve was required.[42]

EVIDENCE FOR GONADOTROPIN-RELEASING HORMONE AGONIST/ANTAGONIST (TABLE 7.2)[43]

In the initial trials, Cochrane library suggested that the use of antagonist was associated with significantly lower chance of pregnancy compared to agonists.[44] But the explanation given by the German registry was that antagonist were used in poor responders as well as patients having multiple failures and aged patients. So, the results of antagonists in terms of clinical pregnancy were poor.[45] In 2011, Cochrane group published that there was

TABLE 7.2: Comparison of agonists and antagonists.

GnRH agonist	GnRH antagonist
Molecular effects	
Downregulation of receptors	Inhibition of receptors without any activation
Desensitization of pituitary	Competitive antagonism
Flare-up response initially followed by downregulation	Immediate suppression
Slowly reversible response	Rapid reversible response
Clinical implications	
Longer IVF regimen	Shorted IVF regimen
Time consuming and more expensive	Less time and less expensive
More injections, inconvenient to patient	Fewer injections increases patient compliance
No endogenous LH surge	Induction of endogenous LH

(GnRH: gonadotropin-releasing hormone; IVF: in vitro fertilization; LH: luteinizing hormone)

no significant difference in clinical pregnancy rate in the antagonist group and agonist group. The recent meta-analysis suggested the use of antagonist is justified because of equivalent pregnancy rate with agonist and increased safety in antagonist cycles.[46,47] Pregnancy rates were the same with flexible protocols as compared to long protocols. Similarly even fixed protocols of antagonist had same clinical pregnancy rates.[48] It is clear from this publication that GnRha era has come to an end.

Antagonists are administered in later half of follicular phase and so profound suppression of pituitary does not occur. So, this is very useful in poor responders. Antagonist is the drug of choice in poor responders. This protocol is as effective as short, ultrashort or microdose protocol.[12] GnRH antagonist versus long protocol was studied in meta-analysis which analyzed that antagonist protocol gives higher oocytes yield.[49] Addition of letrozole also decreases cancellation and total gonadotropin dosage.[50]

RECENT ADVANCES IN ANTAGONIST USAGE

- It can be used in modified natural cycle or mild stimulation IVF.[51]
- Agonist trigger with freeze all policy can completely abolish OHSS.[37]
- Reinitiation of antagonist in case of severely established OHSS is possible.[52]
- Long-acting FSH can be used in antagonist cycles making stimulation more simplified.

DOSAGE OF GONADOTROPINS

The starting dose of 150 IU is generally considered optimum for typical normal responding patient. Pregnancy rates are not increased by using higher doses.[53] Stimulation can be started from day 2 or 3 while in mild stimulation it is to be started from day 5. There is no need to increase the dose of FSH from the day of antagonist initiation. There is no increase in pregnancy rate by increasing gonadotropin dosage.[54,55] The addition of LH at the time of initiation of antagonist has not given increased pregnancy rates in 3 meta-analysis.[56,57] LH is added only in subgroup of patients as discussed in the chapter on LH.

ADDITION OF LUTEINIZING HORMONE IN OVULATION INDUCTION

Low LH levels in antagonist cycles are not the indication of addition of LH.[58] Clomiphene citrate with FSH or human menopausal gonadotropin (HMG) in antagonist protocol had lower pregnancy rate and were not cost-effective too.[59]

LUTEAL SUPPORT IN ANTAGONIST CYCLE

Formerly it was believed that antagonist cycle does not require luteal support, but because of gonadotropin stimulation irrespective of analog used all patients required luteal support.[60] But E2 supplementation did not increase the pregnancy rate.[61]

CARRY HOME MESSAGE

- Agonist can be used as a trigger in antagonist cycle.
- Incidence of OHSS is extremely rare.
- Pregnancy rate is the same as agonist cycle in spite of low E2 level with antagonist.
- The treatment cost is reduced because of lesser number of days of stimulation in antagonist cycle.
- Antagonist is very useful in mild stimulation protocol, poor responders or modified natural cycles.

- Luteal support is a must in all antagonist cycles.

REFERENCES

1. Porter RN, Smith W, Craft IL, et al. Induction of ovulation for in-vitro fertilization using buserelin and gonadotropins. Lancet. 1984;2:1284-5.
2. Lemey A, Maheror F. Development and application of LHRH agonist (Buserelin) as a new therapeutic approach for endometriosis. Fertil Steril. 1984;41:863-74.
3. Pelletier G, Dube D, Guy J, et al. Binding and internalization of a luteinizing hormone-releasing hormone agonist by rat gonadotrophic cells. A radioautographic study. Endocrinology. 1982;111:1068-76.
4. Albuquerque LE, Saconato H, Maciel MC. Depot versus daily administration of gonadotrophin releasing hormone agonist protocols for pituitary desensitization in assisted reproduction cycles. Cochrane Database Styst Rev. 2005;25(1):CD002808.
5. Broekmans FJ, Bernardus RE, Berkhout G, et al. Pituitary and ovarian suppression after early follicular and mid-luteal administration of a LHRH agonist in a depot formulation: Decapeptyl CR. Gynecol Endocrinol. 1992;6:153-61.
6. Lahat E, Raziel A, Friedler S, et al. Long-term follow-up of children born after inadvertent exposure to long acting gonadotrophin releasing hormone agonist in early pregnancy. Hum Reprod. 1999;14:2656-60.
7. Nelson SM, Yates RW, Lyall H, et al. Anti-Müllerian hormone based approach to controlled ovarian stimulation for assisted conception. Hum Reprod. 2009;24:867-75.
8. Akagbosu FT. The use of GnRH agonists in infertility. In: Brinsden R (Ed). A Textbook of In Vitro Fertilization and Assisted Reproduction, 2nd edition. USA: Parthenon Publishing; 1999. pp. 83-9.
9. Tan SL. Luteinizing hormone–releasing hormone agonist for ovarian stimulation in assisted reproduction. Curr Opin Obstet Gynecol. 1994;6:166-72.
10. Biljan MM, Mahutte NG, Dean N, et al. Effects of pretreatment with an oral contraceptive on the time required to achieve pituitary suppression with gonadotrophin-releasing hormone analogues and on subsequent implantation and pregnancy rates. Fertil Steril. 1998;70(6):1063-9.
11. Cedrin-Durnerin I, Bulwa S, Herve F, et al. The hormonal flare up following gonadotrophin-releasing hormone agonist administration is influenced by a progesterone pretreatment. Hum Reprod. 1996;11:1859-63.
12. Kahraman K, Berkar B, Atabekoglu CS, et al. Microdose gonadotropin-releasing hormone agonist flare up protocol versus multiple dose gonadotropin-releasing hormone antagonist protocol in poor responders undergoing intracytoplasmic sperm injection-embryo transfer cycle. Fertil Steril. 2009;91(6):2437-44.
13. Filicori M, Flamigini C, Cognigni GE, et al. Different gonadotropin and leuprorelin ovulation induction regimen markedly affect follicular fluid hormone levels and folliculogenesis. Feril Steril. 1996;65:387-93.
14. Pantos K, Meimeth-Damianaki M, Vaxevanaglou T, et al. Prospective study of modified GnRH long protocol in an IVF program. Fertil Steril. 1994;64:709-13.
15. Frydman R, Belaisch-Allart J, Parneix I, et al. Comparison between flare up and down regulation effect of luteinizing hormone-releasing hormone agonists in in vitro fertilization program. Fertil Steril. 1988;50:471-5.
16. Maheshwari A, Caserta D, Siristatidis CS, et al. Gonadotropin-releasing hormone agonist protocols for pituitary suppression in assisted reproduction. Cochrane Database Syst Rev. 2011;(8):CD006919.
17. Arslan M, Bocca S, Mirkin S, et al. Controlled ovarian hyperstimulation protocols for in vitro fertilization: two decades of experience after the birth of Elizabeth Carr. Fertil Ateril. 2005;84(3):555-69.
18. School DC, Pijlman B, Stijnen T, et al. Effects of gonadotropin releasing hormone agonist addition to gonadotropin induction of ovulation in polycystic ovary syndrome

patients. Eur J Obstet Gynecol Reprod Biol. 1992;45:53-8.

19. Cedrin-Durnerin I, Bidart JM, Robert P, et al. Consequences on gonadotropin secretion of an early discontinuation of gonadotropin releasing hormone agonist administration in short-tern protocol for in vitro fertilization. Hum Reprod. 2000;15:1009-14.

20. Dirnfeld M, Fruchter O, Yshai D, et al. Cessation of gonadotropin-releasing hormone analogue (GnRH-a) upon down-regulation versus conventional long GnRH-a protocol in poor responders undergoing in vitro fertilization. Fertil Steril. 1999;72:406-11.

21. Fujii S, Sato S, Fukui A, et al. Continuous administration of gonadotropin releasing hormone agonist during the luteal phase in IVF. Hum Reprod. 2011;16:1671-5.

22. Loumaye E, Coen G, Pampfer S, et al. Use of gonadotropin releasing hormone agonist, during ovarian stimulation leads to significant concentration of peptide in follicular fluids. Fetil Steril. 1989;52:256-63.

23. Kolibianakis EM, Albano C, Camus M, et al. Prolongation of follicular phase in in vitro fertilization results in a lower ongoing pregnancy rate in cycles stimulated with recombinant follicle-stimulating hormone and gonadotropin releasing hormone antagonists. Feril Steril. 2004;82:102-7.

24. Chen H, Li J, Cui T. Adjuvant gonadotropin-releasing hormone analogues for chemotherapy induced premature ovarian failure in premenopausal women. Cochrane Database Syst Rev. 2011;(11):CD008018.

25. Janssens RM, Lambalk CB, Vermeiden JP, et al. Dose-finding study of triptorelin acetate for prevention of a premature LH surge in IVF: A prospective, randomized, double-blind placebo-controlled study. Hum Reprod. 2000;15:2333-40.

26. Meldrum DR. Ovulation induction protocols. Arch Pathol Lab Med. 1992;116:406-9.

27. Rivier J. Novel antagonist of GnRH: a compendium of their physicochemical properties, activities, relative potencies and efficacy in humans. In: Insler V, Lunenfeld B (Eds). GnRH Analogues: The State of The Art 1993, 1st edition. New York, USA: Parthenon Publishing; 1993. pp. 13-26.

28. Kolibianakis EM, Venetis CA, Bontis J, et al. Significantly lower pregnancy rates in the presence of progesterone elevation in patients treated with GnRH antagonists and gonadotrophins: a systematic review and meta-analysis. Curr Pharm Biotechnol. 2102;13:464-70.

29. Lee TH, Wu MY, Chen HF, et al. Ovarian response and follicular development for single dose and multiple dose protocols for gonadotropin releasing hormone antagonist administration. Feril Steril. 2005;83:1700-7.

30. Olivennes F, Fanchin R, Bouchard P, et al. Scheduled administration of gonadotropin-releasing hormone antagonist (Cetrorelix) on day 8 of in vitro fertilization cycles: a Pilot study. Hum Reprod. 1995;10(6):1382-6.

31. Borm G, Mannaerts B. Treatment with the gonadotropin releasing hormone antagonist ganirelix in women undergoing ovarian stimulation with recombinant follicle stimulating hormone is effective, safe and convenient: results of a controlled, randomized, multicenter trial. The European Orgalutran Study group. Hum Reprod. 2000;15:1490-8.

32. A double-blind, randomized, dose-finding study to assess the efficacy of the gonadotrophin-releasing hormone antagonist ganirelix (Org 37462) to prevent premature luteinizing hormone surges in women undergoing ovarian stimulation with recombine t follicle stimulating hormone (Puregon). Hum Reprod. 1998;13:3023-31.

33. Ludwig M, Katalinic A, Banz C, et al. Tailoring the GnRH antagonist cetrorelix acetate to individual patient's needs in ovarian stimulation for IVF: results of a prospective, randomized study. Hum Reprod. 2002;17(11):2842-5.

34. Kolibianakis EM, Venetis CA, Kalogeropoulou L, et al. Fixed versus flexible gonadotropin releasing hormone antagonist administration in in vitro fertilization: a randomized controlled trial. Feril Steril. 2011;95:558-62.

35. Escudero E, Bosch E, Crespo J, et al. Comparison of two different starting multiple dose gonadotropin releasing hormone antagonist protocols in a selected group of in vitro fertilization-embryo transfer patients. Fertil Steril. 2004;81:562-6.

36. Kolibianakis EM, Collins J, Tarlatzis BC, et al. Amongst patients treated for IVF with gonadotropins and GnRH analogues, is the probability of live birth dependent on the type of analogue used? A systematic review and meta-analysis. Hum Reprod Update. 2006;12:651-71.

37. Griensinger G, Diedrich K, Tarlatzis BC, et al. GnRH antagonists in ovarian stimulation for IVF in patients with poor response to gonadotropins, polycystic ovary syndrome, and high risk of hyperstimulation: a meta-analysis. Reprod Biomed Online. 2006;13: 628-38.

38. Aboulghar MA, Mansour RT, Amin YM, et al. A prospective randomized study comparing coasting with GnRH antagonist administration in patients at risk for severe OHSS. Reprod Biomed Online. 2007;15:271-9.

39. Fluker M, Grifo J, Leader A, et al. Efficacy and safety of ganirelix acetate versus luprolide acetate in women undergoing controlled ovarian hyperstimulation. Fertil Steril. 2001;75(1):38-45.

40. Griesinger G, Kolibianakis EM, Venetis C, et al. Oral contraceptive pretreatment significantly reduces the ongoing pregnancy likelihood in gonadotropin-releasing hormone antagonist cycles: an updated meta-analysis. Fertil Steril. 2010;94:2382-4.

41. Kolibianakis EM, Papanikolaou EG, Camus M, et al. Effect of oral contraceptive pill pretreatment on ongoing pregnancy rates in patients stimulated with GnRH antagonists and recombinant FSH for IVF: A randomized controlled trial. Hum Reprod. 2006;21:352-7.

42. Homburg R. Controlled ovarian stimulation for IVF and ICSI. Ovulation Induction and Controlled Ovarian Stimulation: A Practical Guide. Switzerland: Springer International Publishing; 2014. pp.143-59.

43. Thakker SK, Allahbadia G, Allahbadia A. GnRH agonists versus GnRH antagonists for ovarian stimulation: pros and cons. In: Allahbadia G, Merchant R (Eds). Manual of Ovulation Induction and Ovarian Stimulation Protocols, 3rd edition. Jaypee Brothers Medical Publishers Ltd.;2016. pp. 181-9.

44. Al-Inany H, Aboulghar M. Gonadotropin-releasing hormone antagonists for assisted conception. Cochrane database Syst Rev. 2001;(4):CD001750.

45. Griesinger G, Felber baum R, Diedrich K. GnRH antagonists in ovarian stimulation: a treatment regimen of clinicians' second choice? Data from the German national IVF registry. Hum Reprod. 2005;20:2373-5.

46. Tarlatzis BC, Fauser BC, Kolibianakis EM, et al. GnRH antagonists in ovarian stimulation for IVF. Hum Reprod Update. 2006;12:333-40.

47. Al-Inany HG, Aboulghar M, Mansour R, et al. Optimizing GnRH antagonist administration: meta-analysis of fixed vs flexible protocol. Reprod Biomed Online. 2005;10:567-70.

48. Al-Inany HG, Youssef MA, Aboulghar M, et al. Gonadotropin-releasing hormone antagonists for assisted reproductive technology. Cochrane Database Syst Rev. 2011;(5):CD001750.

49. Franco JG Jr, Baruffi RL, Mauri AL, et al. GnRH agonist versus GnRH antagonist in poor ovarian responders: a meta-analysis. Reprod Biomed Online. 2006;13:618-27.

50. Ozmen B, Sonmezer M, Atabekoglu CS, et al. Use of aromatase inhibitors in poor responder patients receiving GnRH antagonist protocols. Reprod Biomed Online. 2009;19:478-85.

51. Pelinck MJ, Knol HM, Vogel NE, et al. Cumulative pregnancy rates after sequential treatment with modified natural cycle IVF followed by IVF with controlled ovarian stimulation. Hum Reprod. 2008;23:1808-14.

52. Lainas T, Sfontouris IA, Zorzocilis IZ, et al. Live births after management of severe OHSS by GnRH antagonist administration in luteal phase. Reprod Biomed Online. 2009;19:789-95.

53. Wikland M, Bergh C, Borg K, et al. A prospective randomized comparison of two starting doses of recombinant FSH in combination with cetrorelix in women undergoing ovarian

stimulation for IVF/ICSI. Hum Reprod. 2001;16:1676-81.

54. Propst AM, Bates GW, Robinson RD, et al. A randomized controlled trial of increasing recombinant follicle- stimulating hormone after initiating a gonadotropin releasing hormone antagonist for in vitro fertilization-embryo transfer. Fertil Steril. 2006;86:58-63.

55. Aboulghar MA, Mansour RT, Serour GI, et al. Increasing the dose of human menopausal gonadotropins in the day of GnRH antagonist administration: randomized controlled trial. Reprod Biomed Online. 2004;8:524-7.

56. Baruffi RL, Mauri AL, Petersen CG, et al. Recombinant LH supplementation to recombinant FSH during induced ovarian stimulation in the GnRH antagonist protocol: a meta-analysis. Reprod Biomed Online. 2007;14:14-25.

57. Mochtar MH, Van der V, Ziech M, et al. Recombinant luteinizing hormone (rLH) for controlled ovarian hyperstimulation in assisted reproductive cycles. Cochrane Database Syst Rev. 2007;(2):CD005070.

58. Kolibianakis EM, Collins J, Tarlatzis B, et al. Are endogenous LH levels during ovarian stimulation for IVF using GnRH analogues associated with the probability of ongoing pregnancy? A systematic review. Hum Reprod Update. 2006;12:3-12.

59. Engel JB, Ludwig M, Felberbaum R, et al. Use of Cetrorelix in combination with clomiphene citrate and gonadotropins: a suitable approach to 'friendly' IVF? Hum Reprod. 2002;17:2011-26.

60. Beckers NG, Macklon NS, Eijkemans MJ, et al. Nonsupplemented luteal phase characteristics after the administration of recombinant human chorionic gonadotropin, recombinant luteinizing hormone, or gonadotropin-releasing hormone (GnRH) agonist to induce final oocyte maturation in in vitro fertilization patients after ovarian stimulation with recombinant follicle stimulating hormone and GnRH antagonist co-treatment. J Clin Endocrinol Metab. 2003;88:4186-92.

61. Kolibianakis EM, Venetis CA, Papanilolaou E, et al. Estrogen addition to progesterone for luteal phase support in cycles stimulated with GnRH analogues and gonadotropins for IVF: a systematic review and meta-analysis. Hum Reprod. 2008;23:1346-54.

Hypogonadotropic Hypogonadism

Chaitanya Nagori

INTRODUCTION

Hypogonadotropic hypogonadism is hypothalamo-pituitary failure, ovulatory dysfunction World Health Organization (WHO) group I type of anovulation. It is the condition in which secretions of gonadotropins from the pituitary are so low, that there is no growth of follicles in the ovary and so no estrogen production. The classical finding is very low estrogen level along with anovulation and amenorrhea and no withdrawal bleed with progesterone.

The recent studies have shown that kisspeptin regulate gonadotropin-releasing hormone (GnRh) secretion.[1] It has been documented that central and peripheral administration of kisspeptin increases follicle-stimulating hormone (FSH) and luteinizing hormone (LH) secretion by activating GnRh neurons.

CAUSES OF HYPOGONADOTROPIC HYPOGONADISM

- *Hypothalamic causes*:
  - Extremely low body weight—anorexia nervosa or sudden severe crash dieting
  - Strenuous exercises like dancing and running
  - Kallman syndrome (isolated GnRh deficiency)
  - Psychiatric disorders—anxiety
  - Stress.
- *Pituitary causes*:
  - Surgery—hypophysectomy or trauma
  - Radiation to brain
  - Sheehan's syndrome
  - Pituitary tumors
  - Empty sella syndrome
  - Extrapituitary lesions—tumors like craniopharyngioma, glioma, meningioma, etc.
  - Isolated FSH or LH deficiency.
- *Systemic diseases (chronic illnesses)*:
  - Renal failure
  - Cirrhosis
  - Beta thalassemia
  - Sarcoidosis and tuberculosis
  - Meningoencephalitis
  - Syphilis.
- Idiopathic.

DIAGNOSIS

- *On history and examination*: Small uterus and ovaries and other signs of hypoestrinism.

- *Blood investigations*: Low estradiol (E2), low LH, low or normal FSH, and thyroid function tests.

DIFFERENTIAL DIAGNOSIS OF HYPOGONADOTROPIC HYPOGONADISM

- Polycystic ovarian syndrome (PCOS)
- Hyperprolactinemia (HPRL)
- Isolated hypothyroidism
- Premature ovarian failure (POF).

MANAGEMENT

Hormone Replacement Therapy

It is given to all the patients of hypogonadotropic hypogonadism after menarche, even when fertility is not a concern. Estrogen and progesterone are given cyclically. It is protective against osteoporosis and cardiovascular diseases. It helps in the development of genital organs. Moreover with this priming, treating her for fertility becomes easier.

Management for Desiring Pregnancy

- Pulsatile GnRH therapy
- Gonadotropins therapy.

Pulsatile Gonadotropin-releasing Hormone Therapy

Gonadotropin-releasing hormone is the neurohormone synthesized by nerve endings in the anterior hypothalamus. It goes to pituitary and releases FSH and LH. It has a very short half-life and is released in a pulsatile fashion. The frequency and amplitude of the pulse is changed by various factors that affect hypothalamus. This is usually assessed by LH pulse that reflects the GnRh release. GnRh is released once in 60 minutes in follicular phase and once in 4 hours in luteal phase. The amount, timing, and pulsatile release of GnRh determine the pattern of ovulatory cycle by release of hormones (FSH and LH) from the anterior pituitary.

When pituitary is intact, GnRh can be given in a pulsatile manner for FSH and LH release in patients with idiopathic hypothalamic failure. This can be done through an infusion pump by subcutaneous or intravenous route. The dose is 15–20 µg subcutaneously or 5–10 µg intravenously every 60–90 minutes. This is an effective therapy for ovulation induction in hypothalamic amenorrhea and may give pregnancy rates of up to 80%. In these patients, the ovulation trigger with human chorionic gonadotropin (hCG) is not required.[2] Infusion pump can be withdrawn in the luteal phase and luteal support can be given till the menstruation or till pregnancy occurs.

This treatment has an advantage over gonadotropin therapy, that it leads to mono-follicular development and therefore the incidence of multiple pregnancy is less than 5% and risk of ovarian hyperstimulation syndrome (OHSS) is rare (Box 8.1). Multiple pregnancies may occur only when hCG is given as an ovulation trigger.[3] It does not even require a fancy expensive monitoring system. But the difficulty about this treatment is fixing and using the infusion pump, which is inconvenient and expensive and may also lead to thrombophlebitis if used for intravenous route (Box 8.2). But if acceptable to the patient, it is a better treatment option in terms of low multiple pregnancies and low OHSS rate. Though, this treatment option is

---

BOX 8.1: Advantages of GnRh therapy.

- High ovulation rate
- Pregnancy rate 80–90%
- Low OHSS
- Low multiple pregnancy rate
- No monitoring required
- Low abortion rate.

not commonly used. It has been replaced by gonadotropin therapy.

Gonadotropin Therapy

This therapy is useful in hypogonadotropic hypogonadism patients of either hypothalamic or pituitary origin. FSH and LH/hCG is a more effective combination in these cases rather than FSH alone.[4]

When only FSH is given, there will be good follicular development but estrogen level will be low and ovulation may not occur. The endometrial development is also inadequate. For both these reasons, oocyte fertilization and conception rates are low.[5]

According to two-cell–two-gonadotropin hypothesis, LH is required to produce androgen from theca cells and these androgens under the influence of FSH will be converted into estrogen. In hypogonadotropic hypogonadism patients, LH is absent or very low and so no androgen is available for estrogen production (Box 8.3).[6,7]

The dose of gonadotropins is very high and response to the ovary is very slow because ovaries are not exposed to endogenous gonadotropins and FSH receptors on ovary are also less.

So, the stimulation is done by either human menopausal gonadotropin (HMG) or FSH and recombinant LH (rLH) or FSH combined with low dose hCG (Box 8.4).

The woman with basal serum level of LH of less than 1.2 IU/L suggests more severe deficiency of LH and would benefit from LH supplementation.[8,9]

In standard protocol, HMG is usually started in the dose of 150 IU daily or 150 IU recombinant FSH (rFSH) with 75 IU rLH for 5 days. If E2 level is increased, same dose is continued, otherwise 33% increase in the dose is done every 5 days.[10] Response is considered optimum when one follicle of 17–18 mm develops or E2 level of more than 400 IU/L is achieved and midluteal progesterone level reaches 25 nmol/L. Ovulation trigger is given with hCG 10,000.[10]

For ovulation trigger, hCG is a must because endogenous LH is absent and in this case GnRh antagonist is of no use. Luteal support with progesterone or hCG 2,000 IU every 3–4 days is a must as endogenous LH is absent.

The dose of LH is as follows:
- The daily dose of 75 IU of rLH is sufficient. High dose more than 225 IU of LH causes atresia of follicles indicating ceiling effect of LH.[4]
- Majority of the patients require only 75 IU of LH, but few patients may require 225 IU LH. Shoham et al. in a randomized double blind, placebo controlled trial, confirmed the validity of 1.2 IU/L as a cutoff and

efficacy of 75 IU as the effective dose for LH supplementation for patients having severe LH deficiency.[11] The rise of E2 due to LH helps in endometrial development, implantation, and pregnancy. Individual FSH and LH injections are better than HMG for monofollicular development. Fixed ratio of FSH and LH in HMG gives multifollicular development. High doses of rLH in final stage of maturation after 11–12 mm allow one follicle to mature and others to undergo atresia, resulting in monofollicular development when FSH and LH are used separately.

- Priming with rLH, 300 IU for 7 days, before FSH stimulation has shown no beneficial effect in terms of follicular development and pregnancy.[12] But pretreatment with LH may require lower dose of FSH and level of LH may remain high during stimulation. This may be due to its effect on pituitary LH secretion in idiopathic hypogonadotropic hypogonadism due to secretion of kisspeptin that is potent stimulator for gonadotropin secretion. The results reported in hypogonadotropic hypogonadism are 89% and 72% after 6 and 7 ovulatory cycles, respectively.[13,14] The ovarian response in hypogonadotropic hypogonadism patients may not be affected so much with age like in other infertile patients.

So the dose schedule options are:

- 7 days HMG 150–225 according to body weight and then increase after 7 days, if no response.
- Step-up + step-down protocol:
  - Day 1–2 (150 mg) and day 3–7 (75 mg). On day 8 onwards according to response, dose is individualized. Normally FSH/LH ratio should be 2:1 in first half and then should be reversed in the second half.[15]

ADDITIONAL STRATEGIES FOR OVULATION INDUCTION IN HYPOGONADOTROPIC HYPOGONADISM PATIENTS (BOX 8.5)

Several patients with hypogonadotropic hypogonadism may not respond to the conventional HMG protocol and may require additional drugs. Those documented are:

- *Growth hormone (GH) or insulin-like growth factor 1 (IGF 1)*: GH deficiency is one of the causes for poor response to HMG in hypogonadotropic hypogonadism patients. GH has a direct effect on follicle maturation and amplifies the action of FSH and LH.[16] Adding GH to the patients not responding to HMG results in development of more follicles and ovulation. It also reduces the daily dose and treatment duration with HMG.[16] GH deficiency may also be the causative factor in patients with unexplained infertility or poor responders.
- *Pretreatment with estrogen*: Patients with hypogonadotropic hypogonadism, who do not conceive with conventional protocol with HMG may respond well and give good pregnancy rates by adding estrogen and progesterone cyclically. In one study, 22 out of 30 patients conceived with this protocol.[17]

In hypoestrogenic environment, HMG seems to be less effective and so prior treatment with estrogen and progesterone combination results in high estrogen environment and gives better pregnancy rates. It promotes cervical mucus and endometrium for better response to

BOX 8.5: Additional strategies.

- Additional of growth hormone or IGF I
- Pretreatment with estrogen
- Pretreatment with estrogen and progesterone.

> **BOX 8.6:** Recent advances in treatment.
> - Long-acting FSH
> - Exogenous kisspeptin
> - ERK and ERK-2 gene mutation.

gonadotropins.[16] Adding conjugated estrogen with HMG also gives better pregnancy rates.

RECENT ADVANCES IN OVULATION INDUCTION IN HYPOGONADOTROPIC HYPOGONADISM PATIENTS (BOX 8.6)

- *Long acting compounds*: Daily injection of gonadotropins is not accepted by the patients and it increases stress and treatment burden. Long-acting drugs may be preferred to the same. Follitropin alpha, long-acting FSH can replace daily FSH injections for first 7 days of ovulation induction.[18]
- *Kisspeptin/GPR54 complex*: Exogenous kisspeptin GPR 54 stimulates hypothalamo-pituitary-gonadal axis in normal females.[19] Particularly if it is given during preovulatory period, rise in LH is pronounced.[16] Kisspeptin may be a promising drug in future for ovulation induction in hypogonadotropic hypogonadism patients. It causes lower incidence of OHSS. Oral GPR54 agonist has been developed and it will have an advantage over gonadotropin injections.
- ERK1 and ERK2 signal regulated kinases have been found out between LH surge and ovulation.[20] It leads to decrease in cyclic adenosine monophosphate (AMP) between cumulus and oocytes. Cyclic AMP represses the resumption of meiosis and maturation of oocyte. So, reduction of cyclic AMP results in resumption of meiosis and ovulation. These *ERK1* and

ERK2 gene mutation may cause infertility. This gene research will help in in vitro maturation and in vitro fertilization (IVF).

CARRY HOME MESSAGE

- Classical features of hypogonadotropic hypogonadism are low estrogen with amenorrhea and anovulation with low FSH and LH levels.
- Hormone replacement therapy is given when fertility is not an issue.
- Pulsatile GnRh therapy and gonadotropin replacement are the options.
- Human menopausal gonadotropin or rFSH and rLH individually can be used, but individual doses are more useful.
- Recombinant luteinizing hormone in high doses can help in monofollicular development in later half of stimulation.
- Pretreatment with estrogen is not much useful.
- Pretreatment with LH reduces FSH dose during stimulation.
- Growth hormone can be used in poor responders.
- Follitropin alpha and long-acting compounds have future hope.
- Kisspeptin regulated GnRh secretion and is the newer research for management.

REFERENCES

1. Dungan HM, Clifton DK, Steiner RA. Minireview: Kisspeptin neurons as central processors in the regulation of gonadotropin-releasing hormone secretion. Endocrinology. 2006;147:1154-58.
2. Homburg R, Eschel A, Armar NA, et al. One hundred pregnancies after treatment with pulsatile luteinizing hormone releasing hormone to induce ovulation. Br Med J. 1989;298:809-12.
3. Braat DD, Schoemaker R, Schoemaker J. Life table analysis of fecundity of intravenously

gonadotropin-releasing hormone treated patients with normogonadotropic and hypogonadotropic amenorrhea. Fertil Steril. 1991;55:266-71.

4. The European Recombinant Human LH Study Group. Recombinant human luteinizing hormone (LH) to support human follicle-stimulating hormone (FSH)-induced follicular development in LH and FSH deficient an ovulatory women: a dose-finding study. J Clin Endocrinol Metab. 1998;83:1507-14.

5. Balasch J, Miro F, Burzaco, et al. The role of luteinizing hormone in human follicle development and oocyte fertility: evidence from in vitro fertilization in a woman with long standing hypogonadotropic hypogonadism and using recombinant human follicle stimulating hormone. Hum Reprod. 1995;10:1678-83.

6. Thompson EL, Patterson M, Murphy KG, et al. Central and peripheral administration of kisspeptin-10 stimulates the hypothalamo-pituitary-gonadal axis. J Neuroendocrinol. 2004;16:850-8.

7. Fevold HL. Synergism of follicle stimulating hormone and luteinizing hormones in producing estrogen secretion. Endocrinol. 1941;28:33-6.

8. Shoham Z, Balen A, Patel A, et al. Results of ovulation induction using human menopausal gonadotropin or purified follicle stimulating hormone in hypogonadotropic hypogonadism patients. Fertil Steril. 1991;56:1048-53.

9. O'dea L, the US Recombinant Human LH Study Group. Recombinant LH in support of recombinant FSH in female hypogonadotropic hypogonadism-evidence of threshold effect. Fertil Steril. 2000;74(Suppl 1):836.

10. Messinis IE. Ovulation induction: a mini review. Hum Reprod. 2005;20:2688-97.

11. Shoham Z, Smith H, Yeko T, et al. Recombinant LH (lutropin alfa) for the treatment of hypogonadotrophic women with profound LH deficiency: a randomized double-blind, placebo-controlled, proof-of-efficacy study. Clin Endocrinol (Oxf). 2008;69:471-78.

12. Balasch J, Fabregues F, Carmona F, et al. Ovarian luteinizing hormone promising preceding follicle stimulating hormone stimulation: clinical and endocrine effects in women with long term hypogonadotropic hypogonadism. J Clin Endocrinol Metab. 2009;94:2367-73.

13. Flukar MR, Urman B, Mackinnon M, et al. Exogenous gonadotropin therapy in World Health Organization groups I and II ovulatory disorders. Obstet Gynecol. 1994;83:189-96.

14. Tadokoro N, Vollenhoven B, Clark S, et al. Cumulative pregnancy rates in couples with an ovulatory infertility compared with unexplained infertility in an ovulation induction programme. Hum Reprod. 1997;12:1939-44.

15. Krause BT, Ohlinger R, Haase A. Lutropin alpha, recombinant human luteinizing hormone for the stimulation of follicular development in profoundly LH-deficient hypogonadotropic hypogonadal women: a review. Biologics. 2009;3:337-47.

16. Hull KL, Harvey S. Growth hormone: roles in female reproduction. J Endocrinol. 2001;168: 1-23.

17. Yildrim M, Noyan V, Tiras MB. Estrogen-Progestogen pre-treatment before HMG induction in hypogonadotropic patients. Int J Gynecol Obstet. 2000;71:249-50.

18. Fauser BC, Mannaerts BM, Devroey P, et al. Advances in recombinant DNA technology: corifollitropin alfa, a hybrid molecule with sustained follicle-stimulating activity and reduced injection frequency. Hum Reprod Update. 2009;15:309-21.

19. Dhillo WS, Chaudhri OB, Thompson EL, et al. Kisspeptin-54 stimulated gonadotropin release most potently during the preovulatory phase of the menstrual cycle in women. J Clin Endocrinol Metab. 2007;92:3958-66.

20. Fan HY, Liu Z, Shimada M, et al. MAPK3/1 (ERK1/2) in ovarian granulosa cells are essential for female fertility. Science. 2009;324:938-41.

Ovulation Induction in Polycystic Ovarian Syndrome

Chaitanya Nagori

INTRODUCTION

Patients with polycystic ovarian syndrome (PCOS) have high antral follicle count (AFC) and also have high stromal vascularity, which both make them more prone to ovarian hyperstimulation syndrome (OHSS). This is one of the most dreaded complications of ovulation induction. Therefore, ovulation induction in PCOS requires careful assessment of patient and a careful consideration before deciding on the ovulation induction protocols. Moreover, insulin resistance, high androgen and high luteinizing hormone (LH), the major components of the PCOS are also challenges for ovulation induction in these patients.

Approximately 20–30% of women in reproductive age group have polycystic ovaries (PCO) and about half of these have signs and symptoms of PCOS. Earliest description of PCO appears to date from 1845 as "sclerocystic ovaries".[1] According to the European Society for Human Reproduction and Embryology/ American Society for Reproductive Medicine (ESHRE/ASRM) consensus 2003[2] (Rotterdam criteria), the diagnosis of PCOS consists of at least two of the three further given criteria.

1. Oligo- and/or anovulation
2. Hyperandrogenism: Biochemical and/or clinical
3. Polycystic ovaries on ultrasound (excluding other causes like congenital adrenal hyperplasia (CAH): This means an ovary that is 10 cc in volume and/or has more than 12 antral follicles.

Polycystic ovarian syndrome, apart from its endocrinal component, as mentioned in the Rotterdam criteria, also has a metabolic component. The chief components of clinical criteria are irregular menstrual cycles due to oligo-ovulation or anovulation, acne, hirsutism and in severe cases acanthosis nigricans due to hyperandrogenemia. Some of these patients may be very obese or absolutely thin lean. Most important among the hormonal criteria are high androgen, high LH and high anti-Müllerian hormone (AMH). Serum prolactin level is high in 30–40% of PCOS due to high estrogen the source of which is peripheral conversion of estrone from high androgen (Flowcharts 9.1 and 9.2).

Polycystic ovaries on ultrasound: An ovary that is 10 cc in volume and/or has more than

Flowchart 9.1: Androgen metabolism.

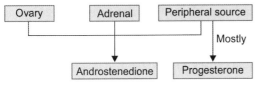

Flowchart 9.3: Serine phosphorylation.

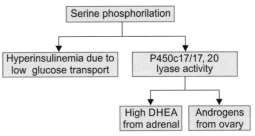

(DHEA: dehydroepiandrosterone)

Flowchart 9.2: Adrenal androgen.

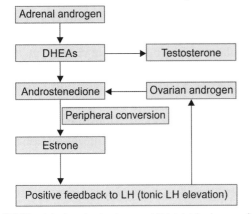

(DHEAs: dehydroepiandrosterones; LH: luteinizing hormone)

- Serine phosphorylation of ovarian and adrenal cytochrome P450c17 enzyme (Flowchart 9.3).
  This activates 17-hydroxylase and 17, 20-lyase activities, that helps in androgen synthesis. This leads to high androgen. About 15% of women with PCO have adrenal hyperandrogenism also.
- Increase in insulin-like growth factor-1 (IGF-1) augments androgen production due to high LH.

CLINICAL PATHOLOGY

- Insulin resistance leads to hyperinsulinemia.
- This increases androgen level directly from ovary and adrenals.
- Indirect rise of androgen is also as a result of high LH.
- Hyperinsulinemia inhibits sex hormone-binding globulin (SHBG) synthesis from liver giving high-free androgen level.
- Hyperinsulinemia and hyperandrogenemia cause anovulation and late sequelae of PCOS.

12 antral follicles according to the Rotterdam criteria. But the recent literature evidences mention that the number of antral follicles may be changed to 26 per ovary in a frank manifestation of PCOS.[3] There are several studies that have mentioned that the volume of 10 cc may be needed to be reconsidered as patients with smaller ovaries have also been found to have PCOS in a considerable percentage of cases.[4] Moreover, a recent study has also mentioned variation in the cutoffs for follicle number and ovarian volume for different age groups.[5]

The metabolic derangements that are commonly seen in patients with PCOS are hyperinsulinemia and hyperlipidemia. Insulin resistance is because of:

- Serine phosphorylation of beta-chain of insulin receptor (Flowchart 9.3).

OPTIONS FOR OVULATION INDUCTION IN PCOS PATIENTS

The comprehensive treatment of PCOS may include correction of both metabolic and endocrinal components. In this chapter, the ovulation induction options are discussed for

PCOS patients. Ovulation induction in PCOS women is different than ovulation induction in non-PCOS women. In PCOS women, fertility is compromised because of oligo-anovulation, but is also compromised due to poor ovum quality due to high LH and in turn high insulin levels. These patients also have a risk of ovarian hyperstimulation due to high androgen levels and they also have a higher abortion rates both due to bad ovum quality and poor endometrial vascularity. This means improving fertility and ovulation induction in these cases should have a holistic approach to decrease, insulin, androgen and LH and also to decrease the risk of OHSS and abortion rates.

Options for ovulation induction in PCOS patients are:

- Weight loss
- Clomiphene citrate
- Letrozole
- Insulin-lowering drugs
- Glucocorticoids
- Gonadotropins
- Gonadotropin-releasing hormone (GnRH) antagonist
- GnRH agonist
- Ovarian drilling
- In vitro fertilization/in vitro maturation (IVF/IVM).

Weight Loss

It is the first line of treatment in obese PCOS patients. Central obesity is more common to cause metabolic changes. These patients typically have a waist-to-hip ratio of 0.7–0.8 which is an android type of obesity. Obesity as is known cannot be judged by just the weight. The best parameter to assess obesity is body mass index (BMI). Normal BMI range is 20–24.9 kg/m^2, whereas when it is between 25 kg/m^2 and 29 kg/m^2, the individual is called overweight.

When BMI is more than 30 kg/m^2, it indicates obesity[6] and BMI of less than 20 kg/m^2 is also considered low and abnormal.

It is the weight loss and decrease in the fat that causes improvement of insulin resistance, decrease in androgen levels and resumption of ovulation. During the initial period of calorie restriction, preferential loss of intra-abdominal fat occurs due to increased lipolysis and its high metabolic activity.[7,8] Only 5% of the total body weight loss is important to induce ovulation.[9] It reduces 30% of visceral fat, this regains reproductive functions in 60–100% of cases. Weight loss reduces hyperinsulinemia, hyperandrogenemia and increases SHBG. It improves the sensitivity for ovulation induction drugs. It also reduces clomiphene resistance. Weight loss decreases the rate of abortions. A retrospective study of 5,019 cycles of IVF revealed that obesity was associated with longer durations and increased amounts of gonadotropin stimulation, increased frequency of cycle cancellation for inadequate response and lower oocyte yields.[10]

Weight loss is an effective way of treating fertility-related complications of PCOS and therefore must be emphasized. Weight loss can be achieved by diet control, exercise, group therapy, behavioral counseling, pharmacological treatment and bariatric surgery. So, it is a teamwork that is required to help the patient to lose weight. But a normal weight PCOS patient may not benefit from weight loss. The role of preconceptional counseling of overweight women was emphasized by 2nd international workshop group and was endorsed by ESHRE and ASRM held in Thessaloniki in Greece in 2007.

Clomiphene Citrate

Clomiphene citrate (CC) induces ovulation in 70–80% of cases with 30–40% pregnancy rate and gives 30% cumulative live birth rate.[11-13] CC acts on hypothalamus to secrete GnRH, which in turn gives follicle-stimulating hormone (FSH) and LH. In PCOS patients, LH is otherwise also high and is a cause of bad oocyte quality. Therefore if on day 8–9 of the cycle LH greater than 10 IU in the first CC treated cycle, it is not used in the subsequent cycle.[14] Patients who do not respond to 150 mg of CC are CC-resistant cases. This occurs in 15–40% of PCOS patients.[15]

Letrozole

This is a very good alternative to CC. It causes borderline hypoestrinism and hyperandrogenism. The mechanism has already been discussed in Chapter 4 in this book. Because of fall in estrogen levels it leads to rise in FSH and LH levels that stimulates follicular development. The resultant rise in estrogen has negative feedback mechanism and it reduces FSH and LH thus allowing monofollicular development. Hyperandrogenism caused by letrozole increases the sensitivity of the follicle to FSH. Letrozole with gonadotropins is a synergistic combination without decreasing pregnancy rate.[16]

There are several reports that indicate that letrozole is better than CC for ovulation induction in PCOS[17,18] and some reports that have shown that letrozole is at least as effective as CC for ovulation induction.[19,20] Advantages of letrozole are in PCOS patients is monofollicular development, lesser incidence of multiple pregnancy, lesser risk of OHSS and lower abortion rates due to fall in LH levels and no effect on cervical mucus and endometrium.

Letrozole or CC + metformin are equally effective for ovulation induction and achieving pregnancy in CC-resistant cases. But letrozole is better tolerated and therefore preferred.[21]

Insulin Lowering Drugs (Insulin Sensitizers)

Insulin resistance in PCOS patients causes hyperinsulinemia, which in turn stimulates theca cells of the ovary to secrete more androgen, through LH. Androgen further recruits more follicles and leads to more LH again establishing a vicious cycle. Hyperinsulinemia in women with obesity contributes to anovulation by increased ovarian androgen secretion.[22] More than half of PCOS patients have insulin resistance. Insulin sensitizers like metformin will reduce the insulin levels and thus will break the cycle and thus helps in correcting the hormonal balance.

Earlier metformin was thought to be a useful drug for ovulation induction in PCOS patients. But recent reports indicate that when metformin is used as the only drug for ovulation induction in PCOS patients, the live birth rate is only 7.2% as compared to that with CC which is 22.5%.[23] Findings of two randomized controlled trials (RCTs) indicated that metformin does not increase live birth rates above those observed with CC alone.[24]

It has also been proved that metformin does not lower the dose of CC required when it is used in combination with CC.[24] CC, therefore, is the most appropriate first line of treatment for ovulation induction in PCOS patients. It is interesting to know that anthropometrical data and metabolic characteristics do not give grounds for adjustment of dose of metformin as its efficacy is not dose-dependent, but side effects are. Therefore, metformin should be preferred in lowest possible doses.[25] ESHRE/ASRM 2007 consensus on the use of metformin as an agent for ovulation induction shows that there is no clear evidence that addition of metformin to CC as a primary therapy for induction of ovulation has a beneficial effect.[26]

Therefore, use of metformin in PCOS should be restricted to women with glucose intolerance and frank type II diabetes.[27] Addition of metformin to gonadotropins has no advantage in improving ovulation rates, pregnancy rates, live birth rates, multiple pregnancy rates or incidence of OHSS (Box 9.1).[28,29]

Metformin in Patients for In Vitro Fertilization

There are several papers that indicate no difference in metformin and nonmetformin group in pregnancy rates in IVF patients.[29,30] Though it is a common practice for gynecologists and endocrinologists to administer or sustain metformin treatment in infertile patients with PCOS scheduled for IVF, irrespective of their basal metabolic status or clinical efficacy of treatment. In patients with PCOS and poor ovarian reserve, metformin worsened the response to gonadotropins and it should be stopped before starting controlled ovarian hyperstimulation for IVF.[31]

In a meta-analysis that evaluated the effectiveness of metformin as a cotreatment during IVF cycles in women with PCOS, metformin reduced the risk of OHSS by approximately 75%.[32] Another study also confirms that in patients with PCOS, who are at a high risk for OHSS and who have been stimulated with gonadotropins for IVF cycles, metformin reduces the risk of OHSS by modulating the ovarian response to stimulation.[33] It reduces the number of small follicles and reduces IGF-1 in follicular fluids.[34] It reduces days of coasting and lowers estradiol (E2) level giving positive impact on fertilization and pregnancy rate.[35] A study by Kjøtrød et al. concludes that metformin (1,000–1,500 mg) treatment for 12 weeks before and during IVF or intracytoplasmic sperm injection (ICSI) in nonobese women with PCOS significantly increases pregnancy and live birth rates compared with placebo.[36]

Metformin after Conception

Safety of metformin in pregnancy has not been established. A large prospective RCT has shown that when metformin is continued in early pregnancy does not decrease the miscarriage rate.[20] Indirect data from a recent meta-analysis has shown no significant benefit of pregestational metformin administration on abortion risk in patients with PCOS, when either used as monotherapy or in combination with other fertility drugs.[37] Metformin crosses the placenta and significant level is found in fetal serum. Therefore, metformin should be stopped after the pregnancy test until more consistent data are available.

Metformin in CC-Resistant Cases

In a meta-analysis, metformin + CC showed higher ovulation rate and pregnancy rate than CC alone in CC-resistant obese PCOS patients.[38] CC with metformin and laparoscopic ovarian diathermy have similar pregnancy rates in CC-resistant cases.[39] This combination results in modest ovulation and should be tried before gonadotropins in developing countries.[21]

Metformin for young patients with PCOS have a long timeline to achieve pregnancy.

BOX 9.1: Metformin and infertility.

- Clomiphene citrate (CC) is better than metformin for ovulation induction
- Combination of CC and metformin does not increase pregnancy rate[24]
- Combination does not lower the dose requirement of CC
- Metformin combined with gonadotropin does not have better outcome than gonadotropin alone
- If given in resistant PCOS patients, it decreases the sensitivity to ovulation induction drugs
- Incidence and severity of OHSS is reduced by 6–12 weeks of pretherapy with metformin
- It does not reduce the abortion rate.[24]

It is a drug of choice in PCOS patients who do not want to conceive immediately. Its action is gradual and within 6 months, it establishes ovulatory cycles by decreasing insulin and androgen level. Other advantage of metformin is that it decreases the incidence of multiple pregnancies with ovulation induction drugs. If the patient does not conceive when on metformin, option of CC remains open for her. A recent meta-analysis revealed that metformin does not result in weight loss among overweight and obese PCOS patients.[17,40] Addition of metformin to lifestyle had no significant benefit on ovulation and circulating androgen levels.[41]

Carry home message for metformin has been shown in Box 9.2.

Other Insulin Sensitizers

Insulin sensitizers, pioglitazone and rosiglitazone and other drugs like acarbose or D-chiro-inositol have not been found superior over metformin and so their routine use for infertile patient has not been established. The safety of all these drugs during pregnancy is still not established.

- Pioglitazone in a dose of 30–50 mg/day and rosiglitazone in a dose of 4–8 mg/day may be used in combination with metformin in

---

BOX 9.2: Carry home message for metformin.

- It has systemic and local effect
- It is used in type II diabetes and decreases hyperinsulinemia
- It decreases lipolysis, hepatic gluconeogenesis and glucose absorption and so decreases the requirement of insulin
- It increases the sensitivity of target cells to insulin
- It acts on theca cells and decreases androgen, which in turn decreases LH level
- Metformin does not cause weight loss[40]
- Lifestyle management is superior over metformin in prophylaxis of diabetes[42]
- Oral contraceptive (OC) pill is superior for menstrual irregularities, endometrial hyperplasia and malignancy.[43]

---

patients who are resistant to metformin.[44] Acarbose is also as effective as metformin in a dose of 100 mg in clomiphene-resistant PCOS.[45]

- D-chiro-inositol in a dose of 1,200 mg/day for 6–8 weeks corrects ovulatory dysfunction. The safety of all these drugs during the pregnancy is still not established. Addition of metformin to lifestyle had no significance benefit on ovulation and circulating androgen levels.[41]

Glucocorticoids

Half of PCOS patients have adrenal component in hyperandrogenism and is evidenced by increased dehydroepiandrosterone sulfate (DHEA-S).[46] This is secreted from zona reticularis of adrenal cortex. These patients are resistant to 150 mg of CC and may also require higher doses of gonadotropins. To improve intraovarian androgen milieu, reduction of circulating and intraovarian androgen is required. Only then and then ovulation may occur. Only adrenal androgen can be reduced effectively with glucocorticoids and so it is extensively tried in the resistant PCOS. Dexamethasone 0.5 mg is given continuously for 3 months as ovarian follicle takes 100 days for complete development. Dose can be titrated with testosterone or DHEA levels.

Dexamethasone 0.5 mg daily can be added for 3–6 months in these patients along with CC. Dexamethasone leads to water retention in patients. Water logging can be reduced by adding diuretics once a week or decreasing the dose of dexamethasone to 0.25 mg or drug may also be discontinued after ovulation. Serious complications are extremely rare and so this drug must be tried in obese CC-resistant PCOS.

Gonadotropins

Gonadotropins are indicated in patients with CC failure with high LH and having

TABLE 9.1: Specific bioactivity of gonadotropins.	
HMG (1950)	8 IU/mg of protein
uFSH (1980)	100–150 IU/mg of protein
uHMG-HP	2,000 IU/mg of protein
uFSH-HP (1982)	9,000 IU/mg of protein
rFSH (1995)	10,000 IU/mg of protein

antiestrogenic effect of CC. It has a higher pregnancy rate than CC + metformin.[21,47] As LH is already high in PCOS patients, in nondownregulated cycles, it is advisable to use FSH as the ovulation inducing gonadotropin in PCOS patient. Bioactivity of highly purified urinary FSH (uFSH-HP) and recombinant FSH (rFSH) is also higher than other preparations and dose required will be also less of these preparations.

Specific bioactivity of gonadotropins has been shown in Table 9.1.

Recombinant FSH does not have inhibiting substances like FSH. It has more basic isoforms, higher consistency and has less batch to batch variations. Because of high bioactivity, the dose requirement is less. Though no significant difference is seen in the live birth rate comparing the uFSH and rFSH.[48]

Recombinant FSH versus Human Menopausal Gonadotropin

Meta-analysis of eight RCTs conforming rFSH with human menopausal gonadotropin (hMG) has shown that rFSH has 50% higher pregnancy rates.[49] The FINVAT report 1999 also showed that the pregnancy rates were higher with rFSH than with hMG. The prospective study of 24,000 assisted reproductive technology (ART) cycles from Germany also showed higher birth rate and lower dosage with rFSH than hMG.[50] But a Cochrane review in 2009 shows a nonsignificant higher live birth rate with hMG as compared to rFSH.[48]

Chronic Low-Dose Protocol

In PCOS patients, gonadotropins are used as chronic low-dose protocol. The incidence of OHSS is reduced from 4.6% to 1% and multiple pregnancy rate is reduced to 5.7% as compared to 22–34% using this protocol. Uniovulatory cycle rate of 70% is achieved with rFSH with chronic low-dose protocol.[51] The basic concept of chronic low-dose protocol is the threshold theory which demands the attainment and maintenance of follicular development with exogenous FSH without exceeding threshold requirement of the ovary.

In chronic low-dose protocol 37.5 IU of rFSH is started from day 5 of the cycle. The same dose is continued for 14 days. Increasing the dose before 14 days loses the advantages of chronic low-dose protocol. Though ovulation monitoring is done during this period and in most of the cases a mature follicle develops within these 14 days. If it does not then the dose of gonadotropin is increased by 37.5 IU for another 7 days. If after that the follicle does not develop again 37.5 IU or even less, rFSH is increased after another 7 days till the mature follicle is achieved.[52] This protocol gives monofollicular development and therefore higher pregnancy rates. Multifollicular development leads to high E2 and progesterone levels, their altered ratios and therefore low implantation rates.

Professor Roy Homburg and Prof. Howles published a study on 2005 stating that if low-dose rFSH is used as the first line of treatment for ovulation induction, the pregnancy rates can be doubled to that of CC. This study showed a clear superiority of low-dose FSH over CC for treating anovulatory patients with PCOS. In first cycle, pregnancy rates are 30% with rFSH as compared to 14% with CC, and in second cycle, it is 50% with rFSH as compared to 32% with CC.[52] This explains that the time to achieve pregnancy is significantly reduced. If cost is not a prohibiting factor, rFSH in a chronic low-dose protocol is to be preferred over CC.

Chronic low-dose protocol is also described as chronic low-dose step-up protocol. In those patients who have high FSH threshold, chronic low-dose step-down protocol is used. This protocol has higher cancellation and complication rate.[53]

Even ultra-low-dose step-up protocol with only 10 IU of rFSH is useful.[54] In patients who have high FSH threshold, chronic low-dose step-down protocol is used. But this regimen has higher cancellation and complication rate.[53] Multifollicular development in PCOS is not because of differential FSH threshold but it is because of availability of more FSH sensitive antral follicles in the cohort as compared to normal ovaries.[55] Chronic ultra-low-dose protocol gave very good results when as small as 8.3 IU of FSH was given in incremental doses. It reduces the cost and gives monofollicular development with low cycle cancellation rates.[56]

Chronic Low-Dose Step-Down Protocol

It activates preovulatory follicles by surpassing FSH threshold. Once the follicles develop, the dose of FSH is reduced because of number of days of FSH in FSH windows decide the number of recruited follicles. So because of shorter half-life of FSH, dose reduction will limit the number of growing follicles. As the follicle grows, sensitivity for FSH increases and so requires lower dose of FSH. This will allow monofollicular development and leads to atresia of other follicles.[57]

How is it given?
About 75–150 IU of FSH is given for 4–5 days initially and minimum 5–7 days are required

to have a steady level of FSH. The dose is decreased as soon as ovarian reaction is seen on US, e.g. 10 mm of follicle, monofollicular development and avoids OHSS. The dose is reduced by 37.5 IU for 2 days and then again reduced by 37.5 IU. Initiation of follicular growth is expected when serum levels of FSH are from 6.5 U/L to 10.4 U/L. This assay is useful in poor responders.[47] It is concluded that monofollicular development and ovulation are achieved more effectively in chronic step-up protocol than step-down protocol.[58] So step-down protocol is second-line backup protocol for PCOS. Estrogen and progesterone injection in luteal phase maintains pregnancy rate.[59]

Multifollicular development in PCOS is common not because of difference of FSH threshold but these contain twice the number of available FSH sensitive antral follicles in the cohort as compared to normal ovary.[55]

We have found a combination of letrozole with rFSH very useful. It is cost-effective as it reduced the consumption of rFSH and also gives monofollicular development. Letrozole is given from day 3 to day 7 and rFSH is started from day 8. This regimen decreases the incidence of OHSS and multiple pregnancies with comparable results as those of rFSH alone.

Gonadotropin-Releasing Hormone Antagonist

In PCOS patients, there is a tonic rise of LH, particularly in thin lean PCOS patients. There is also a possibility of premature LH surge because of high estrogen levels. The advantage of the GnRH antagonist protocol is the growth of fewer follicles, leading to lower peak E2 levels and lower risk of OHSS.[60,61] Moreover, the risk of OHSS is also reduced as there is an option of using GnRH agonist as a trigger. It has also been proved that the dose of gonadotropins required is also less in GnRH antagonist protocols.[62] Antagonist is started when at least one follicle has grown to 14 mm, to prevent LH surge and is continued till follicle matures, i.e. the day of hCG. If antagonist is started early and the LH level is not high at that time, the follicle will regress, as certain amount of LH is required for final stages of maturation of the follicle. Gonadotropin dose does not require increment when antagonist is started. Antagonist also helps in correct timing of intrauterine insemination (IUI). But antagonist is not to be added if premature LH surge is not documented in the previous cycle or there is no proof of raised LH on ultrasound. In IVF cycles, GnRH antagonist can be used as a fixed or flexible protocol. In the fixed protocol, GnRH antagonist is started on day 6 of the stimulation whereas in flexible protocol, it is started when the lead follicle is greater than 13 mm or the serum E2 levels are more than 600 pg/mL. Antagonist used is Ganirelix or Cetrotide 0.25 mg daily. Similar conception rates can be achieved in long agonist and flexible GnRH antagonist protocols.[63] But with antagonist protocol, incidence of severe OHSS is reduced to 50%.[60,61]

- Oral contraceptive (OC) pills pretreatment for 2–3 months was used to decrease LH in PCOS patients but it may be detrimental to cycle outcome in antagonist cycle.[64]
- Micronized E2 2 mg BD for 10 days before the expected menstruation or from midluteal phase may decrease FSH and LH and good cohort of the follicles can be achieved.
- Norethisterone 10 mg/day can be used to schedule the cycle as it decreases LH level.

Stimulation can also be started after 4–5 days of OC pills, 3–5 days of progesterone and 1–2 days after estrogen.[65]

Advantages of antagonist protocol have been shown in Box 9.3.

BOX 9.3: Advantages of antagonist protocol.
- Lower risk of OHSS has 50% compared to agonist protocol
- Gonadotropin-releasing hormone agonist can be used for ovulation trigger
- Gives equivalent pregnancy rates
- It decreases the amount of gonadotropin used
- Estradiol concentration is lower on the day of hCG.

Gonadotropin-Releasing Hormone Agonist

Gonadotropin-releasing hormone agonist is used for ovulation trigger in PCOS patients. It induces a sustained release of LH from the pituitary gland that lasts for 24 hours.[66] (This is effective to induce preovulatory oocyte maturation).[67] The advantage is that the duration of action of GnRH agonist is shorter (24–36 hours) than hCG and is similar to natural surge.[68] It leads to lesser rise in E2 and progesterone levels and therefore gives better implantation rates and chance of OHSS is also reduced. But when agonist is used as a trigger, the chance of luteal phase defect is very high due to lower circulating luteal E2 and progesterone.[69] Some may also have early luteolysis and a short luteal phase.[70] Luteal support is therefore mandatory in these cases.

Gonadotropin-releasing hormone agonist for downregulation is an established treatment in IVF cycles, but should not be used in IUI cycles for the same purpose. This is so because, downregulation in IUI cycles, increases gonadotropin consumption, multiple pregnancy rate and incidence of OHSS, without any benefit. For IVF cycles also the recent studies have shown that downregulation with antagonist is a better option in PCOS patients. It significantly reduces the risk of OHSS, and also prevents supraphysiological levels of estrogen which may be an important cause for implantation failure.

Antagonist + Agonist Protocol

In PCOS patients, GnRH antagonist is used for downregulation and agonist is then used for oocyte trigger. Agonist when used as a trigger has 24–36 hours duration of action. It leads to lower FSH and LH resulting in luteal phase deficiency. Therefore, luteal support with 1,500 IU hCG, every 3rd day can be used[71] along with progesterone. This protocol decreases the risk of OHSS significantly. According to the recent studies, even dual trigger may be given. According to this protocol, agonist trigger is backed by 1,500 IU of hCG on the day of oocyte retrieval.[71] This decreases the chance of luteal phase defect but should not be used when the follicles are plenty. When follicles are plenty "freeze all" policy is most successful.[72]

Ovarian Drilling

Ovarian drilling is an effective tool for ovulation induction for PCOS patients. The advantage of ovarian drilling is that it induces unifollicular development without the risk of OHSS or high-order multiple pregnancies[73] and its beneficial effects can last for up to 9 years.[74] Cochrane review says that 12 months pregnancy rate after drilling and 6 months gonadotropin stimulation both have similar pregnancy rates.

It has also been quoted by Professor Roy Homburg that spontaneous pregnancy can occur after several years of drilling. Ovarian drilling gives 70–80% of ovulation rate and 60% of pregnancy rates.[75]

A Cochrane database analysis of four RCTs comparing laparoscopic ovarian drilling (LOD) with gonadotropin therapy, showed similar cumulative pregnancy rates 6–12 months after LOD and after 3–6 months of gonadotropin therapy.[76]

How Ovarian Drilling Works?

Various explanations have been described in literature as to why drilling works. But the most acceptable theory is that drilling decreases androgen level by destroying ovarian stroma. This decrease in androgen will decrease LH and change FSH/LH ratio. Stein-Leventhal had long back suggested that larger the ovary, larger portion of its stroma needs to be removed to decrease androgen and insulin levels. So, what I have found in my practice, only four punctures do not work in majority of cases. Larger the stromal volume, larger amount of stroma needs to be destroyed and therefore more punctures need to be done to decrease the androgen levels to effective limits. Ovarian drilling leads to destruction of the stromal cells which in turn reduces androgen production, decrease in stromal blood flow, leading to fall in serum levels of vascular endothelial growth factor (VEGF) and IGF-1. On drilling along with the stroma, small follicles are also destroyed, which leads to fall in AMH levels and therefore increases the sensitivity of follicles to FSH.[74,77] Failure of ovarian drilling in women with relatively high power Doppler indices along with high levels of AMH may be due to severity of PCOS in these women. It is possible that the extent of follicle destruction by LOD in these women was not enough to reduce intraovarian AMH to a level consistent with resumption of ovulation.[78] Another study has also shown that adjusted diathermy dose based on ovarian volume for LOD of PCOS has better reproductive outcome compared with fixed thermal dosage.[79] This means that measuring AMH and ovarian stromal three-dimensional (3D) power Doppler blood flow for women with anovulatory PCOS undergoing ovarian drilling may provide a useful tool in evaluating the outcome of ovarian drilling.[80]

Mechanism of action in ovarian drilling has been given in Box 9.4.

Method

It may be done with unipolar cautery, dipping 4 mm into ovarian stroma and has excellent

BOX 9.4: Mechanism of action in ovarian drilling.

- Decreases androgen levels because of destruction of stroma
- Decreases LH level is directly proportional to pregnancy rate after LOD
- Increases FSH level
- Decreases estrogen level and gives feedback to FSH
- Reverses LH/FSH ratio
- Temporary decrease in inhibin level
- Local and systemic effects promote ovulation
- Subcapsular cyst has high androgen rich fluid that is released and decreased androgen levels.

BOX 9.5: Guidelines of experts in Thessaloniki in Greece in 2007 for LOD.

- Laparoscopic ovarian drilling achieves unifollicular development with no risk of OHSS and high order multiple pregnancies
- It is a onetime treatment
- Intensive monitoring is not required
- It is as effective as gonadotropin therapy
- Adhesions formation, destruction of ovarian tissue and surgery-related complications are minimal
- Surgery should be performed by expert personnel.

results similar to laser therapy.[81] Various other methods have been described in literature without added advantage. Newer methods for ovarian drilling that are being tried now are transvaginal hydrolaparoscopic drilling, ultrasound-guided transvaginal ovarian needle drilling (UTND) and laparoscopic ovarian multi-needle intervention (LOMNI). The purpose for trials on these procedures is to ease out the ovarian drilling into a less invasive and a simple procedure.

Guidelines of experts in Thessaloniki in Greece in 2007 for LOD have been given in Box 9.5.

Advantages of Ovarian Drilling

- Ovarian drilling is especially indicated in PCOS patients who are resistant to CC. If ovarian drilling is done before starting gonadotropin therapy, the dose of gonadotropin required can be decreased and risk of OHSS and multiple pregnancy are reduced. As it destroys stroma and decreases the androgen and in turn LH levels, it improves the ovum quality and decreases the risk of abortions, the incidence of which is higher in PCOS patients as compared to non-PCOS patients. Ovarian drilling is a onetime procedure and therefore is a suitable method to facilitate ovulation induction in PCOS patients who cannot repeated come for monitoring or follow-up.
- The mean treatment costs per live birth within 8–12 years after initial treatment are significantly lower per live birth when treatment is started with laparoscopic electrocautery compared with when started with ovulation induction with rFSH, and electrocautery is a rational treatment for clomiphene-resistant PCOS.[75] Laparoscopic electrocautery of the ovaries is as effective as ovulation induction with FSH treatment in terms of live births, but reduces the need for ovulation induction or ART in a significantly higher proportion of women and increases the chance for second child.[82]

Disadvantages of Ovarian Drilling

- In spite of having significantly advantageous, ovarian drilling has been widely blamed for postprocedure ovarian failure. Though the risk is probably exaggerated. Ovarian failure after ovarian drilling is possible only when it is done in an ovary that does not have stromal excess or is not a polycystic ovary. Therefore, it is important and essential to do baseline ultrasound scan prior to laparoscopy and diagnosis of PCO is confirmed and preferable stromal volume is also calculated. Api et al. have concluded in their study that there was no concrete evidence of a decreased ovarian reserve nor premature ovarian failure associated with LOD in women with PCOS.[83]

- *Adhesions*: Pelvic or ovarian adhesions are seen in 40-60% of cases and it does not depend on number of punctures. But it does not change the pregnancy rate and adhesiolysis does not improve pregnancy rates.[84]

Variations in the Method of Ovarian Drilling

Newer methods for ovarian drilling—under trials:

1. *Transvaginal hydrolaparoscopic drilling*: Ovarian drilling by hydrolaparoscopy is an effective treatment in CC-resistant PCOS and it has given 76% pregnancy rates within a period of 7.2 months.[85]
2. *Ultrasound-guided transvaginal ovarian needle drilling*: It gives equivalent results. But safety and efficacy requires further studies.
3. *Laparoscopic ovarian multi-needle intervention*: This was devised by Kaya and associates.[86]
4. Transvaginal ultrasound-guided follicular aspiration of subcapsular cysts without causing significant stromal damage has yielded a 50-85% ovulation rate, thus proving that removal of androgen from follicular fluid helps to decrease LH and reverting LH/FSH ratio.[87]

But LOD gives better results than all other alternative techniques.

Unilateral drilling has been suggested by some workers, with an argument that it has an advantage of a short procedure time, minimized adhesions and ovarian tissue damage, but still induces activity in both ovaries.[87] Though according to other authors, this requires further evaluation.[88] In a latest study, Sunj et al. have shown that unilateral ovarian drilling using thermal doses adjusted to the ovarian volume (60 J/cc) was more effective than bilateral drilling done with constant thermal doses for both ovaries.[89] We have not even seen significant adhesions after drilling during cesarean section of the patients in whom we have done ovarian drilling. Ovarian malignancy after drilling has not been proved.

The major concern though is that how many punctures should be done per ovary. According to Adam Balen and Armar's technique, 4 punctures for 4 seconds at 40 W should be done in each ovary.[90] According to Naether[91] and colleagues, 5–20 punctures for 1 second at 400 W and according to Gjonnaess,[92] 5–8 punctures for 5–6 seconds at 300–400 W. If the above data is closely observed and analyzed, puncture duration is decreased when the power of current (Watts) are increased and number of punctures are less if each puncture is continued for longer time.

In our unpublished study that was conducted from 2002–2009 and total number of patients with PCOS enrolled was 2,733. Out of these 134 patients did not turn up after initial investigations and 2,699 patients were taken for study. Out of these 2,699 patients, 1,566 patients had come after taking treatment for subfertility for more than a year. In all the patients, a baseline ultrasound scan was done on day 2–3 of the cycle to assess the ovarian volume, stromal volume and the number of antral follicles and in these patients insulin resistance was also confirmed prior to the procedure. Depending on the stromal volume value 20–40 punctures with 400 W unipolar

TABLE 9.2: Results of 20–40 punctures with 400 W unipolar cautery in each ovary.

	No drilling	With drilling
Conceived	882 (55.68%)	828 (74.26%)
Not conceived	702	287
Total	1,584	1,115

BOX 9.6: Polycystic ovarian syndrome and assisted reproductive technology (ART).

- Polycystic ovarian syndrome is not an indication for ART
- Treat anovulation as a cause of infertility
- Assisted reproductive technique is indicated for associated pathology
- Assisted reproductive technique is preferred for single embryo transfer and to avoid multiple pregnancies
- Fresh cycle transfer has poor results due to high E2 and progesterone
- Freeze all is the preferred approach.

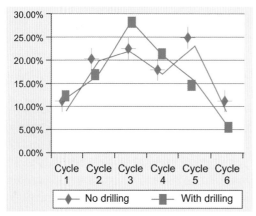

Fig. 9.1: Conception rate against number of treatment cycles.

cautery were done in each ovary and the results are displayed in Table 9.2.

It is seen in Figure 9.1 that the number of cycles for conception are fewer when ovarian drilling was done. And the author would like to emphasize that there was not a single case of ovarian failure in this series.

In Vitro Maturation

In vitro maturation (IVM) is the future for PCOS patients, as it is 100% OHSS-free treatment. The treatment cost is low as consumption of gonadotropins is very low. For this technique, ovulation induction is done with 125 IU/day of FSH (day 3–10 of the menstrual cycle) for 3 days is stopped when the follicle size reaches 10–11 mm. hCG 10,000 IU is given to the patient for final maturation and ovum pick-up is done after 33–38 hours. Period for IVM is 24–48 hours. Thereafter, ICSI is done

on these mature oocytes. The initial study has documented 8.9 oocytes/retrieval, 64% of maturation rate, 45% of fertilization rate after IVF/ICSI, 15.3% pregnancy rate per transfer and 7.3% live birth rate.[62] The challenges may be adequate laboratory conditions and learning skills for the clinical doing the ovum pick-up and also the embryologist.

Polycystic Ovarian Syndrome and ART

Polycystic ovarian syndrome and ART have been shown in Box 9.6.

SUMMARY

- Weight loss is the first line of treatment.
- Clomiphene is the time tested drug.
- Letrozole is an excellent alternative and may be more preferred.
- Adding metformin has no advantage on ovulation induction, though corrects the metabolic component, thus supports the pregnancy better.
- Glucocorticoids may be useful in CC-resistant PCOS patients.
- Chronic low-dose FSH protocol is very effective ovulation induction method for PCOS patients.
- Agonist may be used as an ovulation trigger.

- Antagonists to prevent premature LH surge are very useful in thin lean PCOS both in IUI and IVF cycles.
- Ovarian drilling has excellent results in best hands.
- In vitro maturation is the future.

REFERENCES

1. Dr Thatcher. Defining PCOS—a perspective. The American Infertility Association Newsletter, February 2001.
2. Rotterdam ESHRE/ASRM-Sponsored PCOS Consensus Work Group. Revised 2003 consensus on diagnostic criteria and long-term health risks related to polycystic ovarian syndrome. Hum Reprod. 2004;19(1):41-7.
3. Lujan ME, Jarrett BY, Brooks ED, et al. Updated ultrasound criteria for polycystic ovary syndrome: reliable thresholds for elevated follicle population and ovarian volume. Hum Reprod. 2013;28(5):1361-8.
4. Lam PM, Raine-Fenning N. Role of three-dimensional ultrasonography in polycystic ovary syndrome. Hum Reprod. 2006;21(9):2209-15.
5. Kim HJ, Adams JM, Gudmundsson JA, et al. Polycystic ovary morphology: age-based ultrasound criteria. Fertil Steril. 2017;108(3):548-53.
6. Erel CT, Senturk LM. The impact of body mass index on assisted reproduction. Curr Opin Obstet Gynecol. 2009;21:228-35.
7. Park HS, Lee K. Greater beneficial effects of visceral fat reduction compared with subcutaneous fat reduction on parameters of the metabolic syndrome: a study of weight reduction programmes in subjects with visceral and subcutaneous obesity. Diabet Med. 2005;22:266-72.
8. Smith SR, Zachwieja JJ. Visceral adipose tissue: a critical review of intervention strategies. Int J Obes Relat Metab Disord. 1999;23:329-35.
9. Homburg R. Understanding the problems of treating PCOS. In: Homburg R (Ed). Ovulation Induction and Controlled Ovarian Stimulation: A Practical Guide, 2nd edition. Switzerland: Springer International Publishing; 2014. pp. 65-72.
10. Fedorscak P, Dale PO, Stroreng R, et al. Impact of overweight and underweight on assisted reproduction treatment. Hum Reprod. 2004;19:2523-8.
11. Hammond MG. Monitoring techniques for improved pregnancy rates during clomiphene ovulation induction. Fertil Steril. 1984;42:499-508.
12. Dickey RP, Taylor SN, Curole DN, et al. Incidence of spontaneous abortion in clomiphene pregnancies. Hum Reprod. 1996;11:2623-8.
13. Glyser M, March CM, Mishell DR Jr, et al. A decade's experience with an individualized clomiphene treatment regimen including its effect on the postcoital test. Fertil Steril. 1982;37:161-7.
14. Panda B, Mohapatra L, Sahu MC, et al. Success in pregnancy through intrauterine insemination at first cycle in 300 infertile couples: an analysis. J Obstet Gynecol India. 2014;64(2):134-42.
15. National Collaborating Center for Women's and Children's Health/National Institute for Clinical Excellence. Fertility: assessment and treatment for people with fertility problems. London (UK): RCOG Press; 2004.
16. Ozdemir U, Ozaksit G, Cakir Gungor AN, et al. Letrozole usage adjuvant to gonadotropins for ovulation induction for patients with clomiphene citrate failure. Arch Gynecol Obstet. 2013;288(2):445-8.
17. Begum MR, Ferdous J, Begum A, et al. Comparison of efficacy of aromatase inhibitor and clomiphene citrate in induction of ovulation in polycystic ovarian syndrome. Fertil Steril. 2009;92:853-7.
18. Badawy A, Elnashar A, El-Ashry M, et al. Gonadotropin-releasing hormone agonists for prevention of chemotherapy-induced damage: a prospective randomized study. Fertil Steril. 2009;91:694-7.
19. Badawy A, Abdel Aal I, Abulatta M. Clomiphene citrate or letrozole for ovulation induction in women with polycystic ovarian syndrome: a prospective randomized trial. Fertil Steril. 2009;92:849-52.

20. Casper RF. Letrozole versus clomiphene citrate: which is better for ovulation induction? Fertil Steril. 2009;92(3):858-9.

21. Abu Hashim H, Wafa A, El Rakhawy M. Combined metformin and clomiphene citrate versus highly purified FSH for ovulation induction in clomiphene-resistant PCOS women: a randomized controlled trial. Gynecol Endocrinol. 2011;27(3):190-6.

22. Bohler H Jr, Mokshagundam S, Winters SJ. Adipose tissue and reproduction in women. Fertil Steril. 2010;94:795-825.

23. Creanga AA, Bradley HM, McCormick C, et al. Use of metformin in polycystic ovary syndrome: a meta-analysis. Obstet Gynecol. 2008;111(4):959-68.

24. Legro RS, Barnhart HX, Schlaff WD, et al. Clomiphene, metformin or both for infertility in the polycystic ovary syndrome. N Engl J Med. 2007;356:551-66.

25. Falghesu AM, romualdi C, Di Florio C, et al. Is there a dose-response relationship of metformin treatment in patients with polycystic ovary syndrome? Results from a multicentric study. Hum Reprod. 2012;27(10):3057-66.

26. Moll E, Bossuyt Patrick MM, Korevaar JC, et al. Effect of clomiphene citrate plus metformin and clomiphene citrate plus placebo on induction of ovulation in women with newly diagnosed polycystic ovary syndrome: randomized double-blind clinical trial. BMJ. 2006;332(7556):1485.

27. Nestler JE. Metformin in the treatment of infertility in polycystic ovarian syndrome: an alternative perspective. Fertil Steril. 2008;90(1):14-6.

28. Palomba S, Orio F Jr, Falbo A, et al. Prospective parallel randomized double-blind, double-dummy controlled clinical trial comparing clomiphene citrate to metformin as the first-line treatment for ovulation induction in nonobese anovulatory women with polycystic ovary syndrome. J Clin Endocrinol Metab. 2005;90:4068-74.

29. Costello MF, Chapman M, Conway U. A systematic review and meta-analysis of randomized controlled trials on metformin co-administration during gonadotropin ovulation induction or IVF in women with polycystic ovary syndrome. Hum Reprod. 2006;21:1387-99.

30. Kjotrod SB, von During V, Carlsen SM. Metformin treatment before IVF/ICSI in women with polycystic ovary syndrome; a prospective, randomized, double-blind study. Hum Reprod. 2004;19:1315-22.

31. Palomba S, Falbo A, Di Cello AD, et al. Does metformin affect the ovarian response to gonadotropins for in vitro fertilization treatment in patients with polycystic ovary syndrome and reduced ovarian reserve? A randomized controlled trial. Fertil Steril. 2011;96(5):1128-33.

32. Tso LO, Costello MF, Albuquerque LE, et al. Metformin treatment before and during IVF or ICSI in women with polycystic ovary syndrome. Cochrane Database Syst Rev. 2009;2:CD006105.

33. Palomba S, Falbo A, Carrillo L, et al. Metformin reduces the risk of ovarian hyperstimulation syndrome in patients with polycystic ovary syndrome during gonadotropins-stimulated in vitro fertilization cycles: a randomized controlled trial. Fertil Steril. 2011;96(6):1384-90.

34. Stadtmauer LA, Toma SK, Riehl RM, et al. Metformin treatment of patients with polycystic ovary syndrome undergoing in vitro fertilization improves outcomes and is associated with modulation of insulin-like growth factors. Fertil Steril. 2001;75:505-9.

35. Stadtmauer LA, Toma SK, Riehl RM, et al. The impact of metformin therapy on ovarian stimulation and outcome in 'coasted' patients with polycystic ovary syndrome undergoing in-vitro fertilization. Reprod Biomed Online. 2002;5:112-6.

36. Kjøtrød SB, Carlsen SM, Rasmussen PE, et al. Use of metformin before and during assisted reproductive technology in non-obese young infertile women with polycystic ovary syndrome: a prospective, randomized, double-blind multi-centre study. Hum Reprod. 2011;26(8):2045-53.

37. Palomba S, Falbo A, Orio F, et al. Effect of preconceptional metformin on abortion risk

in polycystic ovary syndrome: a systematic review and meta-analysis of randomized controlled trials. Fertil Steril. 2009;92:1646-58.

38. Wang LL, Ren W, Cheng QF, et al. Therapeutic effect of metformin for clomiphene-resistant infertility patients with polycystic ovary syndrome: a systematic analysis. Zhonghua Fu Chan Ke Za Zhi. 2012;47(9):659-63.

39. Abu Hashim H, El Lakany N, Sherief L. Combined metformin and clomiphene citrate versus laparoscopic ovarian diathermy for ovulation induction in clomiphene-resistant women with polycystic ovary syndrome: a randomized controlled trial. J Obstet Gynecol Res. 2011;37(3):169-77.

40. Lord JM, Flight IH, Norman RJ. Metformin in polycystic ovary syndrome: systematic review and meta-analysis. BMJ. 2003;327:951-3.

41. Ladson G, Dodson WC, Sweet SD, et al. The effects of metformin with lifestyle therapy in polycystic ovary syndrome: a randomized double-blind study. Fertil Steril. 2011;95(3):1059-66.

42. Knowler WC, Barrett-Connor E, Fowler SE, et al. Reduction in the incidence of type 2 diabetes with lifestyle intervention or metformin. N Engl J Med. 2001;346:393-403.

43. Costello MF, Shrstha B, Eden J, et al. Metformin versus oral contraceptive pill in polycystic ovary syndrome: a Cochrane review. Hum Reprod. 2007;22:1200-9.

44. Glueck CJ, Moreira A, Goldeberg N, et al. Pioglitazone and metformin in obese women with polycystic ovary syndrome not optimally responsive to metformin. Hum Reprod. 2003;18:1618-22.

45. Sonmez AS, Yasar L, Savan K, et al. Comparison of the effects of acarbose and metformin use on ovulation rates in clomiphene citrate-resistant polycystic ovary syndrome. Hum Reprod. 2005;20(1):175-9.

46. Lobo RA, Granger LR, Davajan V, et al. An extended regimen of clomiphene citrate in women unresponsive to standard therapy. Fertil Steril. 1982;37:762-6.

47. Van Weissenbruch MM, Schoemaker HC, Drexhage HA, et al. Pharmacodynamics of human menopausal gonadotropin (hMG) and follicle stimulating hormone (FSH). The importance of the FSH concentration in initiating follicular growth in polycystic ovary-like disease. Hum Reprod. 1993;8(6):813-21.

48. Van Wely M, Kwan I, Van der Veen F, et al. Recombinant FSH versus urinary gonadotrophins for ovarian hyperstimulation in IVF and ICSI cycles. A systematic review and meta-analysis. Hum Reprod. 2009;Suppl 1:i134.

49. Daya S, Gunby J, Hughes EG, et al. Follicle-stimulating hormone versus human menopausal gonadotropin for in vitro fertilization cycles: a meta-analysis. Fertil Steril. 1995;64:347-54.

50. Ludwig M, Rabe T, Buhler K, et al. Wirksamkeit von recombinantem humane FSH in Vergleigh zu urinarem hMG nach Downregulation im langen Protokoll – eine Analyse von 24,764 ART-Zyklen in Deutschland. J Reproduction Med Endocrinol. 1994; 4:284-8.

51. Homburg R, Howles CM. Low-dose FSH therapy for anovulatory infertility associated with polycystic ovarian syndrome: rationale, results, reflections and refinements. Hum Reprod Update. 1999;5(5):493-9.

52. Homburg R, Hendriks ML, Konig TE, et al. Clomifene citrate or low-dose FSH for the first-line treatment of infertile women with anovulation associated with polycystic ovary syndrome: a prospective randomized multinational study. Hum Reprod. 2012;27(2):468-73.

53. Van Santbrink EJ, Fauser BC. Urinary follicle-stimulating hormone for normogonadotropic clomiphene-resistant anovulatory infertility: prospective, randomized comparison between low dose step-up and step-down dose regimens. J Clin Endocrinol Metab. 1997;82(11):3597-602.

54. Orvieto R, Homburg R. Chronic ultra-low dose folicle-stimulating hormone regimen for patients with polycystic ovary syndrome: one click, one follicle, one pregnancy. Fertil Steril. 2009;91(4Suppl):1533-5.

55. Van der Meer M, Hompes P, de Boer J, et al. Cohort size rather than follicle-stimulating hormone threshold levels determines ovarian

sensitivity in polycystic ovary syndrome. J Clin Endocrinol Metab. 1988;83:423-6.

56. Orvieto R, Homburg R. Chronic ultra-low-dose follicle-stimulating hormone regimen for patients with polycystic ovary syndrome: one click, one follicle, one pregnancy. Fertil Steril. 2009;91(4 Suppl):1533-5.

57. diZerega GS, Hodgen GD. The primate ovarian cycle: suppression of human menopausal gonadotropin-induced follicular growth in the presence of the dominant follicle. J Clin Endocrinol Metab. 1980;50(5):819-25.

58. Christin-Maitre S, Hugues JN; Recombinant FSH Study Group. A comparative randomized multicentric study comparing the step-up versus step-down protocol in polycystic ovary syndrome. Hum Reprod. 2003;18:1626-31.

59. Engmann L, DiLuigi A, Schmidt D, et al. The use of gonadotropin-releasing hormone (GnRH) agonist to induce oocyte maturation after cotreatment with GnRH antagonist in high-risk patients undergoing in vitro fertilization prevents the risk of ovarian hyperstimulation syndrome: a prospective randomized controlled study. Fertil Steril. 2008;89:84-91.

60. Al-Inany HG, Youssef MA, Aboulghar M, et al. Gonadotrophin-releasing hormone antagonists for assisted reproductive technology. Cochrane Database Syst Rev. 2011;(5):CD001750.

61. Kolibianakis EM, Collins J, Tarlatzis BC, et al. Among patients treated for IVF with gonadotropins and GnRH analogues, is the probability of live birth dependent on the type of analogue used? A systematic review and meta-analysis. Hum Reprod Update. 2006;12:651-71.

62. Navot D, Bergh PA, Laufer N. Ovarian hyperstimulation syndrome in novel reproductive technologies: prevention and treatment. Fertil Steril. 1992;58:249-61.

63. Lainas RG, Sfontouris IA, Zorzovilis IZ, et al. Flexible GnRH antagonist protocol versus GnRH long agonist protocol in patients with polycystic ovarian syndrome treated for IVF: a prospective randomized controlled trial (RCT). Hum Reprod. 2010;25(3):683-9.

64. Kolibianakis EM, Papanikolaou EG, Camus M, et al. Effect of oral contraceptive pill pretreatment on ongoing pregnancy rates in patients stimulated with GnRH antagonists and recombinant FSH for IVF. A randomized controlled trial. Hum Reprod. 2006;21:352-7.

65. Cedrin-Durnerin I, Bstandig B, Parneix I, et al. Effects of oral contraceptive, synthetic progesterone or natural estrogen pretreatments on the hormonal profile and the antral follicle cohort before GnRH antagonist protocol. Hum Reprod. 2007;22(1):109-16.

66. Casper RF, Sheehan KL, Yen SS. Gonadotropin-estradiol responses to a superactive luteinizing hormone-releasing hormone agonist in women. J Clin Endocrinol Metab. 1980;50:179-81.

67. Itskovitz J, Boldes R, Levron J, et al. Induction of preovulatory luteinizing hormone surge and prevention of ovarian hyperstimulation syndrome by gonadotrophin-releasing hormone agonist. Fertil Steril. 1991;56:213-20.

68. Scheele F, van der Meer M, Lambalk CB, et al. Exploring the recovery phase after treatment with gonadotropin-releasing hormone agonist for ovulation induction in polycystic ovarian syndrome: three pilot trials. Eur J Obstet Gynecol Reprod Biol. 1995;62(2):221-4.

69. Itskovitz J, Boldes R, Barlev A, et al. The induction of LH surge and oocyte maturation by GnRH analogue (buserelin) in women undergoing ovarian stimulation for in vitro fertilization. Gynecol Endocrinol. 1988;2(Suppl 2):165.

70. Gonen Y, Balkier H, Powell W, et al. Use of gonadotropin-releasing hormone agonist to trigger follicular maturation for in vitro fertilization. J Clin Endocrinol Metab. 1990;71:918-22.

71. Humadian P, Ejdrup Bredkjaer H, Westergard LG, et al. 1,500 IU human chorionic gonadotropin administered at oocyte retrieval rescues the luteal phase when gonadotropin-releasing hormone agonist is used for ovulation induction: a prospective, randomized, controlled study. Fertil Steril. 2010;93:847-54.

72. Griesinger G, Schultz L, Bauer T, et al. Ovarian hyperstimulation syndrome prevention by

gonadotropin-releasing hormone agonist triggering of final oocyte maturation in a gonadotropin-releasing hormone antagonist protocol in combination with a 'freeze-all' strategy: a prospective multicentric study. Fertil Steril. 2011;95:2029-33.

73. Balen A. Surgical treatment of polycystic ovarian syndrome. Best Pract Res Clin Endocrinol Metab. 2006;20:271-80.

74. Amer SA, Banu Z, Li TC, et al. Long-term follow-up of patients with polycystic ovary syndrome after laparoscopic ovarian drilling: endocrine and ultrasonographic outcomes. Hum Reprod. 2002;17:2851-7.

75. Homburg R. Ovulation Induction and Controlled Ovarian Stimulation: A Practical Guide, 2nd edition. Switzerland: Springer International Publishing; 2014. pp. 109-13.

76. Farquhar C, Vandekerkhove P, Lilford R. Laparoscopic "drilling" by diathermy or laser for ovulation induction in anovulatory polycystic ovarian syndrome. Cochrane Database Syst Rev. 2001;(4):CD001122.

77. Amer SA, Li TC, Leder WL. The value of measuring anti-Mullerian hormone in women with anovulatory polycystic ovary syndrome undergoing laparoscopic ovarian diathermy. Hum Reprod. 2009;92:1586-93.

78. Nardo LG, Gelbaya TA, Wilkinson H, et al. Circulating basal anti-Mullerian hormone levels as predictor of ovarian response in women undergoing ovarian stimulation for in vitro fertilization. Fertil Steril. 2009;92:1586-93.

79. Mahmoud S, Kamal MM, Hamed MD. Laparoscopic ovarian drilling in polycystic ovary syndrome: efficacy of adjusted thermal dose based on ovarian volume. Fertil Steril. 2011;95:1115-8.

80. Elmashad AI. Impact of laparoscopic ovarian drilling on anti-Mullerian hormone levels and ovarian stromal blood flow using three-dimensional power Doppler in women with anovulatory polycystic ovarian syndrome. Fertil Steril. 2011;95(7):2342-6.

81. Donesky B, Adashi E. Surgically induced ovulation in the PCO syndrome: ovarian wedge resection revisited. Fertil Steril. 1995;63:439-63.

82. Nahuis MJ, Lohuis EO, Bayram N, et al. Long-term follow-up of laparoscopic electrocautery

of the ovaries versus ovulation induction with recombinant FSH in clomiphene citrate-resistant women with polycystic ovary syndrome: an economic evaluation. Hum Reprod. 2012;27(12):3577-82.

83. Api M. Is ovarian reserve diminished after laparoscopic ovarian drilling? Gynecol Endocrinol. 2009;25:159-65.

84. Mercorio E, Mercorio A, Di Spiezio Sardo A, et al. Evaluation of ovarian adhesion formation after laparoscopic ovarian drilling by second-look minilaparoscopy. Fertil Steril. 2008;89:1229-33.

85. Gordts S, Gordts S, Puttemans P, et al. Transvaginal hydrolaparoscopy in the treatment of polycystic ovary syndrome. Fertil Steril. 2009;91(6):2520-6.

86. Kaya H, Sezik M, Ozkaya O. Evaluation of a new surgical approach for the treatment of clomiphene citrate-resistant infertility in polycystic ovary syndrome: laparoscopic ovarian multi-needle intervention. J Minim Invasive Gynecol. 2005;12(4):355-8.

87. Balen AH, Jacobs HS. A prospective study comparing unilateral and bilateral laparoscopic ovarian diathermy in women with polycystic ovary syndrome. Fertil Steril. 1994;62(5):921-5.

88. Fernandez H, Morin-Surruca M, Torre A, et al. Ovarian drilling for surgical treatment of polycystic ovary syndrome: a comprehensive review. Reprod Biomed Online. 2011;22:556-68.

89. Sunj M, Canic T, Baldani DP, et al. Does unilateral laparoscopic diathermy adjusted to ovarian volume increase the chances of ovulation in women with polycystic ovary syndrome? Hum Reprod. 2011;28(9):2417-24.

90. Armar NA, McGarrigle HH, Honour J, et al. Laparoscopic ovarian diathermy in the management of anovulatory infertility in women with polycystic ovaries: endocrine changes and clinical outcome. Fertil Steril. 1990;53:45-9.

91. Naether OG, Fischer R, Weise HC, et al. Laparoscopic electrocoagulation of ovarian surface in infertile patients with polycystic ovarian disease. Fertil Steril. 1993;60:88-94.

92. Gjonnaess H. The course and outcome of pregnancy after ovarian electrocautery with PCOS: the influence of body weight. Br J Obstet Gynecol. 1989;96:714-9.

Ovulation Induction in Poor Responders

Chaitanya Nagori

INTRODUCTION

Management of a poor responder is one of the greatest challenges in assisted reproductive technology (ART) management. This is so primarily because there is no clear-cut standard definition of poor responders. Different definitions and consensus include age, ovarian reserve tests, and previous response to gonadotropins as measures to diagnose poor responders. Moreover, the success of an ART cycle is directly related to the number of embryos transferred.[1]

CAUSES OF POOR RESPONSE

There are different causes of poor response, which are as follows:

- Age
- Ovarian surgery
- Advanced endometriosis
- Endometrioma
- Obesity
- Previous pelvic infection
- Smoking
- Postchemotherapy and postradiotherapy
- Family history of early menopause
- Genetic conditions (Turner's)
- Follicle-stimulating hormone (FSH) receptor polymorphism.

Bologna Criteria Consensus

European Society of Human Reproduction and Embryology (ESHRE) consensus definition (2011) states that the presence of two of the three following features is deemed necessary to define poor response:[2]

1. Advanced maternal age (> 40 years) or any other risk factor for poor ovarian reserve.
2. A previous poor response to stimulation (<3 oocytes) or expected poor response when no previous stimulation is done.
3. Abnormal ovarian reserve tests (AFC 5–7 follicles, AMH 0.5–1.0 ng/mL).

Age

Age more than 37 years is the most important predictor of low response. The cohort of follicles decreases giving poor pregnancy rate. All other causes of poor ovarian response are to be considered in young patients.

Bologna criteria have been criticized because of:

- Definition of poor ovarian responder (POR) has also same threshold of three or fewer oocytes.
- Selection of age is arbitrary selection of 40 years.
- Ignorance of oocyte quality and other factors like smoking and medical disorders are not included. So, it is not widely accepted.

Markers for poor ovarian reserve are as follows:
- Anti-Müllerian hormone less than 3 pmol/mL
- Total AFC more than 5
- Less than three developing follicles or three oocytes retrieved after ovarian stimulation are defined as poor responders.[3,4]

All other markers are supportive and are not used routinely.

TREATMENT OPTIONS (BOX 10.1)

Increasing Gonadotropin Dosage

The dose is increased with an idea that it will overcome the effect of aging (decline in AFC). Earlier studies suggested that by increasing the dose of urinary gonadotropins from 300 IU to 450 IU can improve the results in terms of pregnancy rate and less chances of cycle cancellation. But this was not confirmed in other studies.[5,6] Klinkert et al. increased the dose of recombinant FSH (rFSH) to double in women having AFC less than 5, but did not document any benefit. So, increasing the dose of gonadotropin to more than 300 IU does not help in poor responders. Proper diagnosis of poor responders can avoid cancellation and decide correct line of treatment.[7] In a prospective study it was concluded that there was no difference in clinical pregnancy rate per transfer whether the stimulating dose of 300, 450, 600 IU FSH/day in gonadotropin-releasing hormone (GnRH) agonist microdose flare-up protocol.[7] Ovarian response is determined by

> **BOX 10.1:** Treatment options in poor responders.
> - Increase gonadotrophic dose
> - GnRH agonist flare protocol
> - LH supplementation
> - GnRH agonist stop protocol
> - Microdose GnRH agonist in luteal phase
> - Luteal phase FSH + agonist
> - GnRH agonist microdose flare
> - GnRH antagonist
> - Estrogen priming
> - Clomiphene citrate
> - Letrozole
> - L-arginine
> - Growth hormone
> - Glucocorticoids
> - Pre-IVF androgen
> - Natural cycle IVF
> - Aspirin
> - Pyridostigmine
> - Other therapies
> - Donor oocytes
> - Pretreatment OC pills
> - IVM
>
> (FSH: follicle-stimulating hormone; GnRH: gonadotropin-releasing hormone; IVF: in vitro fertilization; IVM: in vitro maturation; LH: luteinizing hormone; OC: oral contraceptive)

number of follicles available for recruitment than by circulating gonadotropin levels. On the contrary higher doses give poor quality oocytes in normal responding ovary.[8] The type of gonadotropin, i.e. rFSH, human menopausal gonadotropin (HMG) or urinary FSH (uFSH) has not shown any statistical difference in pregnancy rate.[9] Step-down regime, is decreasing dose of gonadotropin from 450 IU to 300 IU to 150 IU as follicles develop. This regime gives same results without compromising cycle outcome and also has an economic benefit.[10] Higher dose of FSH also affects endometrial receptivity. Modified natural cycle or with low dose of gonadotropin[11] with oral agents have given the same results like high dose gonadotropins used for ovulation induction. This means higher doses of gonadotropins do not increase the number of oocytes retrieved. In FET cycles results are better than high Gonadotropin cycles. This indicates that high dose affects the endometrial receptivity.

Gonadotropin-releasing Hormone Agonist: Flare-up Protocol or Short Protocol

Initial stimulating effect on endogenous gonadotropin release is observed when agonist is given in the beginning of menstrual cycle. Later on GnRH agonist suppresses the premature luteinizing hormone (LH) surge. So considering this physiological effect, some workers started giving GnRH agonist and gonadotropin from the beginning of the cycle in early follicular phase. Earlier trials did report higher pregnancy rate,[12] others failed to demonstrate improved ovarian response or cycle outcome.[13] GnRH agonist flare-up does not improve results even with prior oral contraceptive (OC) pills. The results of flare-up protocol are similar to antagonist protocol.[14] So, flare-up protocol in poor responders does not improve the result. One of the theories put forward is atresia of the follicles induced by increase in LH and progesterone. FSH that is produced by agonist flare-up is not much bioactive. But in some studies, flare-up protocol has given better results than long protocols.[15] Here GnRH agonist (1 mg leuprolide acetate) is given from the first day and stopped after 3 days and gonadotropins are started from day 3 or 4.

Gonadotropin-releasing Hormone Agonists: Luteinizing Hormone Supplementation

Profound suppression of gonadotropins occurs after midluteal GnRH agonist protocol. Several groups have evaluated outcome by adding 75–150 IU of LH daily from day 6 of stimulation in long protocol as well as flare-

up protocol. Unfortunately this protocol is not beneficial in improving ovarian response and pregnancy rate.[16,17] So addition of LH in poor responders does not improve the outcome.[18] There is a subset of patients in whom LH supplementation can improve the results. They are with profound LH suppression and poor responders.[19] In a study by Humaidan et al., rFSH + rLH gives similar number of eggs like rFSH alone, though pregnancy failure is less with rFSH + rLH combination.[20] In poor ovarian reserve patients, this group has been classified as 'Low prognosis' patients which may be of (a) suboptimal response (4–9 oocytes instead of 10–15 oocytes) or (b) Hyporesponsive who requires higher doses of gonadotropins. This is termed as 'Poseidon criteria' and is discussed in Chapter 14 of this book.

Gonadotropin-releasing Hormone Agonists: Stop Protocols and Reduced Dose

Long luteal GnRH agonist protocol suppresses gonadotropin secretion. If it is continued after menstruation, it profoundly suppresses gonadotropin secretion and may inhibit subsequent response with controlled ovarian hyperstimulation (COH). It has been tried to assess the response after stopping GnRH agonist before starting gonadotropins. A prospective study by Faber et al. showed the pregnancy rate of 24% per transfer and 12.5% cancellation rate with LH surge in only one patient.[21] However, Gracia-Valesco et al. reported that cancellation, pregnancy, and implantation rates are same as long protocol and stop protocol. But higher numbers of mature oocytes are obtained as well as reduced dose of gonadotropins are required with stop protocol.[22] Similar results can be obtained by long protocol of 0.5 mg leuprolide acetate that is reduced to 0.25 mg after downregulation.[23]

Minidose Luteal Phase Gonadotropin-releasing Hormone Agonist

Decreasing dose of GnRH agonist in luteal phase prior to gonadotropin stimulation theoretically will improve the response after stimulation, as suppression will be less. Feldberg et al. tried with triptorelin 0.5 mg before menstruation and then 0.1 mg daily and in another group 0.1 mg before menstruation and 0.05 mg after menstruation. Improved results were observed with decreasing dose.[24] Leuprolide acetate is given as 1 mg in midluteal phase and 0.5 mg after menstruation. Instead if 0.5 mg in midluteal phase and 0.25 mg after menstruation in long protocol improves ovarian response with lesser dose of gonadotropins.[23]

Luteal Phase FSH + GnRH Agonist

Selection of the follicle is done in luteal phase of preceding cycle. So, if FSH is given during the luteal phase, it may give better response in poor responders. In one study, more mature oocytes were obtained when FSH and GnRH agonist were started together in midluteal phase.[25] Further studies are required to assess the efficacy of this protocol.

Dual Stimulation (DuoStim)

It is also very useful in poor responders. Stimulation in follicular phase and after pickup also. Stimulation in luteal phase significantly increases the number of final transferable blastocysts in natural cycle. This strategy may be applied in other situations where obtaining competent oocytes is an urgent need.[26]

Gonadotropin-releasing Hormone Agonist: Microdose Flare

When using microdose flare protocol, lowest dose of agonist is given, that can stimulate endogenous FSH secretion and inhibits LH surge. As low as 25 mg leuprolide acetate can be used to achieve adequate levels of gonadotropins.[27] Pretreatment with oral pills or progesterone can reduce progesterone and raise androgen. In one study, Surrey, et al. introduced 40 mg leuprolide acetate twice daily. This reduced cycle cancellation from 73% to 31.6%. According to this study, when the age was more than 40 years pregnancy rate of 18.2% was achieved.[27,28] So, microdose flare-up protocol is very useful in poor responders. But with natural cycle in vitro fertilization (IVF) and stop protocol results were same like microdose flare-up protocol.[29,30] Comparing microdose flare-up protocol and antagonist protocol, microdose flare-up protocol has higher pregnancy rate.[31,32] But two randomized cohort trials failed to demonstrate any beneficial effect of microdose flare-up protocol when compared with antagonist protocol with regard to number of cycles and pregnancy rates.[6,14]

Gonadotropin-releasing Hormone Antagonist

Gonadotropin-releasing hormone antagonist will inhibits untoward LH surge and progesterone rise. It can be used as a fixed protocol from day 6 of stimulation or when lead follicle is 14 mm in diameter. It does not cause suppression in early follicular phase. Several prospective randomized trials have evaluated antagonist in comparison with alternative regimes in poor responders. Cheung et al. did not get statistical significant difference in pregnancy rates.[31]

No significant difference was seen between antagonist and microdose protocol while some of the studies got better results with microdose flare protocol.[14,30] The main advantage of antagonist is that it does not cause prolonged suppression in early follicular phase, which is the crucial time for poor responders. It also suppresses LH and progesterone rise and so decreases cancellation of cycles. It is the protocol of choice as it decreases the time for stimulation as well as total amount of gonadotropins required. As the results are equivalent with other protocols, antagonist protocol is preferred due to other advantages. In luteal phase antagonist protocol, antagonist is added for 3–5 days before the expected day of menstruation and continued for 4–7 days. Stimulation is started with 300–450 IU and when lead follicle reaches 14 mm, antagonist is restarted till the day of trigger. Here the advantage is that it causes luteolysis before the period. Here, FSH is not sufficiently reduced and cohort of recruitable follicles remains. This has improved the results.[33]

Gonadotropin-releasing Hormone Antagonist with Agonist

In this protocol, agonist is given for 3 days after period and then gonadotropins are given with flexible antagonist protocol or agonist can be given in midluteal phase and stop after menstruation. Then gonadotropin with flexible antagonist protocol is used. None of these regimes has any advantage over antagonist protocol.

Estrogen Priming and Antagonist Treatment

Estradiol administration in luteal phase may induce FSH receptor formation in poor responders and follicles become responsive to gonadotropins in coordination. Estradiol is administered as 0.1 mg transdermal patch or 4 mg daily estradiol valerate in luteal phase. GnRH antagonist is introduced 2 days later and continued for 3 days. Then gonadotropins are given for ovulation induction. Antagonist is reintroduced at a lead follicle size of 14 mm. Ongoing pregnancy rate of 26% was achieved by this protocol.[34] Compared with microdose flare-up protocol, there is not a statistically significant difference in clinical pregnancy rate.[35] Estradiol valerate 4 mg/day can be given from day 21 of luteal phase and continued till day 3 of menstruation or up to the day trigger. This may increase the pregnancy rate in poor responders,[36] but other studies have not shown similar results.[37]

Clomiphene Citrate

Adding clomiphene induces endogenous gonadotropin secretion, that helps in poor responders. These are used in antagonist protocol. In a study comparing long protocol with clomiphene and antagonist protocol, better pregnancy rate was observed with lower cancellation rate in antagonist protocol.[38] The theoretical disadvantage of effect of clomiphene citrate (CC) on endometrial development must be considered and in other studies, results are disappointing.[39]

Letrozole

It is added with an idea that it increases androgen by preventing aromatization to estrogen. This androgen sensitizes the follicle to FSH and this may help reduce the dose of FSH. Letrozole can be given from day 3 to day 7 in a dose of 2.5 mg. Gonadotropins are given simultaneously. Antagonist protocol is used, but in comparison with microflare protocols, this protocol is inferior considering all aspects[40] though some studies have shown better results with letrozole.[41] Implantation rates may be higher as compared to CC, but lower numbers of matured oocytes are obtained in letrozole with antagonist protocol.[41]

L-arginine

It is based in the function of nitric oxide. L-arginine enhances periovulatory vasodilatation. Dose is 16 g daily. It has been claimed to improve pregnancy rates.[42]

BOX 10.2: Actions of growth hormone.
• It promotes steroidogenesis (recruits follicles) • It promotes gametogenesis • This acts directly or through IGF-1 and by increasing the sensitivity to IGF-2 • It indirectly upregulates LH receptors • It increases progesterone production • DNA repairs capacity in oocyte is increased. (DNA: deoxyribonucleic acid; IGF: insulin-like growth factor; LH: luteinizing hormone)

BOX 10.3: Possible mechanism of DHEA.
• Improves the pool of primordial follicles • Increase IGF-1 during stimulation • Increases steroid production, testosterone, and estrogen • Sensitizes FSH receptors • Effect is cumulative and more antral follicles are exposed to treatment • It modulates the level of AMH expression • It delays the effect of ovarian aging • It may augment endometrial function.[50] (AMH: anti-Müllerian hormone; DHEA: dehydroepiandro-sterone; FSH: follicle-stimulating hormone; IGF-1: insulin-like growth factor 1)

Growth Hormone

It is produced centrally by pituitary and locally by ovary. It increases the local production of insulin-like growth factor 1 (IGF-1) and oocyte competence (Box 10.2). IGF-1 improves response of granulosa cells to FSH, helps in oocyte maturation and steroidogenesis. In a meta-analysis by Kolibiankis, it has been shown that adding growth hormone, decreases the cycle cancellation and improves the pregnancy rates. But the studies included were heterogeneous.[43] Further, well-controlled randomized studies have failed to demonstrate beneficial effect. It is useful in IGF-1 deficiency, i.e. hypogonadotropic hypogonadism. Growth hormone is given in a dose of 4–12 IU subcutaneous from the day of stimulation with gonadotropins. This adds to the cost of the treatment without improving results. Same way growth hormone stimulating factor is also not beneficial in treatment of poor responders.

Glucocorticoids

It stimulates the secretion of growth hormone and IGF-1. Giving dexamethasone 1 mg daily in long protocol causes lower cycle cancellation rate, but no difference in implantation or pregnancy rates has been found.[44]

Pre-in Vitro Fertilization Androgens

Androgen sensitizes the follicle to gonadotropin stimulation. In women, upregulation of FSH receptors before stimulation may enhance follicular responsiveness to exogenous gonadotropins and this allows majority of the antral follicles to develop into dominant or mature follicles rather than undergoing atresia. This increase in FSH receptors increases LH receptors also in the later phase, giving good oocyte maturation.[45] Dehydroepiandrosterone (DHEA) is secreted from zona reticularis of adrenal cortex and ovarian theca cells. It is a prohormone in ovarian steroidogenesis. It may reduce aneuploidy rate and so may decrease miscarriage rate.[46] In two randomized controlled trials, transdermal testosterone application was done. 12.5 mg transdermal testosterone gel is applied for 21 days in the cycle preceding controlled ovarian stimulation (COS) with antagonist. The dose can be 20 mg/kg/day given 5 days prior to stimulation.[47] It did not show improvement in oocytes, embryo quality, implantation rate or pregnancy rates.[48,49] DHEA supplementation, especially above the age of 35 years is associated with decreased miscarriage rate in women with diminished ovarian reserve (DOR). DHEA may improve pregnancy rates, but the effect of DHEA on oocyte quality has not been adequately studied (Box 10.3). There is no statistical improvement in ovarian response markers, ovarian response to low dose gonadotropins or IVF outcome in pretreatment DHEA in poor responders.

Natural Cycle In Vitro Fertilization

In this protocol, no gonadotropins are given. Only hCG is given when the follicle matures and pickup is done after 34–35 hours. Pregnancy rate of 17% pertransfer can be achieved.[50] This has a very low pregnancy rate with only one embryo available for transfer and many a times no ovum is retrieved. Early LH surge is very common in natural cycle. The number of cycles tried to give the pregnancy are too many and has a psychological impact on the patient. Ovum donation may be preferred to this in most cases.

Mild Ovarian Stimulation

In poor responder groups, mild ovarian stimulation is more cost-effective and patient friendly than conventional IVF and should be considered for poor responders over 37 years of age.[51] Modified natural cycle is also a good option for young poor responders or older patients.

Aspirin

This is to improve the blood supply and the results are disappointing.[52] Aspirin has three modes of actions: (1) Increases capillary blood flow to endometrium, (2) anti-inflammatory effect, and (3) reduces uterine contractions. But results are not improved as the uterine artery resistance remains unaffected.[53]

Pyridostigmine (Growth Hormone Releasing Factor)

It is given in a dose of 120 mg/day. It is acetylcholinesterase inhibitor. It leads to increase in acetylcholine, which increases the growth hormone. It is given from day 21 of

previous cycle till the day of trigger. Compared with placebo, it showed better pregnancy rates.[54] But other studies showed limited success.

Acupuncture

Current literature does not provide sufficient evidence that adjuvant acupuncture improves IVF clinical pregnancy rates.[54]

Ovum Donation

It can be offered in poor responders as an alternative or incase of failure of retrieving eggs.

Pretreatment with Oral Contraceptive Pills

It has several advantages, which are as follows:
- It produces estrogen environment.
- It increases sex hormone-binding globulin (SHBG) and decreases androgen level helping in preventing apoptosis.
- It decreases LH and so there is follicular synchronization.
- It decreases progesterone rise during preovulatory period.
- It decreases FSH and LH and thus downregulates pituitary.

CARRY HOME MESSAGE

- Poor responders should be correctly identified by Bologna criteria.
- Increasing gonadotropin dosage is not useful.
- Long protocol and flare-up protocol are not useful in poor responders.
- Microdose protocol gives better results.
- Gonadotropin-releasing hormone antagonist with estrogen priming is good alternative.
- Addition of letrozole rather than CC can improve pregnancy rates.

- Growth hormone simply increases the cost of treatment.
- Aspirin, pyridostigmine, glucocorticoids, acupuncture may have a supportive effect but have to still prove their role in improving pregnancy rates.
- Oral contraceptive pills may help some patients by reducing LH in the patients.
- Pre-IVF androgen does not give better results in oocytes and fertilization rate, but decreases abortion rate.

REFERENCES

1. Asch R. Repeated cryopreservation and storage of embryos: a successful alternative for poor responders. In Vitro Fertilization and Assisted Reproduction. 1997. pp. 61-4.
2. Land J, Yarmilinskaya MI, Dumoulin JC, et al. High dose hMG stimulation in poor responder does not improve in vitro fertilization outcome. Fertil Steril. 1996;65(5):951-65.
3. Pandian Z, McTavish AR, Aucott L, et al. Interventions for 'poor responders' to controlled ovarian hyperstimulation (COH) in in-vitro fertilization (IVF). Cochrane Database Syst Rev. 2010;(1):CD004379.
4. Karande VC, Jones GS, Veeeck LL, et al. High dose follicle stimulating hormone stimulation at the onset of the menstrual cycle does not improve the in vitro fertilization outcome in low responder patients. Fetil Steril. 1990;53:486-9.
5. Klinkert ER, Broekmans FJ, Looman CW, et al. Expected poor responders on the basis of an antral follicle count do not benefit from higher starting dose of gonadotrophins in IVF treatment: a randomized controlled trial. Hum Reprod. 2005;20:611-5.
6. Schmidt DW, Bremmer T, Orris JJ, et al. A randomized prospective study of microdose leuprolide versus ganirelix in in vitro fertilization cycles for poor responders. Fertil Steril. 2005;83:1568-71.
7. Berkkanoglu M, Ozgur K. What is the optimum maximal gonadotropin dosage used in micro-dose flare up cycles in poor responders? Fertil Steril. 2010;94(2):662-5.
8. Ben-Rafael Z, Benadiva CA, Ausmanas M, et al. Dose of human menopausal gonadotropin influences the outcome of an in vitro fertilization program. Fertil steril. 1987;48:964-8.
9. Eskandar M, jaroudi K, Jambi A, et al. Is recombinant follicle-stimulating hormone more effective in IVF poor responders than human menopausal gonadotropins? Med Sci Monit. 2004;10(1):16-9.
10. Cedrin-Durnerin I, Bstandig B, Herve F, et al. A comparative study of high fixed-dose and decremental-dose regimes of gonadotropins in a minidose gonadotropin-releasing hormone agonist flare protocol for poor responders. Fertil Steril. 2000;73:1055-6.
11. Youssef MA, van Wely M, Al Inany H, et al. A mild ovarian stimulation strategy in women with poor ovarian reserve undergoing IVF: a multicenter randomized non-inferiority trial. Hum Reprod. 2017;32(1):112-8.
12. Katayama KP, Roesler M, Gunnarson C, et al. Short-term use of gonadotropin releasing hormone agonist (leuprolide) for in vitro fertilization. J In Vitro Fert Embryo Transf. 1988;5:332-4.
13. Gindoff PR, Hall JL, Stillman RJ. Ovarian suppression with leuprolide acetate: comparison of luteal, follicular, and flare up administration in controlled ovarian hyperstimulation for oocyte retrieval. J In Vitro Fert Embryo Transf. 1990;7:94-7.
14. Akman MA, Erden HF, Tosun HB, et al. Comparison of agonistic flare up protocol and antagonistic multiple-dose protocol in ovarian stimulation of poor responders: result of prospective randomized trial. Hum Reprod. 2001;16:868-70.
15. Barri P. Management of poor responders. In Vitro Fertilization and Assisted Reproduction. 1997. pp. 265-73.
16. Barrenetxea G, Agirregoikoa JA, Jimenez MR, et al. Ovarian response and pregnancy outcome in poor responder women: a randomized controlled trial on the effect

of luteinizing hormone supplementation in in vitro fertilization cycles. Fertil Steril. 2008;89:546-53.

17. Fabregues F, Creus M, Penarrubia J, et al. Effects of recombinant human luteinizing hormone supplementation on ovarian stimulation and the implantation rate in down-regulated women of advanced reproductive age. Fertil Steril. 2006;85:925-31.

18. Hill MJ, Levy G, Levens ED. Does exogenous LH in ovarian stimulation improve assisted reproduction success? An appraisal of the literature. Reprod Biomed Online. 2012;24(3):261-71.

19. Levi DP, Navarro JM, Schattman GL, et al. The role of LH in ovarian stimulation. Exogenous LH: let's design the future. Hum Reprod. 2000;15(11):2258-65.

20. Humaidan P, Chin W, Rogoff D, et al. Efficacy and safety of follitropin alfa/lutropin alfa in ART: a randomized controlled trial in poor ovarian responders. Hum Reprod. 2017;32:544-55.

21. Faber BM, Mayer J, Cox B, et al. Cessation of gonadotropin-releasing hormone agonist therapy combined with high dose gonadotropin stimulation yields favorable pregnancy results in low responders. Fertil Steril. 1998;69:826-30.

22. Gracia-Valesco JA, Isaza V, Requena A, et al. High dose of gonadotropins combined with stop versus non-stop protocol if GnRH analogue administration in low responder IVF patients: a prospective, randomized, controlled trial. Hum Reprod. 2000;15:2292-6.

23. Olivennes F, Raghini C, Fanchin R, et al. A protocol using a low dose of GnRH agonist might be the best protocol for patient a with high FSH concentrations on day 3. Hum Reprod. 1996;11(6):1169-72.

24. Feldberg D, Farhi J, Ashkenazi J, et al. Minidose gonadotrophic-releasing hormone agonist is the treatment of choice in poor responders with high follicle-stimulating hormone levels. Fertil Steril. 1994;62:343-6.

25. Ubaldi FM, Capalbo A, Vaiarelli A, et al. Follicular versus luteal phase ovarian stimulation during the same menstrual cycle (DuoStim) in a reduced ovarian reserve population results in a similar euploid blastocyst formation rate: new insight in ovarian reserve exploitation. Fertil Steril. 2016;105(6):1488-95.

26. Deaton JL, Bauguess P, Huffman CS, et al. Pituitary response to early follicular-phase minidose gonadotrophic-releasing hormone agonist (GnRHa) therapy: evidence for a second flare. J Assist Reprod Genet. 1996;13:390-4.

27. Surrey ES, Bower J, Hill DM, et al. Clinical and endocrine effects of a microdose GnRH agonist flare regimen administered to poor responders who are undergoing in vitro fertilization. Fertil Steril. 1998;69:419-24.

28. Detti L, Williams DB, Robins JC, et al. A comparison of three downregulation approaches for poor responders undergoing in vitro fertilization. Fertil Steril. 2005;84:1401-5.

29. Demirol A, Gurgan T. Comparison of microdose flare-up and antagonist multiple-dose protocol for poor responder patients: a randomized study. Fertil Steril. 2009;92(2):481-5.

30. Schoolcraft WB, Surrey ES, Minjarez DA, et al. Management of poor responders: can outcomes be improved with novel gonadotropin-releasing hormone antagonist/letrozole protocol? Fertil Steril. 2008;89(1):151-6.

31. Cheung LP, Lam PM, Lok IH, et al. GnRH antagonist versus ling GnRH agonist protocol in poor responders undergoing IVF: a randomized controlled trial. Hum Reprod. 2005;20:616-21.

32. Nilsson L, Andersen AN, Lindenberg S, et al. Ganirelix for leuteolysis in poor responder patients undergoing IVF treatment: a Scandinavian multicenter 'extended pilot study'. Acta Obstet Gynecol Scand. 2010;89(6):828-31.

33. Dragisic KG, Davis OK, Fasouliotis SJ, et al. Use of a luteal estradiol patch and a gonadotrophic-releasing hormone antagonist suppression protocol before gonadotrophic stimulation for in vitro fertilization in poor responders. Fertil Steril. 2005;84:1023-6.

34. Shastri S, Schoyer K, Barbieri E, et al. Stimulation of the young poor responder: our experience with luteal estradiol/GnRH antagonist suppression versus a standard protocol. (LP microdose Lupron). Fertil Steril. 2008;90 Suppl.1:S32.

35. Chang EM, Han JE, Won HJ, et al. Effect of estrogen priming through luteal phase and stimulation phase in poor responders in in vitro fertilization. J Assist Reprod Genet. 2012;29(3):225-30.

36. Aghahosseini M, Aleyassin A, Khodaverdi A, et al. Estradiol supplementation during the luteal phase in poor responder patients undergoing in vitro fertilization: a randomized clinical trial. J Assist Reprod Genet. 2011;28(9):785-90.

37. D'Amato G, Caroppo E, Pasquadibisceglie A, et al. A novel protocol of ovulation induction with delayed gonadotrophic-releasing hormone antagonist administration combined with high-dose recombinant follicle-stimulating hormone and clomiphene citrate for poor responders and women over 35 years. Fertil Steril. 2004;81:1572-7.

38. Homburg R. Management of poor responders. Ovulation Induction and Controlled Ovarian Stimulation: A Practical Guide, 2nd edition. Switzerland: Springer International Publishing; 2014. pp. 159-68.

39. Schoolcraft W, Surrey E, Minjarez D, et al. Management of poor responders: can outcomes be improved with a novel GnRH antagonist/letrozole protocol? Fertil Steril. 2009;89:151-6.

40. Yaralli H, Esinler I, Polat M, et al. Antagonist/letrozole protocol in poor ovarian responders for intracytoplasmic sperm injection: a comparative study with the microdose flare up protocol. Fertil Steril. 2009;92(1):231-5.

41. Battalgia C, Salvatori M, Maxia N, et al. Adjuvant L-arginine treatment for in vitro fertilization in poor responder patients. Hum Reprod. 1999;14:1690-7.

42. Kolibianakis E, Venetis C, Diedrich K, et al. Addition of growth hormone to gonadotropins in ovarian stimulation of poor responders treated by in vitro fertilization: a systematic review and meta-analysis. Hum Reprod Update. 2009;15:613-22.

43. Keay SD, Lenton EA, Cooke ID, et al. Low dose dexamethasone augments the ovarian response to exogenous gonadotropins leading to a reduction in cycle cancellation rate in a standard IVF program. Hum Reprod. 2001;16:1861-5.

44. Barad G, Gleicher N. Effect of dehydroepiandrosterone on oocyte and embryo yields, embryo grade and cell number in IVF. Hum Reprod. 2006;21:2845-9.

45. Gliecher N, Weghofer A, Barad DH. Dehydroepiandrosterone (DHEA) reduces embryo aneuploidy: direct evidence from preimplantation genetic screening (PGS). Reprod Biol Endocrinol. 2010;10(8):140.

46. Kim CH, Howles CM, Lee HA. The effect of transdermal testosterone gel pre-treatment on controlled ovarian stimulation and IVF outcome in low responders. Fertil Steril. 2011;95(2):679-83.

47. Massim N, Cedrin-Durnerin S, Coussieu C, et al. Effects of transdermal testosterone application on ovarian response to FSH in poor responders undergoing assisted reproduction technique- a prospective randomized double-blind study. Hum Reprod. 2006;21:1204-11.

48. Fabregues F, Penarrubia J, Creus M, et al. Transdermal testosterone may improve ovarian response to gonadotropins in low-responder IVF patients: a randomized clinical trial. Hum Reprod. 2009;24:349-59.

49. Gibson DA, Simitsidellis I, Kelepouri O, et al. Dehydroepiandrosterone enhances decidualization in women of advanced reproductive age. Fertil Steril. 2018;109(4):728-34.

50. Mohsen IA, El Din RE. Minimal stimulation protocol using letrozole versus microdose flare-up GnRH agonist protocol in women with poor ovarian response undergoing ICSI. Gynecol Endocrinol. 2013;29(2):105-8.

51. Fraterelli JL, McWilliams GD, Hill MJ, et al. Low dose aspirin use does not improve in vitro fertilization outcomes in poor responders. Fertil Steril. 2008;89(5):1113-7.

52. Lambers MJ, Hoozzemans Da, Schats R, et al. Low dose aspirin in non-tubal IVF patients with previous failed conception: a prospective randomized double blind placebo-controlled trial. Fertil Steril. 2009;92:923-9.

53. Chung-hoon K, Hee-Dong C, Yoon-Seok C. Pyridostigmine cotreatment for controlled ovarian hyperstimulation in low responders undergoing in vitro fertilization–embryo transfer. Fertil Steril. 1999;71:652-7.

54. El-Toukhy T, Sunkara SK, Khairy M, et al. A systematic review and meta-analysis of acupuncture in in vitro fertilization. BJOG. 2008;115(10):1203-13.

11 Mild Stimulation in ART

Chaitanya Nagori

INTRODUCTION

It was the belief of assisted reproductive technology (ART) consultants that greater the number of eggs retrieved, pregnancy rate will be more. So larger doses of gonadotropins were used for several years after ART practice started and most commonly long protocol was used. But this protocol is expensive and takes longer duration for stimulation leading to more chances of ovarian hyperstimulation syndrome (OHSS) and multiple pregnancy.

Robert Edwards was the first person to advocate lower doses of gonadotropins i.e. milder stimulation, patient friendly, and safe approach in 1996. The balance between patient comfort, cost and live birth rate is very important and therefore this concept gradually became popular. The concept of natural cycle in vitro fertilization (IVF) or minimal stimulation is very common in Japan and USA and some parts of Europe.

There are three groups of patients who can be benefitted by mild IVF:
1. Patients with limited income particularly in developing countries.
2. Patients with low ovarian reserve.
3. Patients who do not want hormonal stimulation or cannot be given hormonal stimulation due to medical disorders.

In group 1, tubal infections are common in lower socioeconomic class in developing countries and the only option left to them for fertility is ART. Natural cycle IVF is affordable to them. In group 2, eggs can be retrieved and collected over several cycles with mild stimulation and are cryopreserved. In these patients with advanced age preimplantation genetic screening (PGS) can be done or single embryo transfer can be done later on.

International Society of Mild Approaches in Assisted Reproduction (ISMAAR) defines mild IVF cycle, either as:
- Gonadotropins are administered at lower dose and/or shorter duration throughout the cycle in which gonadotropin-releasing hormone (GnRh) antagonist is given as cotreatment, or
- Stimulation with oral compounds, either alone or in combination with gonadotropins and GnRh antagonist.[1]

Ovulation induction and luteal support are the part of this protocol where the aim is to collect between 2–7 eggs.[2]

VARIOUS PROTOCOLS

Natural Cycle In Vitro Fertilization

In natural cycle IVF, results are very poor, especially in older patients.[3] Pregnancy rate of approximately 7% is quoted in several papers.[4] About 4–11 natural cycles produce same live birth rate as one conventional cycle. It is frustrating for the patient to accept negative results for several cycles. Therefore, it is not a preferred protocol.

Natural cycles are patient friendly, cheap and safe, and no drugs are used but premature luteinizing hormone (LH) surge is very common. This may lead to cancellation of cycles in up to 20%. In many oocyte retrievals, one may not get a single ovum.

Though some authors have quoted that natural cycle IVF in poor responders is as effective as controlled ovarian hyperstimulation (COH) in terms of pregnancy rate and implantation rate with lower expense and better compliance.[5] Pregnancy rate per cycle and per transfer was 10% and 16–18%, respectively according to these studies. This has been proved also in meta-analysis by Daya S et al.[6] This natural cycle IVF can be used for patients with breast cancer, kidney transplant, liver transplant, and thrombophilia.

Modified Natural Cycle

Initial reports of modified natural cycle using mild stimulation and GnRh antagonist has also given disappointing results. In this protocol, GnRh antagonist is started when size of the lead follicle is 14 mm and at the same time gonadotropin (75–300 IU) is also started. It reduces the cycle cancellation as it prevents LH surge. Here endogenous FSH rise is taken as advantage. Ovulation trigger is done by 10,000 IU hCG or recombinant hCG (rhCG) 250 μg. The pregnancy rate was 8.3%.[7] So the results are disappointing in spite of safe and patient friendly protocol and results are not significantly different from those of natural cycle. Modified natural cycle is used in poor responders and advanced age patients.

Delayed Low Dose FSH with Antagonist (Mild IVF Cycle)

According to this protocol, FSH stimulation is started on day 5–7 in a dose of 150 IU. Antagonist is given for prevention of LH surge, along with endogenous FSH in this protocol, but multiple pregnancy rate is not reduced,[5] therefore single embryo transfer is preferred. Cumulative pregnancy rate for 12 months and standard protocols are the same.[5] The quality of the egg is superior and implantation rate is better as compared to long protocol. Because E2 level is low, the detrimental effect on endometrium, oocyte and embryo is not observed. It is less expensive and gives similar pregnancy rate.

Clomiphene Combined with Gonadotropins

In this protocol, clomiphene citrate (CC) is given in early phase of the cycle and then combined with gonadotropins. This decreases the requirement of gonadotropins and also the risk of OHSS. The results are similar to the conventional antagonist protocol.[8] If CC is given before day 6 of the cycle, it helps in ovulation induction, but has a negative effect on the endometrium.[9] Instead if it is given after 6 days of menstrual cycle, it has inhibitory effect on LH surge and ovulation and probably no effect on endometrium. Therefore in premature LH surge, if CC is given around the time of ovulation, it can improve the quality of oocytes and maturation. In these cases CC is given from day 7. Agonist trigger is preferred in these cycles to prevent functional ovarian cysts. It does not cause luteal phase defect in natural cycles and corpus luteum is adequately functional to support the luteal phase. CC being antiestrogenic does not allow positive feedback of estrogen to release LH and so there is no progesterone surge.[10]

Aromatase Inhibitors with Gonadotropins

Aromatase inhibitors have a dual property. These chemicals prevent androgen to estrogen conversion by aromatization, leading to low estrogen that is beneficial for endogenous FSH production. Increased androgen level sensitizes the preantral and antral follicles to FSH. Letrozole 2.5–5 mg with gonadotropins give promising results. It keeps estrogen close to physiological range and that improves implantation rate. Letrozole increases integrin expression and improves endometrial receptivity.

Low Dose Gonadotropins

In poor responder women, there is a fair evidence that clinical pregnancy rate after IVF are not different when compared to mild stimulation protocol, when using low dose gonadotropin protocol (≤150 IU/day) to conventional gonadotropin protocol.[11]

MILD VERSUS CONVENTIONAL PROTOCOL

- Dose requirement in mild protocol is less and so the cost is low and less monitoring is required.
- In mild stimulation, lesser number of follicles are produced (<8) and this gives better implantation rate.[12]
- Endometrial receptivity is high because of lower estradiol (E2) in mild protocol. Otherwise high E2 alters uterine relaxing property of progesterone and prevents implantation.

- Abnormal and mosaic embryos are more common with conventional protocol. This is because of increased meiotic segregation errors in early embryonic cleavage division.[13] Therefore aneuploidy rate is higher with conventional protocol.
- Twin pregnancy rate is very low with mild stimulation.
- Incidence of OHSS is low with mild stimulation.
- Mild stimulation is more patient friendly.
- In poor responders, natural cycle IVF or mild stimulation has an advantage.

DISADVANTAGES OF MILD STIMULATION

- It may give mono or bifollicular development in 15–20% of patients that may lead to cycle cancellation and gives lower pregnancy rate.
- Less embryos available for cryopreservation.
- In some cases as LH is suppressed the pregnancy rates are low. In these cases hCG or human menopausal gonadotropin (HMG) or recombinant LH (rLH) is to be added.[14]
- Lower pregnancy rate can cause psychological problem.

REFERENCES

1. Schipper I, Hop WC, Fauser BC. The follicle stimulating hormone (FSH) threshold/window concept examined by different inventions with exogenous FSH during the follicular phase of the normal menstrual cycle: duration, rather than magnitude, of FSH increase affects follicle development. J Clin Endcrinol Metab. 1998;83:1292-98.
2. Nargund G, Fauser BC, Macklon NS, et al. Rotterdam ISMAAR Consensus group on terminology for ovarian stimulation for IVF. Hum Reprod. 2007;22:2801-4.

3. Verberg MFG, Macklon NS, Nargund G, et al. Mild ovarian stimulation for IVF. Hum Reprod Update. 2009;15:13-29.

4. Pelinck MJ, Hoek A, Simons AH, et al. Efficacy of natural cycle IVF: a review of the literature. Hum Reprod Update. 2002;8:129-39.

5. Heijen EM, Eijkemans MJ, De Klerk C, et al. A mild treatment strategy for in vitro fertilization: a randomized no-inferiority trial. Lancet. 2007;369:743-9.

6. Daya S, Gunby J, Hughes EG, et al. Natural cycles for in vitro fertilization: cost effectiveness analysis and factors influencing outcome. Hum Reprod. 1995;10:1719-24.

7. Pelinck MJ, Vogel NE, Hoek A, et al. Cumulative pregnancy rates after three cycles of minimal stimulation IVF and results according to subfertility diagnosis: a multicenter cohort study. Hum Reprod. 2006;21:2375-83.

8. Gibreel A, Maheshwari A, Bhattacharya S. Clomiphene citrate in combination with gonadotropins for controlled ovarian stimulation in women undergoing in vitro fertilization. Cochrane Database Syst Rev. 2012;(11):CD 008528.

9. Wallace KL, Johnson V, Sopelak V, et al. Clomiphene citrate versus letrozole: molecular analysis of the endometrium in women with polycystic ovarian syndrome. Fertil Steril. 2011;96(4):1051-6.

10. Teramoto S, Kato O. Minimal ovarian stimulation with clomiphene citrate: a large scale retrospective study. Reprod Biomed Online. 2007;15(2):134-48.

11. Youssef MA, van Wely M, Al-Inany H, et al. A mild ovarian stimulation strategy in women with poor ovarian reserve undergoing IVF: a multicenter randomized controlled trial. Hum Reprod. 2005;20:611-5.

12. Verberg MFG, Eijkemans MJC, Maklon NS, et al. The clinical significance of the retrieval of a low number of oocytes following mild ovarian stimulation for IVF: a meta-analysis. Hum Reprod Update. 2009;15:5-12.

13. Baart EB, Martini E, Eijkemans MJ, et al. Milder ovarian stimulation for in-vitro fertilization reduces aneuploidy in human pre-implantation embryo: a randomized controlled trial. Hum Reprod. 2007;22(4):980-8.

14. Takahashi K, Mukaida T, Tomiyama T, et al. GnRH antagonist improved blastocyst quality and pregnancy outcome after multiple failures of IVF/ICSI-ET with a GnRH agonist protocol. J Assist Reprod Genet. 2004;21(9):317-22.

Ovulation Trigger

Chaitanya Nagori

INTRODUCTION

Appropriate timing, adequate duration and adequate amplitude of midcycle surge are the prerequisites for human female fertility. This midcycle follicle-stimulating hormone (FSH) and luteinizing hormone (LH) surge causes ovulation. In human being, only LH surge can cause ovulation but in animals both FSH and LH surge are mandatory to induce ovulation. The role of FSH surge in human has not been adequately understood till date.

FUNCTIONS OF LUTEINIZING HORMONE SURGE

Functions of LH surge are:
- It induces mucinification of cumulus oophorus allowing oocyte release.
- It provokes the resumption of oocyte meiosis, which is arrested at prophase of first meiotic division and is converted to metaphase II. This is essential for fertilization.
- Luteinizing hormone surge triggers follicular rupture. It induces shift from estradiol secretion to progesterone secretion from granulosa cells.
- LH surge upregulates growth factors like vascular endothelial growth factor (VEGF) and fibroblast growth factor. It stimulates cytokines involved in implantation.

Midcycle surge is governed by gonadotropin-releasing hormone (GnRH), estrogen, progesterone and peptide hormones like gonadotropin surge attenuating factor. Mural granulosa cells have LH receptors. LH stimulates epidermal growth factor in granulosa cells. These then act on cumulus cells that trigger oocyte maturation.

NATURAL LUTEINIZING HORMONE SURGE

Oocytes before LH surge are arrested at the prophase of the first meiotic division. LH surge reinitiates the arrested meiosis and triggers ovulation. Normal midcycle LH surge lasts for 48.7 ± 9.3 hours.[1]

Luteinizing hormone surge has three phases:
1. Rapid ascending phase—14 hours
2. Peak plateau—14 hours
3. Long descending phase—20 hours.

Luteinizing hormone surge is greater than FSH surge. The LH level reaches 10–20 times higher than the basal LH level. The mean peak value is 46 ± 16 IU/L. LH pulse frequency remains the same as in the early proliferative phase but the amplitude is high. Though the duration and amplitude of LH are different in different individuals. The sudden endogenous LH surge is due to positive feedback mechanism to high estrogen level, i.e. 150 pg/mL/follicle. The increased amplitude of LH and FSH pulse is thought to be facilitated by positive feedback of estrogen on kisspeptin neurons in anteroventral periventricular nuclei of the hypothalamus and upregulation of GnRH receptors in anterior pituitary. The serum progesterone starts rising after 12 hours of LH surge and plateaus up to ovulation and once again starts rising after ovulation. Ovulation occurs after 36 hours of onset of LH surge. So, progesterone increases in two steps. Same way androstenedione and testosterone surge also occur twice and four times respectively at the time of LH surge.[1]

Seibel et al. found that oocyte starts maturing after 18 hours of onset of LH surge and majority of oocytes retrieved after 25 hours reach meiosis after injection of human chorionic gonadotropin (hCG).[2] So, the threshold level of resumption of meiosis is 14–18 hours and to obtain the oocytes with metaphase II after aspiration, requires at least 28 hours after onset of the surge.

The threshold amplitude of LH surge for oocyte maturation is quite low. Only 5% of LH peak concentration is required for meiosis and sufficient luteinization. The rest is required for triggering ovulation.[3] This means that actually in assisted reproductive technology (ART) because ovum pick-up is done, very low dose of LH instead of 10,000 hCG may suffice. This will drastically reduce the incidence of ovarian hyperstimulation syndrome (OHSS), but no actual study data is available on ART with low-dose LH or hCG.

SEQUENCE OF HORMONAL EVENTS AT MIDCYCLE

1. Onset of LH and FSH surge occurs abruptly.
2. It is associated with estrogen peak.
3. It occurs 12 hours after the estrogen peak.
4. Duration of FSH and LH surge is 48 hours.
5. LH surge has ascending limb lasting for 14 hours and is associated with rise in progesterone and decline in estradiol.
6. Then it has a plateau of 14 hours.
7. Descending limb lasts for 20 hours associated with progesterone rise. This is after 36 hours of onset of FSH and LH surge.
8. The level of LH, 100 IU and FSH, 25–30 IU is considered normal.

INDICATIONS OF SURROGATE LUTEINIZING HORMONE SURGE

- Hypogonadotropic hypogonadism (WHO I)
- Hypothalamic-pituitary dysfunction (WHO II).

Here correct timing and amplitude of LH surge is absent after FSH induced follicular growth.[4] Multiple follicular development prevents LH surge in stimulated cycles. It is said that gonadotropin surge inhibiting factor, inhibin and other nonsteroidal factors prevent FSH and LH surge which is otherwise induced by estrogen. GnRH analog can counter this surge.[5]

- Pretreatment with GnRH agonist (GnRHa) prevents LH surge and so surrogate LH surge is required.
- In patients undergoing intrauterine insemination (IUI), it is required to time

IUI. Moreover, it lasts for 2 days giving better pregnancy rate. Routine use of hCG, i.e. surrogate LH surge is not found beneficial unless some intervention is to be done like IUI.[6,7]

OVULATION TRIGGER

Ovulation trigger can be given by:
1. Human chorionic gonadotropin
2. Gonadotropin-releasing hormone agonist
3. Recombinant LH.

Human Chorionic Gonadotropin Surge

Characteristics of Human Chorionic Gonadotropin Surge

- It has two to four times more binding affinity than LH.
- It has a biological half-life of more than 24 hours as compared 60 minutes for endogenous LH. This is so because beta-subunit of hCG is highly glycosylated and has a longer half-life.
- It stimulates the secretion of VEGF, which causes OHSS.
- Subcutaneous or intramuscular routes have same serum levels and same pregnancy rates.[8]
- Human chorionic gonadotropin is used for ovulation trigger since about 30 years. It activates the same receptors as of LH on corpus luteum.
- Bioavailability is less in obese women after giving hCG and so for obese women 10,000 IU is the standard dose for trigger instead of 5,000 IU.
- No difference in oocyte yield is found with 5,000 IU or 10,000 IU of hCG.[9]
- Delayed hCG administration in agonist or antagonist cycle, gives poor pregnancy rate according to some studies but others have similar results.

Indications of Human Chorionic Gonadotropin

- *Gonadotropin therapy*: Endogenous FSH and LH surge is attenuated in women treated with exogenous gonadotropins in spite of high estradiol levels. So, exogenous hCG is required for final maturation.[10,11]
- To plan IUI at a particular time.
- WHO group I where only hCG can be used.
- Agonist cycle in ART.

Advantages

When hCG is used, it causes high levels of estradiol and progesterone and leads to normal luteal phase. The effect of hCG lasts for 5–8 days. So, it initiates and maintains progesterone production more efficiently than natural LH surge and there are less chances of luteal phase defects (LPDs).

Side Effects

- Because of longer half-life, hCG results in sustained luteotropic effect, development of multiple corpora lutea with very high estradiol and progesterone levels compared to spontaneous cycles. These high levels of estradiol and progesterone are detrimental for implantation. Because of multiple corpora lutea, there is supraphysiological level of progesterone in early luteal phase. Progesterone level reaches peak about 3 days after the oocyte collection. While in natural cycle, progesterone reaches to peak in midluteal phase. So, the high progesterone on 3 days after ovum pick-up may be detrimental for implantation. This explains why frozen embryo transfer gives better results.
- Human chorionic gonadotropin trigger over stimulates corpora lutea and produces more estradiol that decreases endogenous LH and this can cause luteal phase defect.[12,13]

- Multiple follicular rupture causes multiple pregnancies.
- Sustained effect of hCG causes OHSS in patients having excessive response to gonadotropins. hCG stimulates VEGF which is the direct cause of OHSS.[14]
- But it is very frustrating to withhold hCG to avoid OHSS and multiple pregnancy and will be waste of time and money as well as number of cancelled cycles will be in high proportion.
- Human chorionic gonadotropin rise after subcutaneous injection is slower than intramuscular injection and slower than GnRHa trigger.

Therefore, in cases with high chance of OHSS, GnRHa is given as ovulation trigger, instead of hCG in antagonist cycle.

Recombinant Human Chorionic Gonadotropin

- It has a structure similar to that of hCG.
- Absorption, distribution and metabolism are the same like hCG.
- It is in a pure form and is theoretically safe.
- Maximum concentration is reached within 12–24 hours and biological half-life is 38 hours.
- Efficacy and safety is same according to the Cochrane review.[15]
- No difference in OHSS rate.
- Efficacy of recombinant hCG (rhCG) is similar to urinary hCG (uhCG) clinically.
- Adverse reactions are not documented.
- The accepted dose of uhCG is 5,000–10,000 IU. The rhCG dose is 250 µg that has the same activity as that of 6,500 IU of uhCG. rhCG has no allergic reaction and there is no failure of ovulation. It has ease of administration for patients and improved efficacy for ovulation and luteal phase support.

Gonadotropin-Releasing Hormone Agonist

Characteristics

- It produces LH surge as efficiently as hCG for oocyte maturation and this was first suggested by Itskovitz in 1988.[16]
- It produces FSH surge also with LH surge, in contrast to hCG, but role of FSH surge has not been established in humans. It has already been established in rats.[17] Both the surges are higher than with hCG surge.
- There is no difference in oocyte maturation and ovulation.
- LH surge due to GnRHa is 24–36 hours as compared to natural surge, which is 48 hours in length, and hCG surge is for 6 days.
- It has only two phases. It has a short ascending limb of more than 4 hours and long descending limb of greater than 20 hours.[18]
- The initial rise is because of flare-up. It leads to LH surge with high peak value and shorter duration than natural LH and hCG.
- Multiple doses do not prolong surge.
- The inhibition of surge is due to gonadotropin surge attenuating factor and inhibin that is induced by estradiol and this inhibition is replaced by GnRHa.
- It can induce LH surge in antagonist cycle indicating that pituitary response to GnRHa is preserved.[19]
- Vascular endothelial growth factor and other substances like angiopoietin 2 (destabilizing factor) are significantly decreased in follicular fluid after GnRHa trigger. This plays major role in decreasing OHSS.[20] GnRHa trigger increases antiestrogenic factors and helps in decreasing the risk of OHSS.

Advantages

- Estradiol and progesterone levels are lower but that can be managed by replacement.

Instead if the levels are supraphysiological, these are detrimental for implantation.[12,13]

- Short duration of surge of 24–36 hours is more physiological and only few follicles are converted into corpus luteum.[21]
- It reduces the risk of OHSS because of complete luteolysis[22] and decreased expression of VEGF.
- Pituitary response to GnRHa is preserved even in antagonist cycle. OHSS-free clinics concept use antagonist to prevent premature LH surge with agonist trigger.[23] Here GnRHa replaces antagonist and gives flare-up effect and releases FSH and LH from pituitary.
- For donors, it is the best accepted protocol.
- As it causes FSH surge. FSH surge promotes formation of LH receptors in luteinizing granulosa cells, nuclear maturation and cumulus expansion.[24] It is useful in luteinized unruptured follicle (LUF).
- More MII oocytes are recovered with GnRHa than hCG trigger according to some studies.[25,26] But other studies do not find difference.

Disadvantages

Gonadotropin-releasing hormone agonist trigger causes direct pituitary downregulation resulting in reduced levels of LH, insufficient to sustain adequate corpus luteal activity. This will lead to reduced luteal phase progesterone level that will not allow optimum implantation.[27] It causes short luteal phase and LPD in all cases because of short duration of LH surge. This shorter duration of LH cannot rescue luteal function because of reduced amount of FSH and LH. The same amount can complete meiosis. Serum LH is less than 2 IU/mL after 4 days. So, it is not the direct effect on corpus luteum. Withdrawal of LH for ≥ 3 days causes luteolysis and so corpus luteal viability can be preserved only for 3 days without LH support.

- Even with luteal supplementation, 25% will still have luteal insufficiency.
- Minimum 600 mg progesterone/day is required which adds the cost in IUI cycles.
- Cannot be used in WHO group I patients.
- Cannot be used in downregulated patients.
- It has lower circulatory estradiol and progesterone in luteal phase than hCG.
- More MII oocytes are recovered with GnRHa than hCG trigger.
- There is a reduced live birth rate and ongoing pregnancy rate with GnRHa trigger than hCG trigger in antagonist protocol in spite of progesterone support[28] in some studies lower implantation rate due to lower oocyte maturation and reduced oocyte and embryo competence is documented.
- Inadequate response:
  - There is suboptimal response after trigger with GnRHa trigger in patients having basal level of LH less than 1–2.2 IU/mL.[29]
  - When LH less than 15 IU/mL after 10–12 hours of the trigger with GnRHa this is suboptimal response. The lower LH on the day of trigger also gives suboptimal response. This is common when progesterone is used to prevent LH surge. Adding 1,000–1,500 IU of hCG is very useful.[29] Dual trigger with trigger doses up to 5,000 IU does not improve the results.
  - Patients with higher body mass index (BMI) give suboptimal response whereas lower BMI less than 22 kg/m^2 also give poor response.
  - When progesterone level is less than 3.5 ng/mL, the response of GnRHa is inadequate. Progesterone level should be between 5 and 10 ng/mL (3,800 IU).
  - High total dosage of gonadotropin can give inadequate response. This

inadequate response is because of hypothalamic failure.

Contraindications of GnRHa Trigger

- *Hypothalamic dysfunction*: In these patients in spite of GnRHa trigger, endogenous surge is absent or very low. So, oocyte maturation does not occur. So, these are not the good candidates for GnRHa trigger.
- Women who have long-term suppression of hypothalamus and pituitary may have failed or may have suboptimal response because they may not be able to mount an optimal LH surge after GnRHa trigger.[30]
- Patients having low FSH and LH basal levels.
- Low LH on the day of trigger.
- Long-term oral contraceptions.[30]

How to Treat Luteal Phase Defect?

- Progesterone and/or estradiol replacement can be done. Luteal phase support with vaginal progesterone 600 mg/day and oral estradiol 4 mg/day has given poor results. Only progesterone vaginal or intramuscular without estrogen has also given poor results. Pregnancy rate is 7.9% compared to 30% with hCG.[31] Serum progesterone level greater than 20 ng/mL and E2 greater than 200 pg/mL should be maintained.[32] Intramuscular progesterone 50 mg with estradiol 6 mg is given for 10 weeks.
- Humaidan's group administered 1,500 IU of hCG on the day of oocyte retrieval after agonist trigger.[26] It has given equivalent pregnancy rate as hCG trigger and decreases pregnancy loss. In this study, no case of OHSS occurred when follicles were less than 25 in number of 11 mm size. This idea came with observation that if E2 greater than 4,000 IU pregnancy rates are

high with agonist trigger and here the LH is high on the day of the trigger. This high LH may rescue few corpus lutea and improve implantation. But if E2 is less than 4,000 IU, there may be benefit with 1,000–1,500 IU of hCG without OHSS.

- Even in normal responders freeze all policy and transfer in the next cycle is also acceptable[33] but pregnancy rates are the same.
- Freeze all is the policy for suspected OHSS cases but occasional patients including oocyte donors may get OHSS due to mutation in FSH, LH or GnRH receptors.[26]
- Garcia-Velasco has report 50% pregnancy rate in patients of high-risk OHSS, when after freezing, embryos were transferred in next cycle.[33,34]

Indications of GnRHa Trigger

- Polycystic ovarian syndrome (PCOS) patients, when multiple follicles develop.
- In ART cycles where agonists are not used for downregulation.
- Those who do not want a fresh embryo transfer.
- Fertility preservation.
- For those who want preimplantation genetic screening (PGS)/PGF as this automatically means frozen transfer.
- Prematurely elevated progesterone level.
- Oocyte donors.
- Risk of OHSS.

Dosage

There are various regimens:

1. Single subcutaneous injection 500–1,000 μg of luprolide acetate.
2. Two injections 12 hours apart of 500–1,000 μg of luprolide acetate.
3. Intranasal buserelin 50–200 pgm. Triptorelin 0.2 mg. It is found that higher

doses do not improve number and quality of oocytes.[34] Unfortunately which compound, which dose and when to give is not standardized.

Recombinant Luteinizing Hormone

- The biological half-life is 1 hour and terminal half-life is 10–12 hours which is quite low than hCG which is 5 hours and 30 hours respectively.
- Recombinant human LH (rhLH) of 2,500–5,000 IU can induce adequate follicular maturation, corpus luteal formation and pregnancy without development of OHSS. It more closely mimics natural LH surge than hCG.[35]
- Implantation rate is significantly higher than hCG because of better quality of embryos.
- It is extremely costly and ampoules of 75 IU only are available. Whereas the dose required for trigger is 15,000 IU (750 µg)–30,000 IU (1,500 µg).

Recent Advances

- *Orally active analog of LH*: Low molecular weight (LMW)—LH agonist has similar mode of action but shorter half-life than hCG. It abolishes the possibility of OHSS as it has no action on vascular changes and does not induce production of VEGF.[36]
- *Dual trigger (Flowchart 12.1)*:
  - FSH + hCG: Adding 450 IU of FSH along with 10,000 hCG trigger improved fertilization rate. But there was no statistical difference in critical pregnancy rate with controls.[37] The idea is to have FSH surge along with LH surge.
  - Agonist + hCG: In the study of high risk of OHSS patients, 4 mg of leuprolide acetate and hCG (1,000–2,500 IU) gave the pregnancy rate of 53%.[38] hCG in dual trigger helps in meiosis of follicles but granulosa cells are refractory during this period and so it does not help in luteal support. It may cause OHSS.

With routine use of 5,000 IU of hCG, 0.2 mg of decapeptyl was given. The pregnancy rate was 36% as compared to hCG alone which had only 22%.[29]

The benefit of LH surge is that it promotes LH receptor formation in luteinizing granulosa cells, resumption of meiosis and cumulus

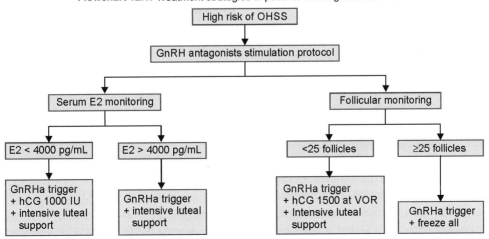

Flowchart 12.1: Treatment strategies in patients with high risk of OHSS.

expansion. The oocyte yield is always better with FSH and LH dual surge than only hCG. It is observed that when LH surge is less than 15 mIU/mL are likely to have lower oocyte retrieval rate and poor cycle outcome. Lower LH level on the day of trigger also is a risk factor for suboptimal response. Adding 1,000 IU of hCG with agonist, i.e. dual trigger in high responders with E2 less than 4,000 pg/mL improves live birth rate without OHSS. But if E2 greater than 4,000 IU, only estrogen with progesterone are given to support the luteal phase.[39]

Along with age, false trigger and poor ovarian reserve, suboptimal response to GnRHa may be the cause of empty follicle syndrome.

So suboptimal responders are those, in whom serum LH is less than 15 mIU/mL approximately 10 hours after GnRHa trigger. Suboptimal responders have higher BMI and lower basal FSH and LH levels (<2.27 mIU/mL).[29] Dual trigger for final oocyte maturation improves oocyte retrieval rate of suboptimal responders to GnRHa.[40]

Suboptimal response is detected when there are no eggs retrieved after puncturing many follicles. This is due to hypothalamic cause, when LH level is low. Here we can give hCG trigger and can get good results in terms of ova and pregnancy rate. This is common in patients having low BMI (22 kg/m^2) and baseline LH less than 1 mIU/mL and higher dose of gonadotropins. Whenever there is a failed trigger, LH level is less than 15 mIU/mL and progesterone less than 3.5 ng/mL, 8–12 hours after trigger. It is found that appropriate elevated post trigger progesterone concentration with low LH can still result in successful oocyte retrieval but low progesterone with normal LH concentration greater than 15 mIU/mL might suggest an inadequate response. There is no effect of long-term oral contraceptive (OC) pills for this effect.[41]

- Low-dose hCG 125 IU from day 2 or 6 daily up to throughout luteal phase has given good results.[42]

CARRY HOME MESSAGE

- Luteinizing hormone surge is mandatory for ovulation.
- Follicle-stimulating hormone surge is useful but its role is not understood.
- Human chorionic gonadotropin surge is required in controlled ovarian hyperstimulation (COH) and IUI cycles.
- In IVF, because of risk of OHSS, hCG is not favored.
- Human chorionic gonadotropin surge does not required luteal support.
- Gonadotropin-releasing hormone agonist as ovulation trigger avoids OHSS.
- It causes LPD that requires judicious luteal support.
- 1,500 IU of hCG can rescue corpus luteum in agonist trigger when given at the time of pick up or IUI.
- Recombinant LH for trigger is very costly.
- Dual trigger with agonist and hCG is beneficial.

REFERENCES

1. Hoff JD, Quigley ME, Yen SS. Hormonal dynamics at midcycle: a reevaluation. J Clin Endocrinol Metab. 1983;57:792-6.
2. Seibel MM, Smith DM, Levesque L, et al. The temporal relationship between the luteinizing hormone surge and human oocyte maturation. Am J Obstet Gynecol. 1982;142:568-72.
3. Peluso JJ. Role of amplitude of gonadotropin surge in the rat. Fertil Steril. 1990;53:150-4.
4. Seibel MM, Kamrava MM, McArdle C, et al. Treatment of polycystic ovary disease with chronic low dose follicle stimulating hormone. Biochemical changes and ultrasound correlation. Int J Fertil. 1984;29:39-43.

5. Kol S, Lewit N, Itskovitz J. Ovarian hyper-stimulation: effects of GnRH analogues. Ovarian hyperstimulation syndrome after using gonadotropin-releasing hormone analogue as a trigger of ovulation: causes and implications. Hum Reprod. 1996;11(6):1143-4.

6. Clark L, Stranger J, Brinsmead M. Prolonged follicle stimulation decreases pregnancy rates after in vitro fertilization. Fertil Steril. 1991;55:1192-4.

7. Tan SL, Balen A, el Hussein E, et al. A prospective randomized study of the optimum timing of human chorionic gonadotropin administration after pituitary desensitization in in vitro fertilization. Fertil Steril. 1992;57:1259-64.

8. Elkind-Hirsch KE, Bello S, Esparcia L, et al. Serum human gonadotropin levels are correlated with body mass index rather than route of administration in women undergoing in vitro fertilization-embryo transfer using human menopausal gonadotropin and intracytoplasmic sperm injection. Fertil Steril. 2001;75:700-4.

9. Shaltout AM, Eid MS, Shohayeb AA. Does triggering ovulation by 5000 iu of hCG affect ICSI outcome? Middle East Fertil Soc J. 2006;11:99-103.

10. Ferrareti AP, Garcia JE, Acosta AA, et al. Serum luteinizing hormone during ovulation induction with human menopausal gonadotropin for in vitro fertilization in normally menstruating women. Fertil Steril. 1983;40:743-7.

11. Schenken RS, Hodgen GD. Follicle-stimulating hormone induced ovarian hyperstimulation in monkeys: blockage of luteinizing hormone surge. J Clin Endocrinol Metab. 1983;57:50-5.

12. Gidley-Baird AA, O'Neill C, Sinosich MJ, et al. Failure of implantation in human in vitro fertilization and embryo transfer patients: the effects of altered progesterone/estrogen ratios in human and mice. Fertil Steril. 1986;45:69-74.

13. Forman R, Fries N, Testart J, et al. Evidence for an adverse effect of elevated serum estradiol concentrations on embryo implantation. Fertil Steril. 1988;49:118-22.

14. Christenson LK, Stouffer RL. Follicle-stimulating hormone and luteinizing hormone/chorionic gonadotropin stimulation of vascular endothelial growth factor production by macaque granulosa cells from pre- and periovulatory follicles. J Clin Endocrinol Metab. 1997;82:2135-42.

15. Youssef MA, Al-Inany HG, Aboulghar M, et al. Recombinant versus urinary human chorionic gonadotrophin for final oocyte maturation triggering in IVF and ICSI cycles. Cochrane Database Syst Rev. 2011;(4):CD003719.

16. Itskovitz J, Boldes R, Barlev A, et al. The induction of LH surge and oocyte maturation by GnRH analogue (buserelin) in women undergoing ovarian stimulation for in vitro fertilization. Gynecol Endocrinol. 1988;2(Suppl 1):165.

17. Moor RM, Osborn JC, Cran OG, et al. Selective effect of gonadotropins on cell coupling, nuclear maturation oocytes. Embryol Exp Morphol. 1981;61:347-65.

18. Scheele F, van der Meer M, Lambalk CB, et al. Exploring the recovery phase after treatment with gonadotropin-releasing hormone agonist. Gynecol Reprod Biol. 1995;62(2):221-4.

19. Olivennes F, Fanchin R, Bouchard P, et al. Triggering of ovulation by gonadotropin-releasing hormone agonist in patients pre-treated with GnRH antagonist. Fertil Steril. 1996;66(1):151-3.

20. Cerrillo M, Rodriguez S, Mayoral M, et al. Differential regulation of VEGF after final oocyte maturation with GnRH agonist versus hCG. A rationale for OHSS reduction. Fertil Steril. 2009;91(4 Suppl):1526-8.

21. Emperaire J, Ruffie A. triggering ovulation with endogenous luteinizing hormone may prevent the ovarian hyperstimulation syndrome. Hum Reprod. 1991;6:506-10.

22. Monroe SE, Henzl MR, Martin MC, et al. Ablation of folliculogenesis in women by a single dose of gonadotropin-releasing hormone agonist: significance of time in cycle. Fertil Steril. 1985;43:361-8.

23. Albano C, Smitz J, Camus M. Comparison of different doses of gonadotropin-releasing

hormone antagonist Cetrorelix during controlled ovarian hyperstimulation. Fertil Steril. 1997;67:917-22.

24. Zelinski-Wooten MB, Hutchison JS, Hess DL, et al. Follicle-stimulating hormone alone supports follicle growth and oocyte development in gonadotropin-releasing hormone antagonist-treated monkeys. Hum Reprod. 1995;10(7):1658-66.

25. Humaidan P, Bungum L, Bungum M, et al. Reproductive outcome using a GnRH antagonist (cetrorelix) for luteolysis and follicular synchronization in poor responder IVF/ICSI patients treated with a flexible GnRH antagonist protocol. Reprod Biomed Online. 2005;11(6):679-84.

26. Humaidan P, Ejdrup Bredkjaer H, Westergaard LG, et al. 1,500 IU human chorionic gonadotropin administered at oocyte retrieval rescues the luteal phase when gonadotropin-releasing hormone agonist is used for ovulation induction: a prospective, randomized, controlled study. Fertil Steril. 2010;93:847-54.

27. Yding Anderson C, Vilbour Anderson K. Improving luteal phase after ovarian stimulation reviewing new options. Reprod Biomed Online. 2014;28:552-9.

28. Humaidan P, Papanikolaou EG, Kyrou D, et al. The luteal phase after GnRH-agonist triggering of ovulation: present and future perspectives. Reprod Biomed Online. 2012;24:134-41.

29. Lu X, Hong Q, Sun L, et al. Dual trigger for final oocyte maturation improves the oocyte retrieval rate of suboptimal responders to gonadotropin-releasing hormone agonist. Fertil Steril. 2016;106:1356-62.

30. Meyer L, Murphy LA, Gumer A, et al. Risk factors for a suboptimal response to gonadotropin-releasing hormone agonist trigger during in-vitro fertilization cycles. Fertil Steril. 2015;104(3):637-42.

31. Griesinger G, Diedrich K, Devroey P, et al. GnRH agonist for triggering final oocyte maturation in the GnRH antagonist ovarian hyperstimulation protocol: a systematic review and meta-analysis. Hum Reprod Update. 2006:12(2):159-68.

32. Engmann L, DiLuigi A, Schmidt D, et al. The use of gonadotropin releasing hormone (GnRH) agonist to induce oocyte maturation after cotreatment with GnRH antagonist in high-risk patients undergoing in-vitro fertilization prevents the risk of ovarian hyperstimulation syndrome: a prospective randomized controlled study. Fertil Steril. 2008;89(1):84-91.

33. Aflatoonian A, Oskouian H, Ahmadi S, et al. Can fresh embryo transfers be replaced by cryopreserved-thawed embryo transfers in assisted reproductive cycles? A randomized controlled trial. J Assist Reprod Genet. 2010;27:357-63.

34. Garcia-Velasco JA. Agonist trigger: what is the best approach? Agonist trigger with vitrification of oocytes or embryos. Fertil Steril. 2012;97(3):527-8.

35. Vuong TN, Ho MT, Ha TD, et al. Gonadotropin-releasing hormone agonist trigger in oocyte donors co-related with a gonadotropin-releasing hormone antagonist: a dose finding study. Fertil Steril. 2016;105(2):356-63.

36. Manau D, Fabergues F, Arroyo V, et al. Hemodynamic changes induced by urinary human chorionic gonadotropin and recombinant luteinizing hormone used for inducing final follicular maturation and luteinization. Fertil Steril. 2002;78:1261-7.

37. Van de Lagemaat R, Raafs BC, van Koppen C, et al. Prevention of the onset of ovarian hyperstimulation syndrome (OHSS) in the rat after ovulation induction with a low molecular weight agonist of the LH receptor compared with hCG and rec-LH. Endocrinology. 2011;152:4350-7.

38. Lamb JD, Shen S, McCulloch C, et al. Follicle-stimulating hormone administered at the time of human chorionic gonadotropin trigger improves oocyte developmental competence in in vitro fertilization cycles: a randomized, double-blind, placebo-controlled trial. Fertil Steril. 2011;95(5):1655-60.

39. Shapiro BS, Daneshmand ST, Garner FC, et al. Gonadotropin-releasing hormone agonist combined with a reduced dose of human chorionic gonadotropin for final oocyte

maturation in fresh autologous cycles of in-vitro fertilization. Fertil Steril. 2008;90(1):231-3.

40. Elbaek HO, Laursen R, Povlsen BB, et al. The exogenous progesterone-free luteal phase in IVF—exploring a new concept. Hum Reprod. 2014;29(i326):502.

41. Chen SL, Ye DS, Chen X, et al. Circulating luteinizing hormone level after triggering oocyte maturation with GnRH agonist may predict oocyte yield in flexible GnRH antagonist protocol. Hum Reprod. 2012;27:1351-6.

42. Chang FE, Beall SA, Cox JM, et al. Assessing the adequacy of gonadotropin-releasing hormone agonist leuprolide to trigger oocyte maturation and management of inadequate response. Fertil Steril. 2016;106:1093-100.

13

Progesterone in Ovulation Induction

Chaitanya Nagori

INTRODUCTION

Controlled ovarian stimulation is done for in vitro fertilization-embryo transfer (IVF–ET). There is a marked increase in E2 level due to multifollicular development. Normally, progesterone level sharply rises after the trigger that is given for final oocyte maturation. But, in some of the patients there is premature luteinizing hormone (LH) surge and may lead to cycle cancellation in IVF. This premature LH surges can be prevented by routine use of gonadotropin-releasing hormone agonist (GnRhA) or antagonist in IVF cycles.

There is a subtle increase in serum progesterone at the time of human chorionic gonadotropin (hCG) in some of the patients, in spite of using agonist or antagonist in IVF cycles. The incidence of progesterone rise is as high as 35% in agonist cycle[1] and up to 38% in antagonist cycle.[2] So, this rise of progesterone is not premature luteinization and follicle is not converted into corpus luteum. This is preovulatory progesterone rise, irrespective of LH level.

PHYSIOLOGY

The growing follicle secretes small amount of progesterone, that can be detected 2–3 days prior to the mid cycle surge. It facilitates the follicle-stimulating hormone (FSH) and LH surge.[3] So, progesterone helps in positive feedback mechanism along with estradiol for LH and FSH surge.

In controlled ovarian stimulation, there are multiple follicles that collectively produce more progesterone than the natural cycle, irrespective of agonist or antagonist used. As a response to rise in progesterone from multiple follicles, in later half of the follicular phase, there is endogenous LH rise and is termed as premature luteinization. But in these cases, LH surge occurs before progesterone rise. Progesterone rise occurs in spite of the use of agonist or antagonist, indicates that the cause is different. Therefore, it is called premature elevation of progesterone and not premature luteinization.

PATHOGENESIS

The pathogenesis of this is poorly understood and there are various hypothesis, thought of.

- *Follicular LH level*: Some authors believe that rise in progesterone level is because of rise in LH in follicular phase.[4] In this case, pituitary desensitization is not complete and some amount of LH is always present. This LH stimulates granulosa cells to secrete progesterone in late follicular phase but it cannot trigger the ovulation.[5]
- *Accumulation of hCG from exogenous human menopausal gonadotropin (hMG)*: hMG that is given for ovulation induction, has LH activity due to hCG added to it. This hCG accumulates in serum because of long half-life and this LH activity stimulates granulosa cells to secrete progesterone.[6] These women had higher serum hCG levels and high progesterone in same studies. If this hypothesis is true, recombinant FSH (rFSH) is a better drug than hMG for stimulation as rFSH has no LH like activity and progesterone rise should not occur during stimulation.[7] Pure FSH with no LH activity gives higher rise of progesterone or the same as hMG.
- *Increased sensitivity of LH receptors of granulosa cells to FSH*: It is found that higher the FSH exposure more is the progesterone rise. This progesterone rise is because of increased LH sensitivity of granulosa cells in FSH treated cycles.[2] Highest sensitivity of granulosa cells to FSH is due to increased estradiol levels. This E2 stimulates the granulosa cells continuously in presence of FSH to secrete progesterone. So, higher dose of FSH will cause more follicles to develop, which in turn gives more estrogen level that sensitizes granulosa cells to secrete progesterone level which is high in preovulatory phase. Because of FSH and E2, the follicle develops LH receptors and so more follicles have more LH receptors and more progesterone. So,

exogenous gonadotropins may lead to high progesterone levels.
- *Poor ovarian response and increased LH activity*: Premature progesterone rise is common in poor responder patients with increased LH sensitivity. But it was found that neither recombinant hCG (rhCG) nor recombinant LH (rLH) was responsible for this. It was due to adverse reaction of oocyte-cumulus complex.

CERTAIN FACTS ABOUT PROGESTERONE RISE

- Rise of progesterone is not related to LH level as it may occur in agonist or antagonist cycles also, when LH levels are very low.
- A positive correlation is found with the dose of FSH required for stimulation. Patients who required higher doses had progesterone level of more than 1.5 ng/mL and these patients were more prone to ovarian hyperstimulation syndrome (OHSS) and vice versa.[8] High FSH dose gives high progesterone level irrespective of agonist or antagonist cycle.
- High E2 levels and more number of oocytes collected are directly related to serum progesterone level elevation. This may be due to more FSH as daily dose may give good response. So, initial high FSH dose induces strong steroidogenic activity in granulosa cells that causes rise in progesterone level.
- The LH driven conversion to estradiol by theca cells is prevented by agonist and antagonist. There are more numbers of follicles due to FSH stimulation. During this stage, progesterone is the intermediate product and is not converted to androgen and then estradiol. So, lack of LH activity also increases progesterone level in

follicular phase that causes advancement of endometrium without any effect on embryo. This advancement of endometrium gives reduced implantation.[9,10] So, this is contradictory to the hMG induced progesterone rise hypothesis. In this case when hMG is used, more LH activity will convert progesterone-to-androgen and then to estrogen giving lower progesterone level. So, according to this explanation progesterone level will be lower in hMG cycles rather than rFSH.[11]

- Serum levels more than 1.5 ng/mL have poor pregnancy rate due to endometrial advancement rather than its effect on embryo and irrespective of stimulation or trigger has low birth rate. So, transfer in subsequent cycle of frozen thawed embryo gives better results.[12] These findings have been confirmed by microarrays.

- If the threshold value is considered low as reported in certain studies then there will not be low pregnancy rate with higher values of progesterone and results will be the same.

- If pre-hCG progesterone levels are high, alternative treatment is to give hCG earlier before progesterone rises. This treatment may be beneficial.[13]

- There is contribution from adrenal cortex also for the progesterone rise and there is some role of dexamethasone to suppress it. But the study by Fanchin et al. proved that increase in progesterone seen during controlled ovarian stimulation was unaltered by dexamethasone treatment, thereby confirming that premature progesterone elevation results solely from the effect of exogenous gonadotropin to ovary and number of mature follicles. Therefore estradiol and progesterone correlate on the day of trigger.[14]

- Since premature progesterone elevation commonly is associated with strong ovarian response to controlled ovarian stimulation, this subgroup often produces competent embryos, may override endometrial alterations and maintain good pregnancy rates. These patients are good responders. But, if progesterone is high with weak ovarian response to controlled ovarian stimulation, poor quality embryo cannot compensate for endometrial changes by progesterone and these embryos should be frozen.

- Data obtained by direct immunoassay may often show high progesterone levels but mass spectrometry may show lower levels. So measuring progesterone by different assays may have different results. In direct immunoassay, 17-OH hydroxyprogesterone is also measured along with progesterone and therefore shows high progesterone levels, leading to unrequired cancelled ET in many cycles.

IMPACT OF PROGESTERONE LEVEL ON PREGNANCY

Progesterone level of 1.5 ng/mL is chosen as an arbitrary level. Pregnancy rates are low when progesterone level is more than 1.5 ng/mL irrespective of agonist or antagonist cycle and irrespective of E2 level and total dose of gonadotropin. The patients who had progesterone level less than 1.5 ng/mL had higher pregnancy rates.[15] A meta-analysis by Venetis et al. has concluded that progesterone level does not correlate with cycle outcome.[16] But in this meta-analysis, the threshold value for high progesterone was kept as 0.9 ng/mL. So, the results are conflicting regarding pregnancy outcome. A recent meta-analysis including several thousand IVF-ET cycles observed a detrimental effect on pregnancy

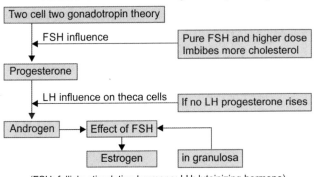

Flowchart 13.1: Two cell two gonadotropin theory.

(FSH: follicle-stimulating hormone; LH: luteinizing hormone)

rate when the progesterone level exceeded 0.8 ng/mL.[17]

BIOCHEMISTRY ON BASIS OF TWO CELL TWO GONADOTROPIN THEORY (FLOWCHART 13.1)

This explains that:

- Progesterone is an intermediate product.
- Higher the FSH, higher is the progesterone level.
- If LH is absent, progesterone is not converted to androgen and progesterone level rises.
- Therefore, hMG-highly purified (HP) will give lesser progesterone rise.

So FSH has got the direct effect on increasing the progesterone level by upgrading 3β hydroxysteroid dehydrogenase (3βHSD), in granulosa cells along with increase in estradiol (Flowchart 13.2).[18] This progesterone goes to theca cells and is converted into androgen. This androgen goes to granulosa cells, where it is converted into estrogen.

EFFECT OF PROGESTERONE ON OOCYTE AND ENDOMETRIUM

The elevated progesterone level may impair the endometrial receptivity. It causes advancement

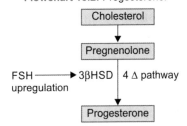

Flowchart 13.2: Progesterone.

(FSH: follicle-stimulating hormone; 3βHSD: 3β hydroxysteroid dehydrogenase)

of the endometrium, endometrial asynchrony, and change in endometrial gene expression.[19] The Bosch et al. group did not find any detrimental effect of high progesterone on oocyte in terms of fertilization, cleavage, or embryo quality. The pregnancy rates were same when embryos of patients with high progesterone levels from donors were transferred to recipients or in the same patient in the subsequent cycle after cryopreservation.

So, it is concluded that low pregnancy rates due to elevated progesterone levels is due to its detrimental effect on the endometrium rather than oocyte or embryo irrespective of trigger or stimulation protocol. But recent two large retrospective analysis have reported different findings.[20,21]

In these studies, the top quality embryos were less when progesterone level was high either in agonist or antagonist cycles.

RESCUE STRATEGIES FOR PROGESTERONE RISE

- Agonist and antagonist protocol does not make difference in pregnancy rate in patients with progesterone rise.
- High doses of FSH increase progesterone rise. But, step-down regime on decrease progesterone rise.
- If the dose of FSH is continued even after 3 follicles of more than 17 mm and delay of hCG causes more progesterone rise.

- Freeze all is most accepted policy.
- If baseline progesterone is high, dexamethasone can reduce the progesterone level.
- In high responders, the critical level of 1.5 ng/mL is higher.

PATHWAY OF STEROID PRODUCTION IN OVARY (FIG. 13.1)

Carry Home Message

- Serum level of 1.5 ng/mL of progesterone is considered as most appropriate threshold irrespective of agonist or antagonist cycle and number of follicles received.
- Progesterone level more than 1.5 ng/mL gives poor pregnancy rate as it affects

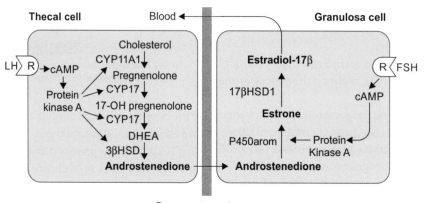

Fig. 13.1: Pathway of steroid production in ovary.
(cAMP: adenosine monophosphate; DHEA: dehydroepiandrosterone: FSH: follicle-stimulating hormone; LH: luteinizing hormone)

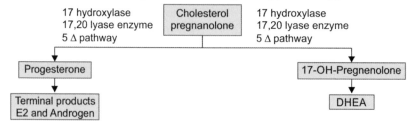

Flowchart 13.3: Progesterone level is high during preovulatory period.

(DHEA: dehydroepiandrosterone)

endometrial receptivity rather than its effect on embryo. In the process of elevation of progesterone level, it may have passed through the normal level and that may lead to endometrial asynchrony and advancement of endometrium.

- Higher progesterone level is seen with rFSH stimulation rather than hMG-HP. This is aggravated by more number of follicles[22] (here absence of LH in rFSH prevents conversion to androgen).
- If progesterone level is more than 1.5 ng/mL, "freeze all" policy should be adopted. The embryos should then be transferred in subsequent cycle.
- When progesterone level is high during preovulatory period, early hCG may be beneficial to the patient (Flowchart 13.3).

REFERENCES

1. Edelstein MC, Seltman HJ, Cox BJ, et al. Progesterone levels on the day of human chorionic gonadotropin administration in cycles with gonadotropin-releasing hormone agonist suppression are not predictive of pregnancy outcome. Fertil Steril. 1990;54:853-7.
2. Ubaldi F, Camus M, Smitz J, et al. Premature luteinization in in vitro fertilization cycles using gonadotropin-releasing hormone agonist (GnRh-a) and recombinant follicle-stimulating hormone (FSH) and GnRH-a and urinary–FSH. Fertil Steril. 1996;66:275-80.
3. Chang RJ, Jaffe RB. Progesterone effect on gonadotropin release in women pretreated with estradiol. J Clin Endocrinol Metab. 1978;47:119-25.
4. Younis JS, Simon A, Laufer N. Endometrial preparation: lessons from oocyte donation. Fertil Steril. 1996;66:873-84.
5. Ubaldi F, Smitz J, Wisanto A, et al. Oocyte and embryo quality as well as pregnancy rate in intracytoplasmic sperm injection are not affected by high follicular phase serum progesterone. Hum Reprod. 1995;10:3091-6.
6. Copperman AB, Horowitz GM, Kaplan P, et al. Relationship between circulating human chorionic gonadotropin levels and premature luteinization in cycles of controlled ovarian hyperstimulation. Fertil Steril. 1995;63:1267-71.
7. Shaw RW, Ndukew G, Imoedemhe DA, et al. Twin pregnancy after pituitary desensitization with LHRH agonist and pure FSH. Lancet. 1985;326:506-7.
8. Bosch E, Labrata E, Crespo J, et al. Circulating progesterone levels and ongoing pregnancy rates in controlled ovarian stimulation cycles for in vitro fertilization—Analysis of over 4000 cycles. Hum Reprod. 2010;25:2092-100.
9. Bosch E, Valencia I, Escudero E, et al. Premature luteinization during gonadotropin–releasing hormone antagonist cycles and its relationship with in vitro fertilization outcome. Fertil Steril. 2003;80:1444-9.
10. Bourgain C, Devroey P. The endometrium in stimulated cycles for IVF. Hum Reprod. Update 2003;9:515-22.
11. Anderson AN, Devrory P, Arce JC. Clinical outcome following stimulation with highly purified hMG or recombinant FSH in patients undergoing IVF: a randomized assessor-blind controlled trial. Hum Reprod. 2006;21:3217-27.
12. Fanchin R, Raghini C, Olivennes F, et al. Premature progesterone elevation does not alter oocyte quality in in vitro fertilization. Fertil Steril. 1996;65:1178-83.
13. Harada T, Yoshida S, Katagiri C, et al. Reduced implantation rate associated with a subtle rise in serum progesterone concentration during the follicular phase of the cycles stimulated with a combination of a gonadotropin-releasing hormone agonist and gonadotrophin. Hum Rerod. 1995;10:1060-4.
14. Fanchin R, Raghini C, Olivennes F, et al. Premature progesterone elevation and androgen elevations are not prevented by adrenal suppression in IVF. Fertil Steril. 1997;67:115-9.
15. Bosch E, Labarta E, Crespo J, et al. Circulating progesterone levels and ongoing pregnancy rates in controlled ovarian stimulation cycles for In vitro fertilization-analysis of over 4000 cycles. Hum Reprod. 2010;25:2092-100.

16. Venetis CA, Kolibianakis EM, Papanikolaou E, et al. Is progesterone elevation on the day of human chorionic gonadotropin administration associated with the probability of pregnancy in in vitro fertilization? A systematic review and meta-analysis. Hum Reprod Update. 2007;13:343-55.

17. Venetis CA, Kolibianakis EM, Bosdou JK, et al. Progesterone elevation and probability of pregnancy after IVF: a systematic review and meta-analysis of over 60,000 cycles. Human Reprod. 2013;19:433-57.

18. Oktem O, Akin N, Bildik G, et al. FSH stimulation promotes progesterone synthesis and output from human granulosa cells without luteinization. Hum Reprod. 2017;32(3):643-52.

19. Smitz J, Anderson AN, Devroey P, et al; Merit Group. Endocrine profile in serum and follicular fluid differs after ovarian stimulation with HP-HMG or recombinant FSH in IVF patients. Hum Reprod. 2007;22:676-87.

20. Huang B, Ren X, Wu L, et al. Elevated progesterone levels on the day of oocyte maturation may affect top quality embryo IVF cycles. PLos One. 2016.11:e0145895.

21. Vanni VS, Somigliana E, Reschini M, et al. Top quality blastocyst formation rates in relation to progesterone levels on the day of oocyte maturation in GnRH antagonist IVF/ICSI cycles. PLoS One. 2017;12:e0176482.

22. Al-Inany HG, Abou-Setta AM, Aboulghar MA, et al. Highly purified hMG achieves better pregnancy rates in IVF cycles but not ICSI cycles compared with recombinant FSH: a meta-analysis. Gynecol Endocrinol. 2009;25:1-7.

Role of Luteinizing Hormone in Ovulation Induction

Chaitanya Nagori

INTRODUCTION

Recent knowledge on luteinizing hormone (LH) has raised lots of controversies regarding its usage in assisted reproductive technology (ART). With the use of gonadotropin-releasing hormone (GnRh) agonist as well as antagonist, LH levels are very low when LH is required for final stages of development of an ova. So use of analogs may be detrimental to the ova. Contradictory thing is growing follicle is more sensitive to LH and dependent on LH on final stages of maturation which is low due to analogs.[1] Some people advocate add-back LH from midfollicular phase in ovarian cycle others have found no benefit of addition of LH. However, addition of recombinant LH (rLH) has shown better oocyte quality.[2]

ROLE OF LUTEINIZING HORMONE (FIG. 14.1)

- Luteinizing hormone is required for follicular steroidogenesis. It helps theca cells to form androgen from the progesterone and pregnanolone.

- It helps in follicular maturation. In the final maturation stage of follicle, only LH is enough for further growth of the follicle.
- It helps in ovulation. LH helps in rupture of the follicle and luteinization of the follicle. The corpus luteum starts secreting progesterone instead of estrogen after ovulation. LH peak prevents growth of the rest of the nondominant follicles.
- Luteinizing hormone stimulates the corpus luteum and maintains luteal phase functions by adequate secretion of progesterone.

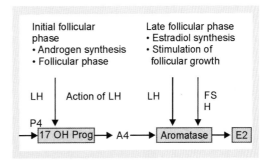

Fig. 14.1: Action of luteinizing hormone. (E2: estradiol; FSH: follicle-stimulating hormone; LH: luteinizing hormone)

PHYSIOLOGY OF LUTEINIZING HORMONE IN OVULATION

Two Cell-Two Hormone Theory[3]

Follicle-stimulating hormone (FSH) draws the cholesterol for its conversion into progesterone. Under the effect of LH, this progesterone is converted into androgen by theca cells. This androgen traverses to granulosa cells in the developing follicle, where due to aromatase activity androgen is converted into estrogen. For final stage of development of follicle, FSH and LH both are required.[4,5]

Basic science, experiment and clinical data have shown that LH is absolutely necessary for normal follicular development and oocyte maturation.[6] Therefore in hypogonadotropic hypogonadism (HH) stimulation with only recombinant FSH (rFSH) gives very poor fertilization rate and exogenous LH is required to optimize ovulation.[6]

At intermediate follicular phase, LH receptors are detected in granulosa compartment[3] and have additive effect afterwards. So LH regulates both theca cells and granulosa cells. FSH and LH also control local production of growth hormones for folliculogenesis. The fluctuation of LH is responsible for change in estrogen level because of change in androgen production. When LH level is low, there will be low estradiol (E2) which will disturb endometrial preparation.

The rise of LH is beneficial as it converts progesterone to androgen that will aromatize to estrogen. So more FSH leads to more production of progesterone from cholesterol and this is detrimental to implantation. So once LH receptors develop, i.e. after 10 mm size of the follicle, dose of FSH can be decreased and further growth of the follicle is taken care of by LH. This is because there is no rise in progesterone, instead it is decreased as it is converted to androgen and later on to estrogen. This high LH also takes care of the luteal phase.[7,8]

THERAPEUTIC WINDOW OF LUTEINIZING HORMONE[6]

Balasch and Fabregues[6] hypothesized that there is a LH ceiling which may be associated with reproductive failure, e.g. polycystic ovary syndrome (PCOS) (Fig. 14.2). During the second-half of the follicular phase, when FSH level decreases, LH dependent phase of

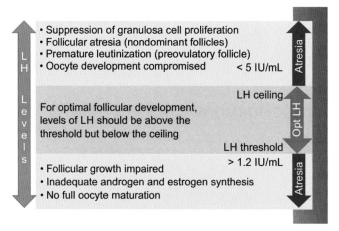

Fig. 14.2: Luteinizing hormone (LH) levels.

follicular development proceeds normally provided LH is above the threshold level and below the ceiling level. But meta-analysis conducted by Mochtar et al. showed no significant difference in pregnancy rates in rLH and rFSH group and only rFSH group.[9] Studies have shown that the level of LH should be between 1.2 IU/L and 5.0 IU/L for optimal follicular development where endogenous LH is suppressed.[4]

Therapeutic aspects of LH can be discussed under following heads:
- Age and LH
- Long protocol and LH
- Antagonist and LH
- Poor responders and LH
- Polycystic ovary syndrome and LH (high LH)
- Follicle-stimulating hormone and LH polymorphism.

Age and Luteinizing Hormone

There is a decline in pregnancy rate after 35 years of age due to less number of ova available and increase in the incidence of aneuploidy. The deoxyribonucleic acid (DNA) content of the oocyte is lower after the age of 35 years. In these patients due to advanced age even with high dose of FSH, there is poor response. More over high FSH dose increases the conversion of cholesterol to progesterone, increasing progesterone level. As there is LH deficiency or less bioactive LH available, progesterone is not converted to androgen. This progesterone excess leads to low implantation rate. Here LH supplementation will convert progesterone to androgen which will be aromatized to estrogen. Low progesterone and high E2, both will favor good endometrial development for implantation. Prof Hill et al. suggest rLH supplementation after the age of 35 years.[10] At Bourn Hall clinic in their stimulation protocol for women over 35 years of age, rLH supplementation is adopted. Cochrane review reiterated the usefulness of rLH in poor responders and advanced aged women at risk of spontaneous abortion.[11] A recent meta-analysis by Hill et al. favors addition of LH in ART in advanced age group.[12]

Criteria to add LH on day 6 of stimulation:[4]
- Luteinizing hormone less than 1.25 ng/mL on day 6 of stimulation
- No follicle more than 10 mm on day 6 of stimulation
- Estradiol less than 200 pg/mL
- Endometrial thickness less than 6 mm.

The disadvantage of LH in elderly people is that ovary has more stromal content and excess LH may have adverse effect because of more sensitivity to stromal tissue. This excessive LH level further damages already aged oocytes. LH level is high in elderly patients, but its bioactivity may be different in different patients. LH may have a ceiling effect on larger follicles. With menopause and advanced age, FSH and LH levels increase and these are biologically less active. Numbers of functioning LH receptors decrease with age. This biologically less active LH causes low estrogen because of low androgen production. Exogenous LH can correct this defect. There is always a discrepancy between immunoactive LH and bioactive LH levels. Bioactivity of LH decreases as age advances. Therefore serum levels of LH cannot decide which patients will require exogenous LH supplementation.

Meta-analysis by Kolibianakis et al. does not support the use of GnRH analogue and also confirms no influence of rFSH + rLH or rFSH treatment.[13] Vuong et al. also does not find any difference when LH was added in women more than 35 years of age. So LH is useful in only subset of patients and that still needs definition.[14]

Alviggi et al. have stated in a systematic review that rLH supplementation is required in:

- Women between age of 35 years and 39 years
- Unexpected hyporesponse to rFSH monotherapy in patients having normal ovarian reserve parameters
- Poor responders with suppressed LH levels due to GnRH analogues, but the role of LH supplementation is controversial.[15]

Long Protocol and Luteinizing Hormone

Long protocol in ART suppresses LH level, though not to zero level. It usually remains between 0.5 IU/L and 2.5 IU/L. Even with this low level of LH, rFSH can produce multiple follicular growth. Even when LH goes to less than 0.5 IU/L there is no difference in pregnancy rates. Only less than 1% of LH receptors are required for normal response. In presence of minimal stimulation by LH, FSH can activate signals modified by IGFs, which sustain androgen synthesis and can have ovarian androgen. Adding LH from day 6 routinely to all patients does not improve the pregnancy rate.[16] This low LH has no adverse effect on ongoing pregnancy rate beyond 12 weeks. There is no cutoff value to identify the women requiring LH supplementation, so LH estimation is of no use. Less than 1% of LH receptors should be occupied to achieve optimum ovarian response.[17] Optimum response is achieved when LH levels are between 0.5 IU/L and 1.5 IU/L.[18] Continuous administration of GnRh agonist helps to maintain small amount of tonic LH secretion because each agonist injection may cause release of a small amount of LH, but its bioactivity is less as compared to normal LH secreted. The reason of differential response to LH between the HH females and normogonadotropic (NG) women could be

that HH stage in NG women is much shorter (2–3 weeks) than in HH women. The normal level of LH before pituitary suppression will prime the small follicles. So follicles are less sensitive to drop in LH level and respond to FSH irrespective of LH levels.

Antagonist Cycle and Luteinizing Hormone

There is a diversified opinion regarding the addition of LH in antagonist cycle. GnRh antagonist is started from day 6 and addition of rLH does not improve IVF outcome, but few reports suggest that by adding LH or human menopausal gonadotropin (hMG) in antagonist cycle improves the results. Meta-analysis by Hillier (2007) proved that adding LH will improve the results,[4] but fall of LH to more than 50% from early to midfollicular phase results in lower birth rate. Low early and midfollicular phase LH had low E2, low oocyte yield, and low embryo development. So LH is to be added if LH level is less than 1.2 IU/L in midfollicular phase.

Luteinizing Hormone in Poor Responders

Luteinizing hormone has an important role in poor responders. There is a subset of patients that are benefited by adding LH. Asia Pacific Fertility Advisory Group[19] in 2011 strongly recommended rLH in cotreatment with rFSH in patients with history of poor response in:

- Suboptimal response to stimulation on day 6
  - No follicle of more than 10 mm in size
  - Endometrial thickness of less than 6 mm
  - Estradiol level less than 200 pg/mL.
- It may be beneficial in females of more than 35 years of age with long agonist or antagonist protocol.[18]

Luteinizing hormone dose of 75 IU is sufficient in most cases, but small percentage of women may require doses of LH up to 150–225 IU. Many studies including one by Musters et al., demonstrated that adding rLH to ovulation induction protocol does not show any difference in top quality embryos or ongoing pregnancy rates.[20] Adding LH is more effective when there is inadequate response to rFSH. Rather than increasing the dose of FSH, rLH is added and that results in more oocyte yield.[21] The ESPART study presents live birth rate was higher in recombinant human FSH (rhFSH)/rLH to rFSH, in spite of the same number of eggs retrieved. The pregnancy outcome failure was significantly lower in rhFSH/rhLH group and is helpful in improving the live birth rate.[22] The reason for better outcome may be because of LH, that may reduce the rate of granulosa cell apoptosis. LH receptors are present in the endometrium during the window of implantation and play an important role in embryo-endometrium crosstalk during implantation. Positive effect of LH on embryo and endometrium helps in implantation in women above 35 years of age.

Luteinizing Hormone in Polycystic Ovary Syndrome

It has already been discussed that high LH can have a ceiling effect on ova and this is observed in PCOS patients. This high LH is associated with reproductive failure. PCOS is a classical example of high LH with poor pregnancy rate and higher abortion rate due to effect of LH on ovum quality and endometrial receptivity. High LH causes follicular atresia, premature luteinization, and poor oocyte quality due to high androgen levels. Preovulatory development of ova is dependent on optimum level of LH, which is above threshold and below ceiling level. LH should be avoided as it

can cause ovarian hyperstimulation syndrome (OHSS). Clomiphene citrate (CC) is the classical example for lower pregnancy rate due to high LH. CC acts on hypothalamus to secrete FSH and LH. This high LH is detrimental to ova. When endogenous LH is elevated, FSH alone is conceptually better.[23]

Follicle-stimulating Hormone and Luteinizing Hormone Polymorphism

Ovarian response to FSH differs from patient to patient due to FSH receptor polymorphism. FSH receptor gene is a marker for ovarian response. FSH receptor gene consists of two single nucleotide polymorphism (SNP) in axon-10 and changes two amino acids at position 307 and 680. Women with 307 Ala and 680 Ser SNPs show reduced response to controlled ovarian hyperstimulation (COH). These patients require higher doses of FSH and are called poor responders.[24] In these cases after the development of follicle of 10–11 mm, LH can be added instead of increasing the dose of FSH for better outcome and lower FSH delivery.

Luteinizing hormone polymorphism: LH receptor gene carries as many as 282 SNPs.[25] In 1991, Petterson and Soderholm identified a common genetic LHβ variant or v-β-LH due to alterations in beta subunit gene leading to changes in amino acid sequence. There is more potency of LH activity of v-β-LH at the receptor site, but its duration of activity is shorter.[26] Presence of v-β-LH increases the requirement of FSH. These are the patients in whom exogenous LH is required for stimulation.[26] It is very common in Japanese patients. Endogenous LH level is not accurate to decide which patients will require LH supplementation.[27] Instead v-β-LH can be used as a marker for ovarian response to rFSH. It helps the clinician to identify the patients who will require LH supplementation.[26] In genuine empty follicle syndrome, there is *LHCGR* gene mutations which is responsible for no ova retrieved on oocyte retrieval. It is inherited in family. So screening of mutation is useful.

Human menopausal gonadotropin or luteinizing hormone: Studies have shown that rLH is better than hMG to be combined with FSH during ovarian stimulation. In hMG, the human chorionic gonadotropin (hCG) i.e. the LH activity may be inconsistent and may affect oocyte maturation and affects pregnancy rates.[28]

Human menopausal gonadotropin: There are controversial results with hMG + rFSH for live birth rates. The only advantage is lesser number of ampoules of rFSH required resulting in lower cost of treatment, but if rLH is added instead of hMG it gives higher birth rates.[29] hCG content is six times greater than that of LH. hCG when is given after follicle size of 10 mm, it has no effect on large follicles, but causes demise of smaller follicles though it has no effect on large follicles.[30]

Disadvantages of hMG are as follows:
- Protein contamination
- Local allergic reaction
- Batch-to-batch inconsistencies
- Supply limitations
- Variable LH quality and bioavailability in different hMG preparations
- Much more hCG than LH activity (at least 10 times).

Characteristics of hCG are as follows:
- Serum half-life is twofold
- More stable
- Slow degradation and high binding affinity to LH receptors
- 1 IU of hCG is six to eight times greater in bioactivity than 1 IU of LH
- Accumulates on daily injections.

COMPARING HUMAN CHORIONIC GONADOTROPIN AND LUTEINIZING HORMONE AT MOLECULAR LEVEL

- Different source
- Different molecular weight
- Different number of AA in beta chain
- Different number of glycosylation sites
- Different half-life.

COMPARING HUMAN CHORIONIC GONADOTROPIN AND LUTEINIZING HORMONE FUNCTIONALLY AND CLINICALLY

- Different effect on cyclic adenosine monophosphate (cAMP)
- Different gene expression
- Luteinizing hormone gives more oocytes/embryo
- Better quality of oocytes/embryo
- Difference in cumulative pregnancy rate with LH.

Administration of low dose hCG 200 IU/day (100–400) replacing rFSH in final days of ovarian stimulation reduces consumption of gonadotropins without differences in oocyte yields and pregnancy outcome.[30] The reason is that developing follicle becomes less dependent on FSH as they acquire LH responsiveness.[31] In a large series[32] rFSH was discontinued when six follicles were larger than 12 mm or E2 was more than 600 ng/L. rFSH was substituted by 200 IU of hCG. There was significant reduction in total dose of FSH, but oocytes retrieved and pregnancy rates were the same.

A meta-analysis by Daya et al. demonstrated use of FSH alone can have better pregnancy rate than hMG,[33,34] but another meta-analysis by van Wely et al. showed better pregnancy rate in the hMG group rather than FSH alone group.[35]

CARRY HOME MESSAGE

- Luteinizing hormone is strictly necessary for meiosis, rupture of follicle, and luteal phase.
- Luteinizing hormone promotes theca cells to produce androgen which is aromatized to estrogen by granulosa cells under the influence of FSH—two cell–two hormone theory.
- Small amount of LH is enough for follicular maturation in agonist downregulated cycles.
- Results are good when LH is more than 1.2 IU/L (threshold) and less than 5 IU/L (ceiling level).
- Adding LH improves the results when the LH level is low.
- Luteinizing hormone receptors develop when follicle is larger than 10 mm in diameter and then LH can takeover the function of FSH.
- With advanced age LH supplementation gives better results because of less bioactive LH or LH polymorphism.
- High LH gives poor pregnancy rate and classical examples are PCOS and CC induced cycles.
- Recombinant LH is more specific than hCG.

REFERENCES

1. Shoham Z. The clinical therapeutic window for luteinizing hormone in controlled ovarian stimulation. Dertil Steril. 2002;77(6):1170-7.
2. Ruvolo G, Bosco L, Pane A, et al. Lower apoptosis rate in human cumulus cells after administration of recombinant luteinizing hormone to women undergoing ovarian stimulation for in vitro fertilization procedures. Fertil Steril. 2007;87(3):542-6.
3. Hillier SG, Whitelaw PF, Smyth CD. Follicular oestrogen synthesis: the 'two-cell two-gonadotropin' model revisited. Mol Cell Endocrinol. 100:51-4.
4. O'Dea L, O'Brien F, Currie K, et al. Follicular development induced by recombinant luteinizing hormone (LH) and follicle stimulating hormone (FSH) in anovulatory women with LH and FSH deficiency: evidence of a threshold effect. Curr Med Res Opin. 2008;24(10):2785-93.
5. Vaskivuo T. (2002). Regulation of apoptosis in the female reproductive system. [online] Available from herkules.oulu. fi/isbn9514266676/isbn9514266676.pdf [Accessed October 2018].
6. Balasch J, Fabregues F. Is luteinizing hormone needed for optimal ovulation induction? Curr Opin Obstet Gynecol. 2002;14(3):265-74.
7. Voutilainen R, Tapanainen J, Chung BC, et al. Hormonal regulation of P450scc (20,22-desmolase) and P450c17 (17 alpha-hydroxylase/17,20-lyase) in cultured human granulosa cells. J Clin Endocrinol Metab. 1986;63(1):202-7.
8. Palermo R. Differential actions of FSH and LH during folliculogenesis. Reprod Biomed Online. 2007;15(3):326-37.
9. Jayaprakasan K. SonoAVC: a novel method of automatic volume calculation. Ultrasound Obstet Gynecol. 2008;31:691-6.
10. Hill MJ, Levens ED, Levy G, et al. The use of recombinant luteinizing hormone in patients undergoing assisted reproductive techniques with advanced reproductive age: a systematic review and meta-analysis. Fertil Steril. 2012;97(5):1108-14.
11. Mochtar MH, Van der Veen, Zeich M, et al. Recombinant luteinizing hormone (rLH) for controlled ovarian hyperstimulation in assisted reproductive cycles. Cochrane Database Syst Rev. 2007;(2):CD005070.
12. Hill MJ, Levens ED, Levy G, et al. Does exogenous LH in ovarian stimulation improve assisted reproduction success? An appraisal of the literature. Reprod Bolmed Online. 2012;24(3):261-71.
13. Kolibianakis EM, Kalogeropoulou L, Griesinger G, et al. Among patients treated with FSH and GnRH analogues for in vitro

fertilization, is the addition of recombinant LH associated with the probability of live birth? A systematic review and meta-analysis. Hum Reprod Update. 2007;13:445-52.

14. Voung TNL, Phung HT, Ho MT. Recombinant follicle-stimulating hormone and recombinant luteinizing hormone versus recombinant follicle-stimulating hormone alone during GnRH antagonist ovarian stimulation in patients aged ≥ 35 years: a randomized controlled trial. Hum Reprod. 2015;30(5):1188-95.

15. Alviggi C, Conforti A, Esteves SC, et al. Recombinant luteinizing hormone supplementation in assisted reproductive technology: a systematic review. Fertil Steril. 2018;109(4):644-64.

16. Kollibianakis EM, Collins J, Tarlatzis B, et al. Are endogenous LH levels during ovarian stimulation for IVF using GnRH analogues associated with probability of ongoing pregnancy? A systematic review. Hum Reprod Update. 2006;12:3-12.

17. Chappel SC, Howles C. Re-evaluation of the roles of luteinizing hormone and follicle stimulating hormone in the ovulatory process. Hum Reprod. 1991;6:1206-12.

18. Wong PC, Qiao J, Ho C, et al. Current opinion on use of luteinizing hormone supplementation in assisted reproduction therapy: an Asian perspective. Reprod Biomed Online. 2011;23(2):81-90.

19. Lahoud R, Al-Jefout M, Tyler J, et al. A relative reduction in mid-follicular LH concentrations during GnRH agonist IVF/ICSI cycles leads to lower live birth rates. Hum Reprod. 2006;21(10):2645-9.

20. Musters AM, van Wely M, Mastenbroek S, et al. The effect of recombinant LH on embryo quality: a randomized controlled trial in women with poor ovarian reserve. Hum Reprod. 2012;27:244-50.

21. De Placido G, Alviggi C, Perino A, et al. Italian collaborative group on recombinant human luteinizing hormone. Recombinant human LH supplementation versus recombinant human follicle-stimulating hormone step up protocol during controlled ovarian stimulation in normogonadotropic women with initial inadequate response to rFSH. A multicenter, prospective, randomized controlled trial. Hum Reprod. 2005;20:390-6.

22. Humaidan P, Chin W, Rogoff D, et al. Efficacy and safety of follicular alfa/lutropin alfa in ART: a randomized controlled trial in poor ovarian responder. Hum Reprod. 2017;32:544-55.

23. Regan L, Owen EJ, Jacobs HS. Hypersecretion of luteinizing hormone, infertility and miscarriage. Lancet. 1990;336:1141-4.

24. Simoni M, Tempfer CB, Destenaves B, et al. Functional genetic polymorphisms and female reproductive disorders: Part I: Polycystic ovarian syndrome and ovarian response. Hum Reprod Update. 2008;14(5):459-84.

25. Themmen AP. An update of pathophysiology of human goadotropin subunit and receptor gene mutations and polymorphisms. Reproduction. 2005;130(30):263-74.

26. Alviggi C, Clarizia R, Pettersson K, et al. Suboptimal response to GnRHa long protocol is associated with a common LH polymorphism. Reprod Biomed Online. 2009;18(1):9-14.

27. Loumaye E, Engrand P, Howles CM, et al. Assessment of the role of serum luteinizing hormone and estradiol response to follicle-stimulating hormone on in vitro fertilization treatment outcome. Fertil Steril. 1997;67:889-99.

28. Carone D, Vizzillo G, Vitti A. Clinical outcomes of ovulation induction in WHO group I anovulatory women using r-hFSH/r-hLH in a 2:1 ratio compared to hMG. Hum Reprod. 2010;25:285-321.

29. Ferraretti AP, Ginarolli L, Magli MC, et al. Exogenous luteinizing hormone in controlled ovarian hyperstimulation for assisted reproduction techniques. Fertil Steril. 2004;82(6):1521-6.

30. Filicori M, Cognigni GE, Tabarelli C, et al. Stimulation and growth of antral ovarian follicles by selective LH activity administration in women. J Clinical Endocrinol Metab. 2001;87:1156-61.

31. Sullivan MW, Stewart-Akers A, Krasnow JS, et al. Ovarian responses in women to recombinant follicle-stimulating hormone and luteinizing hormone (LH): a role of LH in

the final stages of follicular maturation. J Clin Endocrinol Metab. 1999;84:228-32.

32. Van Horne AK, Bates GW Jr, Robinson RD, et al. Recombinant follicle-stimulating hormone (r-FSH) supplemented with low-dose human chorionic gonadotropin compared with r-FSH alone for ovarian stimulation for in vitro fertilization. Fertil Steril. 2007;88:1010-3.

33. Al-Inany HG, Youssef MA, Ayeleke RO, et al. Gonadotropin-releasing hormone antagonists for assisted reproductive technology. Cochrane Database Syst Rev. 2011;5:CD001750.

34. Ludwig M, Katalinic A, Banz C, et al. Tailoring the GnRH antagonist cetrorelix acetate to individual patient's needs in ovarian stimulation for IVF: results of a prospective, randomized study. Hum Reprod. 2002;17:2842-5.

35. Escudero E, Bosch E, Crespo J, et al. Comparison of two different starting multiple dose gonadotropin-releasing hormone antagonist protocols in a selected group of in vitro fertilization-embryo transfer patients. Fertil Steril. 2004;81:562-6.

15 Ovarian Hyperstimulation Syndrome

Chaitanya Nagori

INTRODUCTION

Ovarian hyperstimulation syndrome (OHSS) is the most serious and life-threatening complication of ovulation induction. The incidence of moderate OHSS is 3–6% and severe OHSS is 0.1–2%.[1] Fortunately with acceptance of antagonist used for downregulation with agonist being used as a trigger and "freeze all" policy, the incidence has markedly decreased and has become almost zero in some centers.

Ovarian hyperstimulation syndrome is due to overproduction of ovarian hormones and vasoactive substances that are secreted as a result of uncontrolled ovarian stimulation. These substances increase the permeability allowing the fluids to go to the third space. This accumulation of fluid in the third space is responsible for the signs, symptoms and complications of OHSS.

TYPES OF OHSS

Ovarian hyperstimulation syndrome may be *early-onset* or *late-onset.*

Early-onset OHSS is detected from day 3–7 after ovulation trigger with human chorionic gonadotropin (hCG). But late-onset OHSS appears after 10–12 days after the hCG trigger. Early OHSS is because of excessive drug (gonadotropins) dosages for that particular ovary. Very rarely mutations in follicle-stimulating hormone (FSH) receptor may be stimulated by endogenous hCG and spontaneous OHSS may occur. Late-onset OHSS is because of endogenous hCG secreted by the embryo and as the embryo grows and hCG secretion increases, the OHSS becomes more severe. Late OHSS is present in almost 70% of the patients who had severe OHSS. It cannot be predicted, unlike early OHSS. Moreover, it has equal association with singleton as with multiple pregnancies.[2]

CLASSIFICATION OF OHSS

Classification is extremely useful for the clinician to decide the severity of the condition and also to decide if the patient requires hospitalization and medical or surgical line of treatment. Various classification systems have been described in literature stating mild, moderate and severe variety. But mild

OHSS is very common and does not require any treatment. So the most accepted recent classification was introduced by Rizk and Aboulghar stated only two categories: (1) moderate and (2) severe.[3] This classification is useful in defining clinical groups in relation to prognosis and treatment protocols.

Moderate OHSS

- Patient presents with discomfort, pain, nausea, abdominal distention, but no clinical ascites.
- Though ultrasound shows enlarged ovaries with ascites.
- Hematological and biological profiles are normal.
- Patient can be treated on outdoor basis, provided she can come for the follow-up as and when required, depending on her symptoms.

Severe OHSS

Severe OHSS is divided into grades depending on its severity.

Grade A

- Patient presents with dyspnea, nausea, vomiting, diarrhea, abdominal pain with marked distention.
- Oliguria, ascites and hydrothorax may be clinically detected.
- Ultrasound shows large ovaries and ascites.
- Biochemical profile is normal.
- These patients can be treated as outpatients or may require admission depending on patient's or consultant's comfort.

Grade B

- All signs and symptoms of grade A with increased severity.

- Marked oligouria.
- Increased hematocrit, elevated urea and creatinine, abnormal liver function tests (LFTs).
- Requires admission and vigilant supervision.

Grade C

- Apart from all the signs and symptoms of Grade B, acute respiratory distress syndrome (ARDS).
- Renal shut down.
- Venous thrombosis.
- Requires intensive care unit (ICU) support.

PATHOPHYSIOLOGY OF OHSS

It is extremely important to understand the pathophysiology for prevention and treatment of the disease. It is characterized by ovarian enhancement and shifting of fluid rich in protein especially albumin in third space causing ascites and effusion. Severity of OHSS is directly related to capillary permeability (Flowchart 15.1).

Changes in Ovary

- Bilateral cystic enlargement of the ovary.
- Increased stromal edema.
- Multiple corpora lutea.
- Neovascularization.
- Secretion of vascular endothelial growth factor (VEGF), prorenin, active renin, interleukins, N680, interleukin-1β, 2 and 6, prostaglandins, tumor necrosis factor-α (TNF-α), transforming growth factor-1 (TGF-1), TGF, etc. Most of these substances are angiogenic and are responsible for neovascularization during folliculogenesis and luteinization in the ovary and act through VEGF.

Flowchart 15.1: Clinical pathology of OHSS.

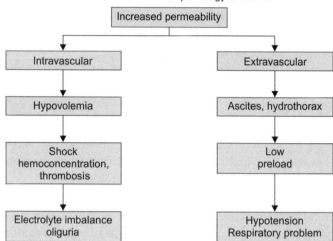

Third Space

There is collection of fluid in third space presenting as ascites, hydrothorax with massive pleural effusion. This fluid shift is due to increased capillary permeability. The shift starts after hCG injection and even before ovum aspiration. VEGF is responsible for increased capillary permeability and fluid shift.[4] Production of VEGF is dependent on hCG, which is given for trigger or on endogenous hCG from embryo. VEGF is secreted by granulosa cells. Intraperitoneal pressure increases beyond the intraluminal pressure of inferior vena cava (IVC). Therefore, blood flow in IVC decreases, leading to decreased preload in the heart, decreased cardiac output causing impairment of respiratory and renal functions. Antidiuretic hormone (ADH) is also increased because of activation of renin-angiotensin mechanism and secretes ADH. This causes oliguria and hemoconcentration. Hypovolemia and hypotension causes arterial constriction. OHSS may be more common in intrauterine insemination (IUI) cycles rather than in vitro fertilization (IVF) as in IVF, all

the follicular fluid containing the causative ingredients of OHSS are extracted out during follicular aspiration.

Vascular permeability factor (VPF): It is similar to VEGF. This causes vascular leakage and is present in corpus luteum. Concentration of VPF is very high in follicular fluid, serum and peritoneal fluid, in patients in whom OHSS develops.[5] It is two times higher in follicular fluid and that indicates ovarian origin. When pregnancy occurs, hCG rescues corpus luteum and there is increase in VPF secretion.

Familial mutations in FSH receptors increase its sensitivity to trophoblastic hCG and can cause OHSS with spontaneous pregnancy. High estradiol (E2) is not responsible for OHSS as when hCG is withheld, high E2 cannot cause OHSS. So estrogen is not having vasoactivity and cannot cause vascular dysfunction.

PREDICTION OF OHSS

Prediction is extremely important for treating the patient and should be done as early as possible. This can be done:

1. Before stimulation
2. During stimulation
3. Before trigger
4. Pregnancy.

Before Stimulation

Clinical

- Young patient.
- Polycystic ovarian syndrome (PCOS)—antral follicle count (AFC) more than 26, increased stromal vascularity.
- Low body mass index (BMI)—thin lean PCOS.
- History of OHSS in previous pregnancy.
- High anti-Müllerian hormone (AMH) greater than 30 pmol/mL or greater than 7 ng/mL. In one study, all cycles were canceled in this scenario.[6]
- Anti-Müllerian hormone greater than 3.36 ng/mL has 90.5% sensitivity and 81.3% specificity for subsequent development of OHSS.[7]

Ultrasound Based

- Follicle number per ovary (FNPO) more than 15.
- Stromal resistance index (RI) less than 0.5.
- Stromal peak systolic velocity (PSV) greater than 10 cm/sec.
- Ovarian volume greater than 10 cc.
- Stromal flow index (FI) greater than 15.
- More follicles of 6–9 mm size.

Follicle-Stimulating Hormone Receptor Genotype

Follicle-stimulating hormone receptor mutations and polymorphisms can cause OHSS when they are activated.[8] To date 744 single nucleotide polymorphisms have been identified in FSH receptor gene. The N680 allele can be associated with hyper-responders who are more prone to OHSS. The significant increase in N680 allele is observed as severity of OHSS increases. So it is concluded that genotype in position of N680 of FSH receptor cannot predict which patient will develop OHSS but it can predict the severity of OHSS amongst the patients who develop OHSS.[9]

Prediction by Bone Morphogenetic Protein-15 Gene

Bone morphogenetic protein (BMP)-15 is related to OHSS which is dose dependent. It is a member of TGF-β. It helps to predict which patients are at a risk of developing OHSS.[10]

Cystic Fibrosis Transmembrane Conductance Regulator

Estradiol upregulates cystic fibrosis transmembrane conductance regulator (CFTR) expression and this phenomenon can cause increase in fluid in peritoneal cavity. So it may provide causative link between hyperestrinism and OHSS.[11]

During Treatment

- Long protocol favors development of OHSS.
- Number of days of gonadotropin stimulation is very important for development of OHSS. These days are always more in downregulated cycles and so these cycles are more prone to OHSS.
- Human chorionic gonadotropin as luteal support.
- Ultrasound prediction:
  - There is a positive correlation between mean number of immature follicles and OHSS.
  - During stimulation, increase in immature follicles and decrease in mature follicles favor severe OHSS (>9 mm follicles, >20 in number).[12]

- Risk of OHSS increases sharply with increase in the volume of the ovary.
  - Stromal volume is important in predicting the risk of OHSS.
- The type of gonadotropin used did not show any significant difference in risk of development of OHSS. Its incidence is same with recombinant FSH (rFSH), urinary FSH and purified human menopausal gonadotropin (hMG).[13] More important is the type of protocol used (chronic low-dose, step-up or step-down protocol). Chronic low-dose protocol has a very low incidence of OHSS.

Before Trigger

- *Estradiol level*: E2 greater than 4,000 pg/mL in assisted reproductive technology (ART) and greater than 1,700 pg/mL in IUI is considered high risk for development of OHSS.
- *Ultrasound findings*: Even when the age of the patient and total number of follicles are similar, the ovarian volume was significantly higher in the patients who developed OHSS (271 ± 87 vs 157.30 ± 54.20 mL).[14] Presence of medium-sized follicles (11–14 mm) more than 5–7 on either side is thought to be a risk factor for development of OHSS. More than or equal to 25 follicles larger than 11 mm in size or more than or equal to 25 oocytes retrieved is a risk factor for OHSS.

Pregnancy

Pregnancy itself is considered a risk factor for development of OHSS.

PREVENTION OF OHSS

- Primary prevention (Box 15.1)
- Secondary prevention (Box 15.2).

BOX 15.1: Primary prevention of ovarian hyperstimulation syndrome.

- GnRH antagonist protocol
- Laparoscopic ovarian drilling
- Insulin sensitizers
- In vitro maturation of ova
- Low-dose gonadotropin protocol
- Natural cycle ART
- Avoid hCG in luteal phase.

BOX 15.2: Secondary prevention of OHSS.

- Withholding hCG
- Coasting
- Reducing the dose of hCG
- GnRH agonist trigger
- Recombinant LH as trigger
- Intravenous albumin
- Intravenous HES
- Glucocorticoids
- Ovarian suppression
- Dopamine agonist
- Freeze all
- Aspirate all follicles
- Intravenous calcium.

Primary Prevention of OHSS

It is by selection of stimulation protocols and drugs that decrease the risk of OHSS.

- *Gonadotropin-releasing hormone (GnRH) antagonist protocol*: Initial studies showed no difference in severe OHSS in antagonist or long protocols. In antagonist protocols, pregnancy rate was also found to be lower.[15] But the two recent meta-analysis comparing agonist and antagonist protocol showed significantly reduced OHSS with antagonist protocol and severity was also less with antagonist protocol.[16,17]
- *Laparoscopic ovarian drilling*: Both ovarian diathermy and laser vaporization performed prior to stimulation reduces the incidence of OHSS. The transvaginal ovarian diathermy can be used in difficult cases. The best results are obtained in thin lean PCOS. Ovarian diathermy should be

reserved for young patients with severe PCOS who tend to hyperstimulation even on a prolonged low-dose FSH regimen.

- *Metformin*: The short-term course of metformin 850 mg BD in PCOS given before the ovum stimulation up to the day of oocyte collection decreases the incidence of OHSS and improves the pregnancy rate.[18,19] But some studies recommend for 2–3 months prior to IVF.
  - In vitro maturation of immature oocytes: This is an alternative management for patients having high risk of OHSS. It totally avoids OHSS.[20]
  - Low-dose gonadotropins: low dose with step-up: Protocol should be used to avoid OHSS. 150 IU urinary FSH should be the starting dose.[21]
  - Natural cycle ART: Completely eliminates OHSS, but has low pregnancy rate.
  - Avoid hCG as a luteal phase support.

Secondary Prevention of OHSS

- *Withholding hCG*: Withholding hCG and canceling the cycle when E2 level is greater than 4,000 pgm/mL can avoid OHSS. Its values are doubling or more every 2–3 days. It is a warning sign of OHSS. This is the common method used to avoid OHSS but there is financial burden on the patient and the patient is never happy in spite of explanation. hCG is the main culprit for OHSS as it promotes secretions of VEGF. And luteinizing hormone (LH) receptors are present on 8–10 mm size of the follicle. So more medium-sized follicles are more dangerous.
- *Coasting*: It is delaying the administration of hCG. It was once most popular method in long protocol to prevent OHSS as it does not require cancellation of the cycle. Ideally coasting starts when lead follicle

is less than 15 mm and E2 level is greater than 1,500 pg/mL lead follicle continues to grow as it already has LH receptors. No further FSH is given for stimulation. Normally follicle continues to grow for 4 days. Coasting should not be done for more than 4 days as it grossly reduces E2 level and pregnancy rates. hCG is given when E2 decreases to less than 3,000 pg/mL, as it reduces OHSS without affecting pregnancy.[16] In agonist cycle, withdrawing agonist and replacing it by antagonist and then giving agonist trigger can reduce OHSS.[22] Antagonist can be continued in high-risk OHSS patients who were downregulated by GnRH agonist (GnRHa). Coasting with GnRHa has no beneficial role in preventing OHSS as discussed in a Cochrane review.[23]

- Mechanism of coasting: It diminishes functioning of granulosa cell cohort, atresia of smaller follicles and reduces VEGF secretion and gene expression. But there is insufficient evidence to recommend coasting for prevention of OHSS according to practice committee of the American Society for Reproductive Medicine (ASRM).
- *Reducing the dose of hCG*: There are no much data available on decreasing dose of hCG but there is general consensus that when E2 is greater than 3,000 pg/mL dose should be halved. The dose between 3,300 pg/mL and 5,000 pg/mL decreases the risk.[24]
- *GnRHa trigger*: In antagonist protocol, GnRHa can be used as the ovulation trigger. Quality of the oocytes is same as of hCG trigger and fertilization and cleavage rates are same. But ongoing pregnancy rates are very low because of luteal phase defects. Though it definitely abolishes occurrence of OHSS. hCG 1,500 IU, on the day of ovum

pick-up can be given to rescue the corpus luteum, if there are less than 24 follicles, which gives good pregnancy rate with extremely low-OHSS rate as suggested by Humaidan et al.[25] Griesinger et al. proposed freeze all embryos and transfer in the subsequent cycle after GnRHa trigger. This gives higher cumulative pregnancy rates.[26] Occasionally moderate OHSS may occur particularly when patient conceives but severe OHSS are not reported with GnRHa trigger.

- *Recombinant LH for ovulation*: Triggering the ovulation with recombinant LH (rLH) decreases OHSS because it does not produce VEGF and so vascular permeability is not increased. But pregnancy rates are low and so optimum dose is under research which would maintain the pregnancy rates along with low risk of OHSS. Ovulating dose is very high and so it is an expensive treatment as multiple doses are required because of its short half-life (20 minutes).[27] rLH is safer than hCG and has long half-life than native LH. So a single peak can cause final maturation. The dose is between 5,000 IU and 30,000 IU of rLH.

- *Intravenous albumin*: Intravenous (IV) albumin prevents third space fluid accumulation and corrects hemodynamic instability by increasing colloidal oncotic pressure. There are various reports in favor of and against the use of albumin for prevention of OHSS. Albumin maintains intravascular volume and prevents hypovolemia, ascites and hemoconcentration. It counters the vasoactive substance released from corpus lutea. In Cochrane review, there is significant reduction in OHSS in albumin group. It is to be given at the time of oocyte retrieval and 48 hours after oocyte retrieval.[28] In established OHSS, albumin always helps to prevent complications that are due to hemoconcentration. But oncotic pressure lasts for only 36 hours and so repeat therapy is needed.

- *Intravenous hydroxyethyl starch solution*: Hydroxyethyl starch (HES) is the volume expander. Six percent HES is used in a dose of 1,000 mL at the time of ovum pick-up and 500 mL is given 48 hours after the first one. HES decreases the incidence of moderate and severe OHSS. Recent Cochrane review states that better results are seen with HES than albumin.[29]

- *Glucocorticoids*: It was thought to be useful because of its anti-inflammatory action during the development of OHSS. But most of the papers have found no protective effect with corticosteroids. It may have inhibitory effect on VEGF gene expression.[30] Aspirin reduces the incidence of OHSS, has grade B evidence according to practice committee of ASRM. ASRM practice committee has also shown that Aspirin + glucocorticoids is also beneficial from stimulation to positive beta-hCG.[31,32]

- *Ovarian suppression*:
  - *GnRH agonist*: Continuous GnRHa after hCG also decreases LH surge and diminishes the occurrence of OHSS. All the embryos are cryopreserved in this case. This is very useful in donation cycles.
  - E2 and hydroxyl progesterone IM after embryo transfer also prevents ovarian secretion and prevents OHSS but it is experimental.
  - Aromatase inhibitors in luteal phase are promising. It decreases luteal E2 concentration and decreases OHSS. It is very useful in donor cycles.

- *Dopamine agonist*: VEGF increases the vascular permeability. VEGF acts by VEGF receptor 2 specific. Inhibition of this receptor can prevent increased vascular permeability which is done by cabergoline or bromocriptine or quinagolide. There are gene expressions of 80 upregulated and 7 downregulated genes in OHSS as compared to controls. Tyrosine hydroxylase is downregulated. So it is the natural inhibitor for angiogenic process. This suggests dopamine can be an antiangiogenic factor and deficit or it can cause OHSS. Dopamine decreases vascular permeability by decreasing VEGF-2 phosphorylation. Dopamine receptor-2 agonist (cabergoline) inhibits VEGF receptor 2-dependent vascular permeability without affecting luteal angiogenesis. It has no luteolytic effect.[27]

The recommended dose is 0.5 mg cabergoline from day of hCG up to 8 days. It does not affect fertilization, cleavage or implantation. Reproductive outcome is not changed.[33] The study of Alvarez et al. showed marked improvement in moderate OHSS but there is no difference in severe OHSS and E2 level also. The non-ergot-derived dopamine agonist quinagolide is promoted now as cabergoline causes vascular disorders in Parkinson's disease. Dose is 50-100-200 μg/daily for 17–21 days till β-hCG is done.

- *Freeze all*: Effective cryopreservation is done in all embryos and so we can avoid late OHSS which is due to pregnancy. The results of fresh transfer and cryopreserved embryos used in next cycle are the same.[34] But the advantage of avoiding pregnancy-induced OHSS is beneficial to the patient. Though still there is insufficient data for this policy and Cochrane review does not support this.[35] OHSS-free clinic will be a reality with embryo freezing. The entire IVF procedure is divided into segments.
  - Segment A: Ovarian stimulation with antagonist protocol and agonist trigger.
  - Segment B: Cryopreservation of embryos and vitrification.
  - Segment C: Embryo transfer after thawing and endometrial preparation by hormone replacement therapy.
- *Aspirate all follicles*: All the follicles larger or smaller should be aspirated to decrease incidence of OHSS.[36] Aspiration of all the follicles from one ovary before hCG was recommended before but much better solutions are available and so aspiration before hCG is not practiced.
- *Intravenous calcium*: 10%, 10 mL of calcium gluconate is given IV in 30 minutes or in 200 mL of normal saline at 1.5 mL/minute on the day of oocyte retrieval and repeated on day 1, 2 and 3 postoocyte retrieval.[37,38] The difference in severity of clinical symptoms is significant. Ascitic fluid volume decreases from day 3 postoocyte retrieval and ovarian size decreases after day 10 of oocyte retrieval. It has no detrimental effects on pregnancy rates. IV calcium reduces the fluid transfer to the third space. IV calcium is better than HES in reducing ascites. It prevents damage and repairs the endothelial cell membrane. It is inexpensive and nontoxic approach that reduces ascites and hematocrit. hCG causes mobilization of calcium from intracellular stores. This is influenced by granulosa cells. hCG and LH receptors are members of a protein-coupled receptor family whose transducers are represented by calcium-dependent kinases and so calcium action in OHSS can be linked to hCG.
- OHSS-free clinic by segmentation of IVF treatment.
  - Segment A: Optimizing ovarian stimulation with antagonist cycle and agonist trigger.

TABLE 15.1: Management of OHSS.

Clinical management	Biochemical monitoring	Ultrasound monitoring
Blood pressure	Blood count	Ovarian size
Heart rate	Hematocrit	Ascites
Respiratory rate	LFT	Pleural effusion
Weight	RFT	Pericardial effusion
Abdominal girth	Electrolytes	Pregnancy status
Intake output chart	Coagulation profile	X-ray chest
	Blood gases	
	Beta-hCG	

- – Segment B: Optimum cryopreservation method or vitrification.
- – Segment C: Embryo replacement in nonstimulated, receptive endometrium.

The patient is treated according to the severity of the condition (Tables 15.1 and 15.2).

Outpatient Management of Moderate OHSS

Patient should report every day by telephone about her condition and she should be called twice a week for assessment.

Assessment:
- Symptoms: vomiting, pain, distention.
- Weight and abdominal girth, vital data.
- Pelvic ultrasound for ovarian size, ascites.
- Urine output, blood tests [blood count, LFT, renal function test (RFT) and coagulation profile, electrolytes].
- Patient should be educated to report for dyspnea, oliguria or neurological symptoms.

Patient should be clearly instructed for:
- No sexual intercourse
- No strenuous activity

- Oral intake of at least 1 L
- Leg exercises should be done to avoid thromboembolism.

Management of Severe OHSS

Outpatient management of severe OHSS can be done for only patients having grade A severe OHSS. Its feasibility depends on comfort of the physician and reliability of the patient. Early and frequent paracentesis is more effective and patient can be treated on outpatient basis.

Hospital Management

All the patients with grade B and C should be admitted. You have to be vigilant as complication can occur at any time.

Clinical Management

- General condition with all vital signs: hypotension, tachycardia due to decrease preload.
- Daily weight assessment and abdominal girth measurement of the patient.
- Intake and output chart (urine output important). Activation of renin-angiotensin mechanism causes increased ADH which causes oliguria. VPF plays an important role.

Biochemical Monitoring

- Blood count greater than 25,000, hematocrit greater than 45% is seen in severe cases.
- Count of 25,000, usually causes a hematocrit of 55%.
- Liver function test.
- Renal function test—creatinine greater than 1.2 mg.
- Serum electrolytes: Na less than 135 mEq/L, K greater than 5 mEq/L.

TABLE 15.2: Symptoms of moderate and severe OHSS.

Symptoms	Moderate OHSS	Severe OHSS grade A	Severe OHSS grade B	Severe OHSS grade C
Discomfort	+	+	+	+
Abdominal pain	+	+	+	+
Nausea	+	+	+	+
Distention	+	+	+	+
Dyspnea	–	+	+	+
Oliguria	–	+	+ <500 cc	+ <500 cc
Vomiting	–	+	+	+
Diarrhea	–	+	+	+
Signs				
Ascites	-ve	+	++	+++
Urine output	Normal	Oliguria	++	+++
Hydrothorax	-ve	+	++	+++
Ultrasound				
Ascites	+	+ve	++	+++
Large ovary	+ >5 cm	+ve	++ >8 cm	+++ >8 cm
Investigations				
hematocrit	<45	Normal	>45	>55
Blood comp	Normal	Normal	WBC >15,000	WBC >25,000
LFT	Normal	Normal	Abnormal	Abnormal
RFT	Normal	Normal	Creatinine >1.5	Creatinine >1.5
Coagulation profile	Normal	Normal		Abnormal
Electrolytes	Normal	Normal		Abnormal
Complications				
Renal failure	–			
Venous thrombosis	–			
ARDS	–			
Treatment		Indoor/outdoor	Indoor	ICU
	Outdoor	depends on patient condition	Expectant management	
		Dr's convenience facility		

- Coagulation profile.
- Blood gases.
- Beta-hCG.
- The frequency of repetition of investigations would depend on the severity of the condition.

On Ultrasound

- Ovarian size
- Ascites
- Pleural and pericardial effusion
- Status of pregnancy.

> **BOX 15.3:** Medical management of OHSS.
> - Antibiotic therapy
> - Volume correction
> - Electrolyte replacement
> - Anticoagulants
> - Diuretics
> - Other drugs
>   - Dopamine
>   - GnRH antagonist
>   - GnRH agonist.

X-ray chest: to exclude hydrothorax.

Invasive monitoring: Central venous pressure and pulmonary artery pressure assessment.

TREATMENT OF OHSS

After OHSS is diagnosed, drugs that are not effective are:
- Prostaglandin synthetase inhibitor
- Antihistamine
- Diuretics
- Danazol
- Volume expanders
- Dopamine
- Anticoagulant therapy
- Abdominal parameters.

On ultrasound:
- Ovarian size
- Ascites
- Pleural and pericardial effusion and status of pregnancy.

Antibiotic Therapy

Before doing any procedure like ascitic tapping or tapping of pleural effusion, antibiotic cover must be given. Hypoglobulinemia in severe cases may also predispose to infections (Box 15.3).

Volume Correction

High oral intake is advised in mild to moderate OHSS. Parental treatment includes IV fluids and plasma expanders in moderate and severe cases.

- *Intravenous fluids*: The motto for IV fluids is to maintain the intravascular volume and electrolyte balance. There is hemoconcentration and to preserve normal renal function, adequate intravascular volume is a must. Fluid should be replaced as crystalline solutions, i.e. normal saline or Ringer's lactate, like in treating hypovolemia, but it should be titrated with urine output to avoid overload. It should be given at a rate of 125–150 mL/hour and urine output of more than 20–30 mL/hour should be monitored.

- *Plasma expanders*: These can be used but gives temporary relief, but otherwise it may increase the third space volume by increasing the intravascular osmotic pressure. Albumin or HES (6%) are the ones commonly used. Albumin should be given in a dose of 50–100 g at 25% concentration every 2–12 hourly till hematocrit falls below 45% and urine output increases. Risks of human blood products must be kept in mind. The reports for the efficacy of these compounds in treating established OHSS are varied in different studies. Though their role for prevention of OHSS is more convincing and can be given at the time of ovum pick-up. Hematocrit should be repeatedly checked when these compounds are administered. Combination of albumin and furosemide works well in patients with oliguria. First the plasma volume is increased by albumin and then if urine output is low, adds furosemide.

Electrolyte Replacement

Electrolyte imbalance should be corrected. Salt and water restrictions are not required during the treatment.[39] Though in cases with ARDS, fluid restriction and dopamine forced diuresis are required. It occurs after fluid overload and so fluids may have to be restricted in severe

OHSS. DNS is always preferred. It is important to avoid hypotonic solution like Ringer's lactate that contains potassium.

Anticoagulants

Venous thrombosis is one of the most serious complications of OHSS and is best prevented. Preventive measures with heparin are extremely beneficial in hypercoagulable states or when there is risk of thromboembolism. Immobilization, pressure on ovaries and ascites, hypercoagulable state due to pregnancy and hyperestrinism all add to the risk of thromboembolism. Heparin as prophylaxis is extremely beneficial for the patient. Though there are diverse views for the use of heparin in severe OHSS, but still should be given in all the patients of congenital thrombophilia or with family history of thrombotic disorders. Prophylaxis is continued for 12–20 weeks depending on the condition of the patient. Hyperestrinism is the precipitating factor along with hypovolemia and hypotension. Arterial thrombosis is more common than venous thrombosis, which occurs later on.

Diuretics

These are contraindicated as will cause more hemoconcentration. This will increase blood viscosity and thromboembolism. The only indication of diuretics in OHSS is pulmonary edema. It may be given in patients with oliguria and only after sufficient hemodilution.
- Abdominal paracentesis may be helpful in these cases.
- GnRH antagonist on 6th day of pick-up after 4 days of OHSS can reduce OHSS. Luteal support is given with estrogen and progesterone.[40]
- GnRHa will also help reduce OHSS.

Dopamine

It is extremely useful in OHSS patients with oliguria as it improves renal circulation. It is required for only 7 days in nonpregnant patients, but if the patient has conceived it may be required for 10–20 days depending on rise in beta-hCG. Recommended dose is 4.32 mg/kg/24 hours.[41] 750 mg tablet of dopamine 8 hourly can be a suitable dose to reduce the severity of OHSS.

Indomethacin

Prostaglandin inhibitors like indomethacin do not cause any clinical improvement in the condition. Instead it may be dangerous due to renal toxicity.[39]

Fluid Aspiration

Indications: Relief of the symptoms, oliguria, tense ascites, rising serum creatinine, hemoconcentration not responding to medical line of treatment, respiratory symptoms. Acute distention of the abdomen, acute abdominal pain, dyspnea, deteriorating respiratory function tests and oliguria are absolute indications (Box 15.4).
- *Transvaginal sonography (TVS)-guided aspiration*: It is a safe and effective procedure. Injury to the ovaries can be avoided and maximum fluid can be aspirated from the dependent pocket. This reduces pressure on the kidney and improves renal perfusion and urine output.

BOX 15.4: Surgical management of ovarian hyperstimulation syndrome (OHSS).

- Aspiration of ascitic fluid and tapping of pleural effusion in severe OHSS
- Dealing with surgical emergencies:
  - Ovarian torsion
  - Ectopic pregnancy
  - Cyst rupture
  - Thromboembolism
  - Pregnancy termination.

It relieves pain, improves respiration and decreases distention. Early and frequent paracentesis are more effective, even on outpatient basis.

- *Abdominal paracentesis*: It has the same advantages as TVS-guided aspiration, but there is a risk of occasional injury to the friable large ovary and may lead to hemoperitoneum. Percutaneous pigtail catheter can be placed to avoid repeated punctures for repeated aspirations. Amount of fluid to be aspirated depends on severity of the symptoms and may vary from 500–4,000 cc. Albumin transfusion may be required to compensate for the protein loss in the aspirated fluid.
- *Autotransfusion of ascitic fluid*: This is a simple and safe procedure. Administration of exogenous fluid is not required. But the disadvantage is reinjection of cytokines in the circulation that may aggravate OHSS. Peritoneovenous shunting in antecubital vein is also recommended.[42]
- *Pleurocentesis*: This gives dramatic improvement in symptoms. Pulmonary thrombosis needs to be excluded before pleurocentesis as a cause of severe pulmonary symptoms.
- Pericardial effusion tapping may be rarely required.

Surgical Treatment

- *Ovarian torsion*: Patient complains of severe unilateral or bilateral abdominal pain. The diagnosis is by ultrasound with Doppler. Whirlpool sign and gradual loss of ovarian vascularity are the signs commonly found on ultrasound, though later may not be seen in all cases or may be seen to variable extent.[16] Early diagnosis can save the ovary. Ovarian unwinding is done by laparoscopy and this regains the ovarian vascularity and perfusion.

- *Ectopic pregnancy*: Due to large ovaries and ascites, the diagnosis is difficult. Rapid deterioration in patient's clinical condition and falling hemoglobin may be indicative.
- *Surgery for ruptured cyst*: Hemostasis is achieved by laparoscopy or open surgery depending on surgeon's expertise. It needs to be differentiated from ectopic pregnancy.
- *Pregnancy termination*: This may be required in very severe cases with marked renal and respiratory symptoms.

RECENT ADVANCES

Vascular endothelial growth factor is the critical modulator of the syndrome. Treatment with VEGF receptor antagonist prevents the capillary permeability in OHSS in rat model.[43] Similarly treatment with *fms*-like tyrosine kinase which binds with VEGF and decreases its availability for endothelial effects have similar results in OHSS in rat model.[44]

REFERENCES

1. Rizk B, Rizk CB, Nawar MG, et al. Ultrasonography in the prediction and management of ovarian hyperstimulation syndrome. In: Rizk B (Ed). Ultrasonography in Reproductive Medicine and Infertility. Cambridge, UK: Cambridge University Press; 2010. pp. 299-312.
2. De Neubourg D, Mangelschots K, Van Royen E, et al. Singleton pregnancies are as affected by ovarian hyperstimulation syndrome as twin pregnancies. Fertil Steril. 2004;82:1691-3.
3. Rizk B, Aboulghar MA. Classification, pathophysiology and management of ovarian hyperstimulation syndrome. In: Brinsden P (Ed). A Textbook of In-Vitro Fertilization and Assisted Reproduction, 2nd edition. Carnforth, UK: The Parthenon Publishing Group; 1999. pp 131-55.
4. Rizk B, Aboulghar M, Smitz J, et al. The role of vascular endothelial growth factor and interleukins in the pathogenesis of severe

ovarian hyperstimulation syndrome. Hum Reprod Update. 1997;3:255-66.

5. Krasnow JS, Berga SL, Guzick DS, et al. Vascular permeability factor and vascular endothelial growth factor in ovarian hyperstimulation syndrome: a preliminary report. Fertil Steril. 1996;65(3):552-5.

6. La Marca A, Guilini S, Tirelli A, et al. Anti-Mullerian hormone measurement on any day of the menstrual cycle strongly predicts ovarian response in assisted reproductive technology. Hum Reprod. 2007;22:766-71.

7. Lee TH, Liu CH, Huang CC, et al. Serum anti-Mullerian hormone and estradiol levels as predictors of ovarian hyperstimulation syndrome in assisted reproductive technology cycles. Hum Reprod. 2008;23:160-7.

8. Rizk B. Genetics of ovarian hyperstimulation syndrome. Reprod Biomed Online. 2009;19:14-27.

9. Daelemans C, Smits G, de Maertelaer V, et al. Prediction of severity of symptoms in iatrogenic ovarian hyperstimulation syndrome by follicle-stimulating hormone receptor Ser680Asn polymorphism. J Clin Endocrinol Metab. 2004;89:6310-5.

10. Moron FJ, de Castro F, Royo JL, et al. Bone morphogenetic protein 15 (BMP15) alleles predict over-response to recombinant follicle stimulation hormone and iatrogenic ovarian hyperstimulation syndrome (OHSS). Pharmacogenet Genomics. 2006;16:485-95.

11. Ajonuma LC, Tsang LL, Zhang GH, et al. Estrogen-induced abnormally high cystic fibrosis transmembrane conductance regulator expression results in ovarian hyperstimulation syndrome. Mol Endocrinol. 2005;19:3038-44.

12. Blankstein J, Shalev J, Saadon T, et al. Ovarian hyperstimulation syndrome: prediction by number and size of preovulatory ovarian follicles. Fertil Steril. 1987;47(4):597-602.

13. Bergh C, Howles CM, Borg K, et al. Recombinant human follicle-stimulating hormone (r-hFSH; Gonal F) versus highly purified urinary FSH (Metrodin HP): results of a randomized comparative study in women undergoing assisted reproductive techniques. Hum Reprod. 1997;12:2133-9.

14. Oyesanya OA, Parsons JH, Collins WP, et al. Total ovarian volume before human chorionic gonadotrophin administration for ovulation induction may predict the hyperstimulation syndrome. Hum Reprod. 1995;10:3211-2.

15. Al-Inany H, Aboulghar M. GnRH antagonist in assisted reproduction: a Cochrane review. Hum Reprod. 2002;17:874-85.

16. Al-Inany HG, Abou-Setta AM, Aboulghar M. Gonadotropin-releasing hormone antagonists for assisted conception. Cochrane Database Syst Rev. 2006;(3):CD001750.

17. Kolibianakis EM, Collins J, Tarlatzis BC, et al. Among patients treated for IVF with gonadotropins and GnRH analogues, is the probability of live birth dependent on the type of analogue used? A systematic review and meta-analysis. Hum Reprod Update. 2006;12:651-71.

18. Tang T, Glanville J, Orsi N, et al. The use of metformin for women with PCOS undergoing IVF treatment. Hum Reprod. 2006;21:1416-25.

19. Moll E, van der Veen F, van Wely M. The role of metformin in polycystic ovarian syndrome: a systematic review. Hum Reprod Update. 2007;13:527-37.

20. Son WY, Yoon SH, Lee SW, et al. Blastocyst development and pregnancies after IVF of mature oocytes retrieved from unstimulated patients with PCOS after in-vivo hCG priming. Hum Reprod. 2002;17:134-6.

21. Polson DW, Mason HD, Saldahna MB, et al. Ovulation of a single dominant follicle during treatment with low-dose pulsatile FSH in women with PCOS. Clin Endocrinol (Oxf). 1987;26:205-12.

22. Martinez F, Rodriguez DB, Buxaderas R, et al. GnRH antagonist rescue of a long-protocol IVF cycle and GnRH agonist trigger to avoid ovarian hyperstimulation syndrome: three case reports. Fertil Steril. 2011;95(7):2432.e17-9.

23. Aboulghar M. Agonist and antagonist coast. Fertil Steril. 2012; 97(3):523-6.

24. Chen D, Burmeister L, Goldschlag D, et al. Ovarian hyperstimulation syndrome: Strategies for prevention. Reprod Biomed Online. 2003;7:43-9.

25. Humaidan P, Bredkjaer HE, Westergaard LG, et al. 1,500 IU human chorionic gonadotropin

administered at oocyte retrieval rescues the luteal phase when gonadotropin-releasing hormone agonist is used for ovulation induction: a prospective, randomized, controlled study. Fertil Steril. 2010;93:847-50.

26. Griesinger G, von Otte S, Schroer A, et al. Elective cryopreservation of all pronuclear oocytes after GnRH agonist triggering of final oocyte maturation in patients at risk of developing OHSS: a prospective, observational proof-of-concept study. Hum Reprod. 2007;22:1348-52.

27. Ludwig M, Katalinic A, Diedrich K. Use of GnRH antagonists in ovarian stimulation for assisted reproductive technologies compared to long protocol. Meta-analysis. Arch Gynecol Obstet. 2001;265:175-82.

28. Aboulghar M, Evers JH, Al-Inany H. Intravenous albumin for preventing severe ovarian hyperstimulation syndrome. Cochrane Database Syst Rev. 2000;2:CD001302.

29. Youssef MA, Al-Inany HG, Evers JL, et al. Intravenous fluids for the prevention of severe ovarian hyperstimulation syndrome. Cochrane Database Syst Rev. 2011;(2):CD001302.

30. Rizk B. Ovarian hyperstimulation syndrome. In: Studd J (Ed). Progress in Obstetrics and Gynaecology. Edinburgh: Churchill Livingstone; 1993. pp. 31-49.

31. Varnagy A, Bodis J, Manfai Z, et al. Low-dose aspirin therapy to prevent ovarian hyperstimulation syndrome. Fertil Steril. 2010;93:2281-4.

32. Revelli A, Dolfin E, Gennarelli G, et al. Low-dose acetylsalicylic acid plus prednisolone as an adjuvant treatment in IVF: a prospective, randomized study. Fertil Steril. 2008;90:1685-91.

33. Youssef MA, van Wely M, Hassan MA, et al. Can dopamine agonist reduce the incidence and severity of OHSS in IVF/ICSI treatment cycles? A systematic review and meta-analysis. Hum Reprod Update. 2010;16(5):459-66.

34. Griesinger G, Schultz L, Bauer T, et al. Ovarian hyperstimulation syndrome prevention by gonadotropin-releasing hormone agonist triggering of final oocyte maturation in a gonadotropin-releasing hormone antagonist protocol in combination with 'freeze-all'

strategy: a prospective multicentric study. Fertil Steril. 2011;95:2029-33.

35. D'angelo, Amso N. Embryo freezing for preventing ovarian hyperstimulation syndrome. Cochrane Database Syst Rev. 2007;(3):CD002806.

36. Zhu WJ, Li XM, Chen XM, et al. Follicular aspiration during the selection phase prevents severe ovarian hyperstimulation in patients with polycystic ovary syndrome who are undergoing in vitro fertilization. Eur J Obstet Gynecol Reprod Biol. 2005;122(1):79-84.

37. Yakovenko SA, Sivozhelezov VS, Zorina IV, et al. Prevention of OHSS by intravenous calcium. Hum Reprod. 2009;24(Suppl 1):i61.

38. Gurgan T, Demirol A, Guven S, et al. Intravenous calcium infusion as a novel preventive therapy of ovarian hyperstimulation syndrome for patients with polycystic ovarian syndrome. Fertil Steril. 2011;96:53-7.

39. Rizk B. Ovarian Hyperstimulation Syndrome: Epidemiology, Pathophysiology, Prevention and Management. Cambridge, UK: Cambridge University Press; 2006.

40. Lainas TG, Sfontouris IA, Zorzovilis IZ, et al. Live births after management of severe OHSS by GnRH antagonist administration in the luteal phase. Reprod Biomed Online. 2009;19(6):789-95.

41. Aboulghar MA, Mansour RT, Serour GI, et al. Ultrasonically guided vaginal aspiration of ascites in the treatment of severe ovarian hyperstimulation syndrome. Fertil Steril. 1990;53:933-5.

42. Koike T, Araki S, Minakami H, et al. Clinical efficacy of peritoneovenous shunting for the treatment of severe OHSS. Hum Reprod. 2000;15:113-7.

43. Gomez R, Simon C, Remohi J, et al. Vascular endothelial growth factor receptor-2 activation induces vascular permeability in hyperstimulated rats, and this effect is prevented by receptor blockade. Endocrinology. 2002;143:4339-48.

44. McElhinney B, Ardill J, Caldwell C, et al. Preventing ovarian hyperstimulation syndrome by inhibiting the effects for vascular endothelial growth factor. J Reprod Med. 2003;48:243-6.

Luteal Phase Defect

Chaitanya Nagori

INTRODUCTION

Luteal phase starts from ovulation and ends at the onset of menstruation or when the pregnancy is diagnosed. The dominant follicle after ovulation is converted into corpus luteum and it is one of the most hormonally active glands in the body. Progesterone secretion from corpus luteum is the hallmark of luteal phase.

Luteal phase defect (LPD) is defined as inadequate corpus luteal function in the latter half of the ovulatory cycle. It is due to insufficient endogenous progesterone production or suboptimal response of endometrium to normal progesterone level. LPD is also known as luteal phase insufficiency or corpus luteum insufficiency or inadequate luteal phase. LPD is associated with infertility, early pregnancy loss, short cycles and premenstrual spotting.

Role of progesterone in luteal phase has been shown in Box 16.1.

PATHOPHYSIOLOGY

Deficient progesterone secretion from corpus luteum can be due to abnormal folliculogenesis, leading to unhealthy follicle that secretes low levels of estradiol (E2); therefore, inadequate luteinizing hormone (LH) surge. Inadequate LH surge may cause luteinization but ovulation might not occur and produces unhealthy corpus luteum, producing low level progesterone.

So, adequate LH surge is a must for a healthy corpus luteum. It is the most vascular organ. Blood flow to corpus luteum is 6–10 mL/g/minute.[1] Daily progesterone production from corpus luteum is 25–50 mg, and is secreted in pulses, every 90 minutes. Progesterone and E2 secretion from corpus

---

BOX 16.1: Role of progesterone in luteal phase.

- Brings about secretory changes for implantation
- Vasodilatation for improved flow in endometrium
- Downregulates ERs, LIF and beta-integrin
- Decidualization with pinopode formation
- Upregulation of IGF-1, interleukin, Hoxa genes, cytokines, EGF, TGF, VEGF, mucin I, integrins, selectins, immunoglobulins, etc.
- Relaxes uterine musculature
- Improves endometrial receptivity.

(ERs: estrogen receptors; LIF: leukemia inhibitory factor; IGF-1: insulin-like growth factor-1; EGF: epithelial growth factor; TGF: transforming growth factor; VEGF: vascular endothelial growth factor)

luteum correlates with LH pulse. Average E2 production is 0.6 mg/day in luteal phase. Corpus luteum secretes estrogen under the influence of LH and insulin-like growth factor-1 (IGF-1) and not follicle-stimulating hormone (FSH). Decline in steroidogenic acute regulatory (StAR) protein expression decreases steroidogenesis and luteolysis.[2]

Corpus luteum has two types of cells. The large cells develop from granulosa cells and secrete progesterone in the first half of luteal phase under the influence of LH pulse. The small cells develop from theca interna and produce progesterone after the stimulation of human chorionic gonadotropin (hCG).[3,4]

Estrogen induces progesterone receptors. Progesterone acts through its own receptors and produces mediator protein known as "progesterone-induced blocking factor" (PIBF). PIBF produces asymmetrical antibodies, i.e. T helper cell type 2 (Th2) and natural killer (NK) cells for protection.

If PIBF is inadequate, Th1 and lymphokine-activated killer (LAK) cells are produced which are cytotoxic and reject the embryo.[5] So the acceptance or rejection depends on the estrogen and progesterone.

Pathway

This StAR protein is not present in granulosa cells and appears after LH peak only. Before preovulatory period, this protein expression is on the theca cells and converts cholesterol into androgen (Flowchart 16.1).

LUTEAL PHASE PHYSIOLOGY

Preovulation LH surge is the stimulus for the luteinization. LH from pituitary continues to act through endocrine feedback during entire luteinization process. In patients with luteal

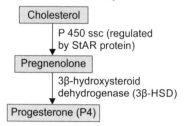

Flowchart 16.1: Pathway of cholesterol.

phase less than 10 days, lower levels of FSH and LH are found in proliferative phase. Long follicular phase cycles do not have short luteal phase in majority of cases. Day 3 high estrone-3-glucuronide (ETG) and pregnanediol 3-alpha glucuronide (PDG) are predictors of short early luteal phase. Here LH is increased in about half the cycles. Luteal phase has three phases. The first is a modulated luteinization process whereas second and third are relatively less modulated processes of progesterone and luteolysis.

- Duration is 12–14 days.
- Progesterone peak is 6–8 days after ovulation. Progesterone is secreted in pulses.
- Luteinizing hormone peak decides the quality of corpus luteum.
- Pulsatile LH is necessary for corpus luteum function.
- Steroidogenic acute regulatory protein governs cholesterol transport for progesterone production.
- Corpus luteum is refractory to LH in later half.
- Human chorionic gonadotropin can rescue corpus luteum by StAR and vascular endothelial growth factor (VEGF) after implantation.
- Minimum required levels of progesterone are not confirmed.
- Luteal phase E2 is LH dependent and not FSH dependent.[2]

- Hyperprolactinemia—luteolysis of corpus luteum
- Obesity—abnormal folliculogenesis
- PCOS—due to premature LH surge
- Anorexia nervosa—abnormal FSH and LH secretion
- Endometriosis—immunological cause
- Athletes—abnormal LH surge
- Extremes of age—abnormal folliculogenesis
- Postpartum due to low LH
- Stress—disturbed GnRH secretion
- Infections.

CAUSES OF LUTEAL PHASE DEFECT IN NON-IVF CYCLES

Hypothalamic-pituitary dysfunction disturbs gonadotropin-releasing hormone (GnRH) pulsatility which in turn disturbs the secretion of FSH and LH which causes poor folliculogenesis and LPDs.

The causes of LPD have been shown in Box 16.2.

RESCUE OF CORPUS LUTEUM IN INFERTILE PATIENT

Human chorionic gonadotropin from embryo restores StAR protein expression to late corpus luteum and induces progesterone production and production of VEGF that causes angiogenesis.

Implantation occurs between day 8 and day 10 after LH surge. Miscarriage rate is very high if implantation is late because unhealthy embryo produces less hCG and inadequate rescue signals in spite of normal corpus luteum. So low progesterone in early pregnancy is because of low hCG produced by unhealthy embryo and progesterone supplementation does not work.[6] Placental steroidogenesis starts at 7 weeks. Corpus luteum starts reducing after 5 weeks of pregnancy but remains active up to 11 weeks. 17-hydroxyprogesterone (17-OHP) is secreted by corpus luteum only and starts regressing after 5 weeks along with regressing vascularity.

After 5 weeks, even hCG does not increase neoangiogenesis and this indicates that hCG-induced rescue for corpus luteum is temporary.[7]

DIAGNOSIS OF LUTEAL PHASE DEFECT

- *History*: Short luteal phase of less than 13 days from the LH surge to menstruation may be indicative of LPD. Patient may have premenstrual spotting, infertility and early abortions. But history is not conclusive, for diagnosis of LPD.
- *Basal body temperature (BBT) chart*: Absence or inadequate thermogenic shift in BBT chart indicates LPD. Its utility is questioned and presently it has no place in diagnosis of luteal phase abnormality.
- *Endometrial biopsy*: Noyce criteria for dating of endometrium are very popular since about six decades. Though endometrial histology is an indirect marker of progesterone action, there is interobserver variation and also intercycle variability. There is no consensus whether biopsy should be taken in one or two or three cycles. Biopsy taken in the latter half of the luteal phase indicates total progesterone effect rather than progesterone secretion on that day. The most interesting thing is that out of phase endometrial histology is also seen in fertile patients and patients who conceive.[8] So endometrial histology is not used as a criteria for diagnosis of LPD.
- *Serum progesterone*: Progesterone secretion starts after 30 minutes of LH surge. In early luteal phase, progesterone secretion is nonpulsatile but in mid and late luteal phase, its secretion becomes pulsatile. Therefore, single assessment does not reflect the actual progesterone secretion. It was reported that three readings between day 5 and day 9 postovulatory should be

taken and cutoff of 30 ng/mL was thought to have a sensitivity of 100% and specificity of 80%.[9] Normal progesterone level in mid luteal phase is 10 ng/mL. But there are no studies to confirm these findings. Histology of the endometrium does not correlate with progesterone level. So progesterone does not differentiate normal and defective luteal phase. Serum progesterone greater than 3 ng/mL only documents ovulation. But it is not used for diagnosis of LPD.

- *Ultrasound*:
  - Correlation of corpus luteum resistance index (RI) and serum progesterone.
  - Corpus luteum Doppler shows high resistance flow (RI 0.58 ± 0.4) (Figs. 16.1A and B).
  - Bilateral high resistance intraovarian flow, and same in both ovaries, unlike normal luteal phase that shows low resistance in the dominant ovary.
  - Increased resistance in spiral artery RI (0.72 + 0.06) (Figs. 16.2A and B).
- *New promising tests*:
  - Daily salivary progesterone measurement.
  - PIBF measurement.

Currently no tests can stamp the diagnosis of LPD and differentiate fertile from infertile patients.[6]

Controversies in Diagnosis

- Luteal phase defect can exist with normal progesterone levels.[10]
- There may be no correlation of endometrial histology and serum progesterone.
- Pregnancy can continue with lower serum progesterone levels.
- Serum progesterone and endometrial biopsy are not related tests.
- Some papers say that E2:P ratio is more important than only progesterone levels.[11]
- No tests can stamp the diagnosis.
- The timing of embryo transfer depends on the duration of exposure rather than blood levels.[12]

THERAPY FOR LUTEAL PHASE DEFECT

- Ovulation induction
- Human chorionic gonadotropin supplementation
- Progesterone supplementation.

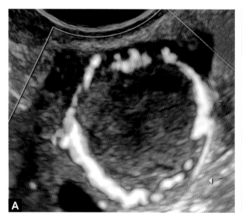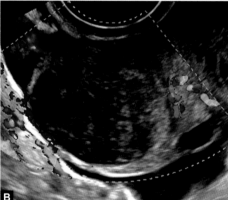

Figs. 16.1A and B: (A) Normal corpus luteal flow as a complete ring of color; (B) Scanty corpus luteal flow of corpus luteal inadequacy—luteal phase defect.

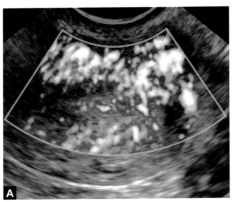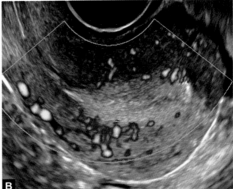

Figs. 16.2A and B: (A) Normal secretory endometrial flow; (B) Scanty secretory endometrial flow—luteal phase defect.

Ovulation Induction

Inadequate luteal function is because of inadequate follicular development. Ovulation induction will lead to development of better cohort of follicles and high E2, that induces LH and progesterone receptors and corrects LPD. Progesterone gives the better pregnancy rates.[13]

Clomiphene citrate: Clomiphene acts on hypothalamus and pituitary to secrete FSH and LH that leads to development of follicles and secretes more estrogen. High estrogen causes upregulation of LH and progesterone receptors. Therefore, in clomiphene-stimulated cycles, LPD is not common. In spite of estrogen receptors being occupied by CC, multiple follicles develop and there is no abnormality of LH or progesterone secretion because of high E2 level. LPD found in clomiphene citrate (CC) cycle is due to high LH, particularly in polycystic ovarian syndrome (PCOS) patients, that is detrimental to ovum leading to abnormal folliculogenesis, and is responsible for LPD. Adding estrogen to clomiphene is not proved to improve the pregnancy rate. Clomiphene, letrozole or gonadotropins can be used for ovulation induction.

Human Chorionic Gonadotropin Supplementation

In a normo-ovulatory female, in unstimulated cycle, administration of hCG in luteal phase does not downregulate LH secretion in luteal phase.[14]

It stimulates theca lutein cells to produce more progesterone and other steroids that are required for the maintenance of normal pregnancy. hCG also increases the placental protein 4 and relaxin that are required for implantation. It is administered every 3–4 days. It is given in the dosage of 2,000 IU on day 3, 7, 10 or 5,000 IU on day 5–9 postovulatory. It is an excellent drug in non-in vitro fertilization (IVF) patients and in poor responders in IVF also. But if the pretrigger E2 is more than 1,600 IU in intrauterine insemination (IUI) cycle and more than 4,000 IU in IVF cycle, hCG is not given as a trigger for the risk of ovarian hyperstimulation syndrome (OHSS). In these cases, agonist is given as a trigger. In these cases, hCG 1,500 IU is given at the time of IUI or at the time of ovum pick-up (OPU) to rescue the corpus luteum, if the number of follicles are not more than 25 of more than 11 mm in diameter. It gives equal pregnancy rates as hCG trigger and avoids OHSS.[15,16]

It can be used safely even in IVF cycles especially in poor responders. But now since antagonist can be used to suppress LH surge and agonist can be used for ovulation trigger, hCG in these patients can be used in the dose of 1,500 IU every fourth day as a luteal phase support.

Disadvantages

- It should not be given when E2 is more than 1,600 pg/mL in IUI cycles and more than 4,000 pg/mL in IVF cycles because of development of OHSS and multiple pregnancies.
- When there are more follicles, it will increase E2 and may change E2:P which may decrease implantation but this is only theoretical assumption.
- Even the low dose of hCG as 1,500 IU is given, every 3 days after agonist trigger, can cause OHSS.[15]
- Prolonged hCG exposure in proliferative phase may affect endometrial receptivity.[17] During natural menstrual cycle, LH in luteal phase seldom exceeds 5–10 IU/mL, which is capable of eliciting progesterone level in excess of 25–35 nmol/L. So supraphysiological levels of LH/hCG is not required in luteal phase. Endogenous Progesterone is very high due to multiple corpus lutea and exogenous progesterone results in concentration of <75 nmol/L only.

Microdose supplement 100–150 IU/day of hCG throughout the luteal phase without using any exogenous progesterone is sufficient. The progesterone level thus achieved is similar to that achieved when ovulation trigger is given by 6500 IU hCG and progesterone support. When this microdose hCG is used with agonist trigger, hCG levels remains within physiological limits, i.e. 5–10 IU/mL. The only difficulty is the delivery of microdose.[18]

Progesterone Supplementation

Progesterone has an important role in inducing or in facilitating LH surge and is also required for full responsiveness of pituitary to GnRH.[19,20]

Role of Progesterone

- Secretory endometrial transformation and receptivity depends solely on duration of exposure to adequate progesterone concentration provided that sufficient estrogen priming has already occurred during follicular phase.[21] *It causes local vasodilatation for better perfusion.*
- It causes quiescence of uterine muscles by inducing nitric oxide synthesis in decidua.[22]
- Uterine relaxing property of progesterone prevents expulsion of the embryo during and after embryo transfer.[23]
- Though progesterone is being given to support pregnancy, it has been shown by Kyrou et al. in a study on recombinant FSH (rFSH)/antagonist cycles, that withdrawal of progesterone supplementation in early pregnancy, with normally increasing beta-hCG levels on 16th post-embryo transfer day had no clinical impact on ongoing pregnancy rates.[24] Prolongation of progesterone supplementation in early pregnancy has no influence on pregnancy outcomes in GnRH agonist (GnRHa) cycles also.[25]
- Older patients and those with endometriosis might need longer progesterone support due to progesterone resistance.[26]
- Luteal phase defect occurs in stimulated cycles due to multiple follicular development that leads to supraphysiological levels of progesterone from multiple corpora luteum. This gives a negative feedback to LH and causes LPD.[27] Therefore, progesterone supplement is required for first 2 weeks after embryo transfer. Once trophoblast

starts secreting hCG, progesterone secretion is stimulated from corpus lutea by endogenous hCG. hCG injection given for ovulation trigger supports luteal phase for first 8 days.[28]

Different Progesterones

Synthetic progesterones: These are medroxyprogesterone acetate and dydrogesterone. These are not commonly used as luteal support. Vaginal micronized progesterone is significantly more effective than oral dydrogesterone in creating "in-phase secretory endometrium".[29,30] But Ganesh et al. have found oral dydrogesterone to be a promising drug for luteal support in women undergoing IVF.[31] It has also been confirmed in another study that dydrogesterone is as effective as micronized vaginal progesterone for luteal support.[32]

Natural progesterones:
- Not commonly used routes:
  - Intranasal
  - Sublingual
  - Rectal.
- Commonly used routes:
  - Oral
  - Intramuscular (IM)
  - Vaginal routes.

Oral progesterones:
- It causes drowsiness, flushing and nausea and it has selective and hypnotic effect because of metabolites.
- It causes fluid retention.
- Efficacy changes with food particle size and its vehicle. Bioavailability is only 10% when taken orally.
- Extensive first pass hepatic metabolism and therefore multiple doses required. It has poor intestinal absorption.
- It is ineffective in inducing an in-phase secretory endometrium.[33]

- It has lower pregnancy rate.
- Slow-release (SR) EROMAT is a new technology. The drug is released gradually in a controlled manner over a span of 16–24 hours in the distal part of the gastrointestinal tract allowing lymphatic absorption of intact drug into systematic circulation and direct entry of the drug through the mucosal lining of colon into systemic circulation. The dose of sustained release progesterone capsule is 300 mg daily. This has less side effects compared to conventional oral preparation.

Oral progesterone and dihydrogesterone failed to foster predecidual transformation in absence of endogenous progesterone.[34] Because of the failed acid test, uncertainty remains as to whether these synthetic drugs will be actually effective in assisted reproductive technology (ART) patients. Use of dihydrogesterone for endometrial support in donor cycles failed to affect predecidual transformation. Hence, its use in luteal phase support is not beneficial.

Intramuscular progesterone:
- It gives high serum concentrations, adequate endometrial secretory features and satisfactory pregnancy rates, comparable to vaginal progesterone.
- Daily injections are uncomfortable and very painful and may result in inferior secretory endometrial histology.
- It can cause inflammation at injection site leading to redness, pain and even sterile abscess at injection site because of the preservative (Benzyl alcohol) used.
- Rarely it may also cause acute eosinophilic pneumonia.
- It is not preferred in favor of vaginal progesterone.

Subcutaneous (SC) aqueous progesterone preparations are also available now, in which progesterone is combined with cyclodextrin, a starch residue, and is given as 25 mg or 50 mg doses twice a day and has shown results comparable with IM progesterone.[35] Gillian et al. have proved that SC injection of water soluble progesterone 25 mg is safe and as effective as vaginal progesterone gel and remains an option for those, who do not want vaginal progesterone on cultural, personal or medical reasons.[36] Transdermal progesterone is not the option because the skin is rich in 5 reductase, which will inactivate progesterone. Another reason is that daily E2 production is 0.5 mg/24 hours, while that of progesterone is 25 mg/24 hours. Such large doses are difficult to deliver by transdermal patches.

3. Vaginal progesterone: Vaginal progesterone is highly effective and predictable. In spite of subnormal serum progesterone levels, there is high tissue concentration of progesterone. This is because of the direct transport of the drug from vagina to uterus—first uterine pass effect (FUPE). This results from countercurrent exchange that affects upper one-third of vagina.[37,38] This is a vein to artery exchange.

Advantages of vaginal progesterone:
- Stable plasma concentration and consistent tissue levels.
- First uterine pass effect with targeted delivery into endometrium.
- Minimal side effects.

Vaginal progesterone application is now most accepted route. Progesterone because of its first pass effect reaches in high concentration to uterus.[39] So in spite of low serum levels, endometrial secretory transformation is adequate. It gives high implantation rate and low early pregnancy loss.[40]

Progesterone absorption changes with estrinization, formations like tablets, suppositories, cream, oil-based solution or gel. But better steady state serum progesterone concentrations are achieved with vaginal formulations.[41]

Progesterone vaginal effervescent tablets: This is a new delivery system of progesterone. Disintegration of tablet occurs in 7–10 minutes. It increases absorption. Twice a day dosage can achieve higher concentration of progesterone and reach steady state within 24–32 hours and maintain mean concentration above 10 ng/mL.[42]

As explained in Figure 16.3, the absorption of progesterone occurs by passive diffusion as well as paracellular transport which results in greater concentration and prolonged blood levels. CO_2 opens up tight junctions of the cells and so paracervical absorption is increased.

Advantage of effervescent tablet:
- Greater bioavailability
- Effective systemic absorption
- Avoids hepatic first pass metabolism
- Higher concentration in endometrium
- Lower doses are required
- Less fluctuation in serum levels
- Healthy vaginal environment because of acidic pH
- As efficient as other vaginal progesterone
- Less irritation and discharge.

Vaginal progesterone rings are also available now. These rings once inserted would release 10–20 nmol/L of progesterone for 90 days. Compared to 50 mg/day IM progesterone, this product has shown comparable or better implantation rate.[43]

Progesterone gel: It contains 90 mg (8%) of progesterone. It contains micronized progesterone in emulsion system which also contains water soluble polymer, "polycarbophil" having mucin like actions. It is as effective as vaginal tablets. There is no substantial difference in ongoing pregnancy

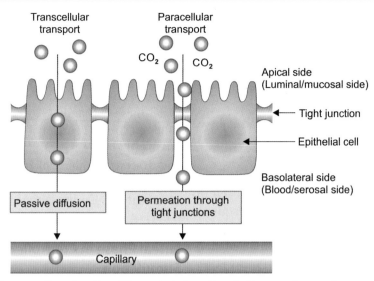

Fig. 16.3: Diagrammatic explanation of the vaginal absorption of effervescent progesterone vaginal tablets.

rate between vaginal progesterone gel and vaginal micronized progesterone tablets.[44] But vaginal gel has given higher pregnancy rates than IM progesterone below the age of 35 years in IVF patients and after the age of 35 years, pregnancy rates were same for both the gel and the IM progesterone group.[45] Its dosage schedule is once a day, so acceptance is very good. Only disadvantage of this preparation is its high cost.

Progesterone combinations:
- Progesterone + E2: No role except in long protocol where it may improve implantation.[46]
- Progesterone + ascorbic acid: No role.[47]
- Progesterone + prednisolone: No role.[48]
- Progesterone + aspirin: No role.[49]

Prednisolone and aspirin might have role in recurrent IVF failures.

Exogenous gonadotropins affect the ovaries to produce more E2. This leads to negative feedback to hypothalamic-pituitary-ovarian (HPO) axis and may lead to abnormal LH pulsatility and abnormal progesterone secretion from corpus luteum.[50] Though progesterone is important for pregnancy, elevated progesterone level on the day of trigger, affects pregnancy rates adversely. Progesterone level of 1.5 ng/mL is a threshold for poor ovarian responders, greater than 1.75 ng/mL is associated with low ongoing pregnancy rates for intermediate responders and 2.25 ng/mL can be applied for high responders.[51] This progesterone level is elevated in superovulated cycles as each mature follicle secretes a trace of progesterone. Endometrium is exposed to progesterone before hCG injection leads to decreased endometrial receptivity.[52] A systematic review and meta-analysis suggest that luteal phase support improved the likelihood of clinical pregnancy and live birth in gonadotropin-stimulated IUI cycles.[53]

GONADOTROPIN-RELEASING HORMONE AGONIST AS LUTEAL SUPPORT

- Gonadotropin-releasing hormone agonist increases LH secretion from pituitary.

- It acts directly on endometrium through locally expressed GnRH receptors.[54]
- Agonist increases serum hCG, by acting on embryos, E2 and progesterone levels in luteal phase of agonist and antagonist cycles.[55]
- But adverse effects on oocytes and embryo need evaluationally larger studies.

Gonadotropin-releasing hormone agonist is used for luteal support as it stimulates to release LH from the pituitary. It is used in combination with progesterone. It is given after 6 days after oocyte retrieval or 3 days after embryo transfer. It increases implantation and pregnancy rate in ART.[56] Pirard et al. introduced daily injection of GnRHa (nafarelin 200 µg twice a day) for 14 days for luteal support giving similar results.[54]

Cochrane meta-analysis demonstrated significantly higher pregnancy rate when progesterone luteal support was combined with GnRHa compared with progesterone alone without influencing the miscarriage rate or multiple pregnancy rate.[57] GnRHa acts on corpus luteum, endometrium and embryo by secretion of LH. Buserelin 200 µg twice a day or leuprolide acetate 1 mg as a single or multiple diseases can be given as a luteal support. It avoids OHSS in hyper-responders.

LUTEAL SUPPORT IN VARIOUS SITUATIONS

- Luteal phase in natural cycle
- Luteal phase in controlled ovarian stimulation
- Luteal phase in hCG trigger
- Luteal phase in IUI
- Luteal phase in IVF
- Luteal phase in agonist trigger
- Luteal phase with prolonged hCG exposure
- Luteal phase and recurrent pregnancy loss (RPL).

Luteal Phase in Natural Cycle

Endogenous LH is sufficiently enough to secure the functions of corpus luteum. High level of E2 and small rise of progesterone is responsible for FSH and LH surge in mid cycle. These FSH and LH surge last for about 48 hours. The LH surge has short ascending phase of 14 hours, a peak plateau of 20 hours and descending phase of 20 hours. This LH surge is sufficient to maintain luteal phase and so routine use of progesterone in luteal phase is not justified in natural unstimulated cycles.[2]

Luteal Phase in Controlled Ovarian Stimulation

It is an established fact that luteal phase is defective in all stimulated cycles.[28] In controlled ovarian stimulation, there are multiple follicles which grow giving supraphysiological levels of E2 and progesterone which inhibits LH secretion by the pituitary by negative feedback at hypothallamopituitary axis level for LH release which causes early demise of corpus luteum and fall in progesterone level.[58] Moreover, agonist or antagonist has already suppressed LH in follicular phase and therefore endogenous LH is very low. Adequate LH is important for maintenance of corpus luteum. So luteal phase support is required in all the patients when agonists or antagonists are used. Endogenous LH is also important for secretion of other growth factors and cytokines and leukemia inhibitory factor (LIF) for implantation. Exogenous hCG helps to rescue corpus luteum. In gonadotropin stimulation, there is advancement of histology in late proliferative phase, earlier shift into implantation window and asynchrony if the maturation of mid and late luteal phase due to high E2, i.e. altered E2/P ratio.[59]

Human chorionic gonadotropin administration and removal of granulosa cells may decrease the steroid production. Stimulated IVF cycles are associated with defective luteal phase in almost all patients.[60] High E2 does not increase uterine contractions (5/minute). But high E2 because of controlled ovarian stimulation causes some degree of resistance to the uterine quiescent effect of progesterone that can be countered by exogenous progesterone.

Luteal Support in Intrauterine Insemination

Progesterone support is beneficial for patients undergoing gonadotropin stimulation for IUI. But progesterone supplementation is not useful in clomiphene citrate-induced cycles. So endogenous luteal function depends on stimulation protocol.[53,61] Supraphysiological levels of steroids due to gonadotropins cause negative feedback to LH causing premature luteolysis and defective progesterone.[50] Efficacy with progesterone gel for luteal support in IUI was proved in the first published study.[62]

Luteal Phase in hCG Trigger

In follicular phase, LH is low because of agonist or antagonist as well as high E2 and progesterone giving negative feedback to pituitary for LH. However, early luteal phase function of LH is covered by bolus of hCG (5–1,000 IU), which is routinely used for trigger. hCG also secures growth factor and cytokines for implantation.

Human chorionic gonadotropin produced by the implanting embryo is detected as early as 8th day after ovulation that takes care of the luteal phase. Luteal phase support with progesterone is mandatory during overlapping period after ovarian stimulation for IVF to sustain early pregnancy.[63] On day 5 after OPU, LH levels are low because of negative feedback of high progesterone and exogenous hCG. It is crucial to have certain amplitude and frequency of LH during luteal phase. So progesterone supplementation is required.

Luteal Support in In Vitro Fertilization

Luteal support is mandatory in all IVF cycles.

Former belief that granulosa cells are removed during OPU is disproved.[64]

- GnRH agonist suppresses LH and FSH and causes LPD in almost all cases in long protocol. Prolonged suppression of LH results in lack of support to corpus luteum (Box 16.3).[65]
- Human chorionic gonadotropin for ovulation trigger suppresses LH in stimulated IVF cycles.[66] This is not the case in nonstimulated cycles.
- Antagonist cycles can reduce luteal phase length and may compromise pregnancy rate. Therefore, luteal support is mandatory.[67]
- Supraphysiological levels of steroids secreted by large number of corpora lutea during early secretory phase causes LPD by suppressing LH by negative feedback mechanism. High E2 does not cause increase in uterine contractions but causes some degree of resistance to uterine quiescence by endogenous progesterone, which can be countered by exogenous progesterone.
- Corpus luteum requires constant LH stimulation for performing physiological functions and withdrawal of LH causes luteolysis.[68]

> **BOX 16.3:** Causes of suppression of luteinizing hormone in IVF.
>
> - GnRh agonist
> - GnRH antagonist
> - High level E2
> - hCG trigger.

- Supraphysiological E2 may cause defect in endometrial receptivity but it is not proved by other studies but high E2 causes low progesterone by feedback mechanism.
- Pituitary gonadotropins remain suppressed up to 2–3 weeks after discontinuation of agonist. This prolonged suppression causes luteal phase deficiency in long protocol because of low E2 and progesterone secretion.[69]
- In antagonist cycle, there is a short luteal phase due to deficient LH secretion and causes LPD.[70] The study of donor stimulated cycle with antagonist definitely indicates deficient and abnormal luteal phase.[71] So the existing research strongly suggests luteal phase support in all ART cycles.[72]

Luteal Phase in Agonist Trigger

It is more physiological as it elicits FSH and LH surge on the day following the trigger. It differs from hCG as hCG gives you only LH surge, while agonist gives FSH and LH surge.

But this high LH is not sufficient to stimulate multiple corpus luteum to produce needed steroids. LH is enough for oocyte maturation and ovulation. So it is routine used in oocyte donors. On day OPU + 5, progesterone and E2 levels are very low, which is not the case with hCG trigger. So the luteal phase is extremely disturbed. The reason is that LH had short ascending phase of less than 4 hours instead of regular 14 hours. Increase in the dose of GnRHa does not correct this defect. So it is confirmed that LPD is because of low luteal LH levels. Luteal support with vaginal progesterone, may be insufficient in GnRHa trigger but luteal LH and IM progesterone normalize the endometrial receptivity.[73]

This relative short surge of LH can cause normal oocyte maturation and ovulation but luteal phase length is reduced significantly and there is incomplete luteinization. So luteal support is required under these conditions. Normal progesterone level on OPU + day 5 was 11 ng/mL after 600 mg/day of exogenous progesterone indicates complete luteal insufficiency after agonist. One bolus of 1,500 IU of hCG at the time of IUI or OPU after GnRHa trigger gives equivalent pregnancy rate and low incidence of OHSS, when there are 15–25 follicles of greater than 11 mm. But if you give 2nd bolus then incidence of OHSS is high.[15,74] Optimum receptivity of the endometrium is on day 3–5 of progesterone exposure.[75]

GnRhA trigger is used in freeze all policy and advantage is that PGS can be done for aneuploidy detection and transfer of healthy embryos can be done in the next cycle. The added advantage is that it eliminates the risk of OHSS.

Strategies for supporting luteal phase after GnRhA trigger:
- Exogenous E2 + P support with close monitoring.
- Dual trigger: Agonist + hCG (1000–2500 IU).
- hCG 1500 IU at the time of oocyte retrieval.
- Low dose hCG in luteal phase.
- Luteal phase LH administration.
- *Intensive luteal support:* IM progesterone 25–75 mg/day or micronized progesterone 800 mg/day vaginally with estradiol patch 0.1 mg, 3–4, on alternate days with 2–8 mg or oral estradiol valerate is given. Adjust the dose to keep serum E2 level above 2000 pgm/mL and progesterone level 20 ng/mL by frequent testing. The results are similar to those of hCG trigger and progesterone support.[76]
- *Dual trigger:* Along with GnRhA trigger, hCG 1000–2500 IU is added for rescuing CL by providing additional signal for adequate leutinization. It has given pregnancy rate up to 53% with one case of OHSS.[77] hCG

at the time of ovum pick up gives excellent results but incidence of OHSS is reduced with dual trigger.

- hCG at the time of oocyte retrieval (1500 IU—at pick up.
- *Low dose beta hCG:* 100–150 IU hCG as luteal support has already been discussed. Adding 1000 IU. of hCG may serve the same purpose and can be backed up in case of GnRHa trigger failure.
- *Luteal phase LH administration:* It is very costly but can also reduce the risk of OHSS.

Modified Luteal Phase Support

- Give GnRHa trigger.
- Human chorionic gonadotropin 1,500 IU after IUI or OPU.
- Vaginal micronized progesterone 400 mg BD.
- E2 2 mg, BD supplementation.

This regimen reduces OHSS, gives more eggs with equal live birth rates.[15]

Luteal Phase after Prolonged hCG Exposure in Proliferative Phase

Prolonged exposure to hCG in proliferative phase negatively affects pregnancy rate. hCG downregulates its own receptors in endometrium. Pre-exposure to chronic low-dose hCG renders the cell refractory to active hCG and prevents implantation. Otherwise hCG on day 8 from developing embryo rescues endometrium for implantation process.

Progesterone in Recurrent Pregnancy Loss

According to the American Society for Reproductive Medicine (ASRM) committee report, there is no proven role of adding progesterone or hCG for luteal support, once the pregnancy has been confirmed.[6] But 70% of the women with serum progesterone less than 15 ng/mL completes first trimester after adding progesterone. Check et al. have mentioned in their paper that 60% of pregnancies could be saved with progesterone supplementation even with serum progesterone less than 8 ng/mL. So low progesterone is a correctable cause of miscarriage. Empirical treatment advocated is benign and must be given rather than not treating the patient. It is also narrated in the same paper that need of progesterone supplementation, is seen only in one-third of pregnancies would it not be worthwhile to use such supplementation in every cycle to eliminate 33% miscarriage rate.

ESTRADIOL SUPPLEMENTATION IN LUTEAL PHASE

Estradiol supplementation is mandatory to prepare the endometrium for embryo recipient model. But several papers show that E2 supplementation is not necessary in luteal phase. In an IVF cycle, levels of estrogen and progesterone drop in mid to late luteal phase. It has not been proved that this drop has an effect on clinical pregnancy rates in meta-analysis conducted by Fatemi et al., whether only progesterone or estrogen plus progesterone were added in luteal phase.[78]

Low E2 depletes the progesterone receptors and changes the endometrial receptor dynamics. E2 inhibits reactive oxygen species (ROS)-induced apoptosis of corpus luteum cells. It decreases HOXA-10 expression.

Pregnancy rate is decreased in long protocol because of increased E2 in proliferative phase gives negative feedback and decreases LH secretion that prevents E2 and progesterone production from corpus luteum. So estrogen supplementation (4 mg E2 valerate) is useful in long protocols for higher pregnancy rate.[79]

E2 production in luteal phase is dependent on LH or hCG and not on FSH and so serum LH level assessment is a must and beta-hCG helps in production of E2 in pregnancy. Addition of E2 is different when GnRhA is used as trigger. Here it is always necessary as there is deficiency of LH and CL is not at all stimulated to produce E2 and progesterone.

ONSET OF LUTEAL SUPPORT

Progesterone started on the day of oocyte retrieval decreases uterine contractility on the day of transfer rather than started late. Uterine contractility was higher 4 days after hCG administration than the natural cycle LH surge. Higher E2 level increases uterine contractility and this high E2 causes uterine resistance to the uterine relaxing property of progesterone.[80] The vaginal progesterone causes elective tissue concentration in the uterus through direct transport. There is no harm in starting the luteal support from the day of oocyte retrieval.[57] There is no difference when luteal support is started on the day of hCG, on the day of ovum retrieval or on the day of embryo transfer.[81] The onset of luteal phase support should not be later than day 3 after ovum retrieval. But if it is started before ovum pick up or at the time of trigger, it closes the window of receptivity earlier.

There is endometrial advancement because if increased E2 and progesterone in proliferative phase. Increased E2 is because of high androgen secreted from theca cells, where granulosa cells convert it into estrogen. So progesterone being an intermediate product, it always is high whenever E2 is high in proliferative phase. So even normal progesterone level will appear early and initiate premature secretory changes. This leads to advancement of endometrium. Therefore whether the progesterone is started on the day of hCG or day of OPU or within 3 days of OPU, pregnancy rates are the same.[81]

Vaginal progesterone if it is delayed for a day or two, gives good results as compared to IM progesterone which is given on the day of oocyte retrieval. So the route of administration is also important along with the starting day of the luteal support.[45]

DURATION OF LUTEAL SUPPORT

Prospective randomized controlled trial[82] indicated that prolongation of progesterone supplementation in early pregnancy had no influence on miscarriage rate. Theoretically we can stop progesterone support once beta-hCG is positive, but most of the IVF specialists continue till 10–12 weeks of pregnancy. Caspo et al. have shown that continuation of pregnancy is independent of corpus luteum function as early as 8–10 weeks of pregnancy.[83] The function is taken over by placenta.[84] The study by Graciela Kohls et al. has shown that vaginal progesterone supplementation after ART can be safely withdrawn at 5 weeks of gestation because cycle outcome was similar to conventional luteal support that is given till 8 weeks of gestation.[85] At 5 weeks, hCG level is greater than 1,000 IU/L and that is sufficient to support corpus luteum without a doubt. The circulating level of progesterone is greater than 8 ng/mL at 5 weeks of pregnancy. But in FET cycle, it is continued till the luteo-placental shift, i.e. 9–10 weeks of pregnancy.

PROGESTERONE RESISTANCE

- Endometriosis
- PCOS with androgen elevation.

Progesterone resistance is because of inhibitor progesterone receptor isoform (PR-A) and the absence of the stimulation isoform PR-B.[86] There is pituitary ovarian dysfunction.[87] This is because of impaired follicular growth giving low FSH and LH because of low E2 and causing LPD. It causes abnormal expression of endometrial biomarkers of implantation.[88] But this is a controversial issue.

In case of progesterone resistance, luteal support will not be efficient until the resistance is removed. So before initiating the treatment, progesterone resistance must be dealt with. In endometriosis. ART outcome was improved by 3–6 months of ovarian suppression by GnRHa.[89]

Recently it has been shown that 6–8 weeks with oral contraceptive (OC) pills normalized implantation and pregnancy rates in women suffering from endometriosis.[90] It is doubtful if similar treatment is helpful in PCOS. This is because of androgen excess. OC pills lower the LH and in turn androgen. Whether higher levels of progesterone can counter progesterone resistance or not, is also not proved.

ESTROGEN AND PROGESTERONE IN FROZEN EMBRYO TRANSFERS CYCLES

Indications of Frozen Embryo Transfers

- Prevention of OHSS.
- When preimplantation genetic screening (PGS) or preimplantation genetic diagnosis (PGD) is required.
- When progesterone rises greater than 1.5 ng/mL in proliferative phase.
- Fluid in uterine cavity.
- Patient's choice.
- Clinician's preference, as freezing of embryos and transfer later has shown better results than fresh transfers.

Physiology for Implantation

- Window of implantation is the time when endometrium supports trophoblast-endometrial interaction occurs around 22–24 days of 28 days cycle,[91] i.e. 3–4 days after ovulation and opens for 4–5 days.

- Endometrium is unchanged in thickness in secretory phase but epithelium and vasculature continues to grow and results in dense endometrium.
- During the window of implantation, number of specific proteins and biochemical markers are present that can be known by microarrays.
- Subendometrial wave activity reduces implantation and may cause ectopic pregnancy. These are due to high estrogen levels.
- Progesterone greater than 20 ng/mL on the day of transfer in frozen embryo transfer (FET) cycle gives lower pregnancy rate.
- High pregnancy rates in frozen embryo transfer cycle teaches that all the substances secreted from the ovary except estrogen and progesterone like androgen, peptides are harmful for good endometrial receptivity.

Frozen Embryo Transfer in Various Situations

Natural Cycle Transfer

- In N-FET cycle, E2 and progesterone are derived from the spontaneous follicular development and ovulation. So this method is to be offered to the patients with ovulatory cycles.
- In natural cycle, by urinary LH kit, LH surge is detected and progesterone is started. But in several cases endometrium may be out of phase.[92]
- This may be due to inaccurate determination of ovulation and also due to cycle to cycle variation.
- Embryo transfer is done on LH + day 6.

Modified Natural Cycle with hCG

- Give hCG when follicle is 17–18 mm in size.
- Progesterone support is not required.
- Embryo transfer is done on hCG + day 7.

- Results of NC-FET and mNC-FET are the same.
- Premature LH or progesterone rise is possible and should be measured. But progesterone rise does not change the pregnancy rate in FET cycle and cancellation of cycle because of elevated LH is not done.[93]

GnRH Agonist Downregulation (Programmed FET Regimen)

- It prevents spontaneous follicular development and ovulation.
- After 5 days of progesterone, endometrium mimics that of 20th day of 28 days cycle.
- In 25%, there is delay of endometrial development.
- So mock cycle with microarray or biopsy may be preferred.
- Routinely agonists are not used in FET cycle as it does not have much benefit.

E2 + Progesterone (Programmed FET Regimens)

- Estrogen is given for 2–3 weeks, till endometrium of 8 mm is grown with zone 3–4 vascularity. E2 less than 12 days and more than 28 days increases the abortion rate. The dose of E2 is 4–12 mg/day. Transdermal E2 and oral tablets have the same results.[94]
- Progesterone is added for 3–5 days depending on cleavage stage or blastocyst transfer respectively.
- High doses of estrogen in early phase prevent follicular development.
- If endometrial peristalsis is less than 5/minute on the previous day than the embryo transfer (FET) should be done, otherwise review progesterone dosage.
- Personalized embryo transfer is useful by adding progesterone for 1–3 days in cases

of delayed endometrial maturity. Day 5 transfers give better results than day 6 transfers.

Additional Luteal Support in FET Cycles

- Serum progesterone level on day 7 after 800 mg progesterone perday in woman for FET cycle, 25% of women had P level of less than 9.2 ng/mL and ongoing pregnancy rate was markedly reduced. So, if these findings are correct, we must be sacrificing numerous pregnancies when we use only vaginal progesterone as luteal support.[95]
- In FET cycles apart from vaginal progesterone twice a day, IM progesterone is recommended every third day for better results.[96]
- In natural cycle FET, hCG used as luteal support, does not improve the pregnancy rates.[97]
- NC-FET, mNC-FET and AC-FET give the same results.

CARRY HOME MESSAGE

- Luteal phase defect is because of low progesterone or suboptimal response with normal progesterone.
- Low progesterone may be due to abnormal folliculogenesis in non-IVF patients.
- Low LH is mainly responsible for LPD in IVF cycles.
- No laboratory tests are reliable for diagnosis of LPD.
- Corpus luteum rescue is because of hCG.
- Low progesterone is because of low hCG in unhealthy embryo.
- Duration of exposure of progesterone is important than blood levels.
- Ovulation induction is a very useful luteal support.

- Human chorionic gonadotropin is also an effective luteal support.
- Micronized progesterone is the best.
- Vaginal route is the best route.
- All superovulated cycles require luteal support.
- Agonist and antagonist cycles cause LPD.
- Luteal support should not be started later than 3 days after ovum retrieval.
- Luteal support in natural cycle is not justified.
- 1,500 IU of hCG on the day of IUI or oocyte retrieval, is very useful, when GnRHa is used as a trigger.
- E2 supplementation is given in long protocol for luteal support.
- Endometriosis and PCOS have progesterone resistance.
- Duration of progesterone after positive beta-hCG is controversial.

REFERENCES

1. Niswender GD, Juengel JL, Silva PJ, et al. Mechanisms controlling the function and lifespan of the corpus luteum. Physiol Rev. 2000;80:1-29.
2. Speroff L, Fritz MA. Clinical Gynecologic Endocrinology and Infertility, 7th re-edition. Philadelphia: Lippincott Williams and Wilkins; 2005. pp. 199-242.
3. Hinney B, Henze C, Kuhn W, et al. The corpus luteum insufficiency: a multifactorial disease. J Clin Endocrinol Metab. 1996;81:565-70.
4. Kiriakidou M, McAllister JM, Sugawara T, et al. Expression of steroidogenic acute regulatory protein (StAR) in the human ovary. J Clin Endocrinol Metab. 1996;814:122-8.
5. Daya S. Habitual abortion. In: Copeland LJ (Ed). Textbook of Gynecology. Philadelphia: WB Saunders; 2000.
6. The Practice Committee of the American Society of Reproductive Medicine. The clinical relevance of luteal phase deficiency: a committee opinion. Fertil Steril. 2012;98(5):1112-7.
7. Järvelä IY, Ruokonen A, Tekay A. Effect of rising hCG levels in the human corpus luteum during early pregnancy. Hum Reprod. 2008;23(12):2275-81.
8. Balasch J, Vanrell JA. Corpus luteum insufficiency and fertility: a matter of controversy. Hum Reprod. 1987;2:557-67.
9. Jordan J, Craig K, Clifton D, et al. Luteal phase defect: the sensitivity and specificity of diagnostic methods in common clinical use. Fertil Steril. 1994;62:54.
10. Check JH, Levin E, Bollendorf A, et al. Miscarriage in the first trimester according to the presence or absence of the progesterone-induced blocking factor at three to five weeks from conception in progesterone supplemented women. Clin Exp Obstet Gynecol. 2005;32(1):13-4.
11. Maclin VM, Padwanska E, Binor Z, et al. Progesterone:estradiol ratios at implantation in ongoing pregnancies, abortion, non-conception cycles resulting from ovulation induction. Fertil Steril. 1990;54:238-44.
12. De Ziegher D. Hormonal control of endometrial receptivity. Hum Reprod. 1995;10:4-7.
13. Goldstein D, Zuckerman H, Schwartz M. Correlation between estradiol and progesterone in cycles with luteal phase deficiency. Fertil Steril. 2003;80:654-5.
14. Tavaniotou A, Devroey P. Effect of human chorionic gonadotropins on luteal luteinizing hormone concentrations in natural cycles. Fertil Steril. 2003;80:654-5.
15. Humaidan P, Ejdrup Bredkjaer H, Westergard LG, et al. 1,500 IU human chorionic gonadotropins administered at oocyte retrieval rescues the luteal phase when gonadotropin-releasing hormone agonist is used for ovulation induction: a prospective, randomized, controlled study. Fertil Steril. 2010;93:847-54.
16. Kummer N, Benadiva C, Feinn R, et al. Factors that predict the probability of successful clinical outcome after induction of oocyte maturation with gonadotropin-releasing hormone agonist. Fertil Steril. 2011;96:63-8.
17. Evans J, Salamonsen LA. Too much of a good thing? Experimental evidence suggests

prolonged exposure to hCG is detrimental to endometrial receptivity. Hum Reprod. 2013;28(6):1610-9.

18. Anderson Y, Fisher R, Giorgione V, et al. Microdose hCG as luteal support without exogenous progesterone administration. Mathematical model of hCG concentration in circulation and initial experience. J Assist Reprod Genet. 2016;33:1311-8.

19. Hotchkiss J, Dierschke DJ, Butler WR, et al. Relation between levels of circulating ovarian steroids and pituitary gonadotropins content during the menstrual cycle of rhesus monkey. Biol Reprod. 1982;26:241-8.

20. Mahesh VB, Brann DW. Regulation of the preovulatory gonadotropin surge by endogenous steroids. Steroids. 1998;63:616-29.

21. De Zeigler D, Bergeron C, Cornel C, et al. Effects of luteal estradiol on the secretory transformation of human endometrium and plasma gonadotropins. J Clin Endocrinol Metab. 1992;74:322-31.

22. De ziergler D, Fanchin R. Progesterone and progestins: applications in gynecology. Sterods. 2000;65:671-9.

23. Fanchin R, Righini C, Olivennes F, et al. Uterine contractions at the time of embryo transfer alter pregnancy rates after in vitro fertilization. Hum Reprod. 1998;13:1968-74.

24. Kyrou D, Fatemi HM, Zepridis L, et al. Does cessation of progesterone supplementation during early pregnancy in patients treated with rFSH/GnRH antagonist affect ongoing pregnancy rates? A randomized controlled trial. Hum Reprod. 2011,26(5):1020-4.

25. Anderson AN, Popovic-Todorovic B, Schmidt KT, et al. Progesterone supplementation during early gestation after IVF or ICSI has no effect on the delivery rates: a randomized controlled trial. Hum Reprod. 2002;17:357-61.

26. Bulun S, Cheng YH, Yin P, et al. Progesterone resistance in endometriosis: link to failure to metabolize estradiol. Mol Cell Endocrinol. 2006;248:94-103.

27. Fauser BC, Devroey P. Reproductive biology and IVF: ovarian stimulation and luteal phase consequences. Trends Endocrinol Metab. 2003;14:236-42.

28. Fatemi HM, Popovic-Todorovic B, Papnikolaou E, et al. An update of luteal phase support in stimulated IVF cycles. Hum Reprod Update. 2007;13:581-90.

29. Fatemi HM, Camus M, Kolibiankis EM, et al. The luteal phase of follicle stimulating hormone/gonadotropin-releasing hormone antagonist in in vitro fertilization cycles during supplementation with progesterone or progesterone and estradiol. Fertil Steril. 2007;87:504-8.

30. Fatemi HM, Bourgain C, Donosh P, et al. Effect of oral administration of dydroprogesterone versus vaginal micronized progesterone on secretory transformation of endometrium and luteal endocrine profile in patients with POF. Hum Reprod. 2007;22:1260-3.

31. Ganesh A, Chakravorty N, Mukherjee R, et al. Comparison of oral dydrogesterone with progesterone gel and micronized progesterone for luteal support in 1,373 women undergoing IVF: a randomized clinical study. Fertil Steril. 2011;95:1961-5.

32. Tournaye H, Sukhikh GT, Kahler E, et al. A phase III randomized controlled trial comparing the efficacy, safety, tolerability of oral dydrogesterone versus micronized vaginal progesterone for luteal support in IVF. Hum Reprod. 2017;32:1019-27.

33. Devroey P, Braekmans P, Camus M, et al. Embryo donation in patients with primary ovarian failure. Hum Reprod. 1988;3(Suppl 2):85-7.

34. Chakravorty BN, Shirazee HH, Dam P, et al. Oral dydrogesterone versus intravaginal micronized progesterone as luteal phase support in assisted reproductive technology (ART) cycles: results of a randomized study. J Steroid Biochem Mol Biol. 2005:97:416-20.

35. De Zeigler D, Sator M, Binelli D, et al. A randomized trial comparing the endometrial effects of daily subcutaneous administration of 25 mg and 50 mg progesterone on aqueous preparation. Fertil Steril. 2013;100(3):860-6.

36. Lockwood G, Griesinger G, Comett B, et al. Subcutaneous progesterone versus vaginal progesterone gel for luteal phase support in in-vitro fertilization: a noninferiority randomized controlled study. Fertil Steril. 2014;101:112-9.

37. Cicinelli E, de Ziegler D. Transvaginal progesterone: evidence for a new functional 'portal system' flowing from vaginal to the uterus. Hum Reprod Update. 1999;5:365-72.

38. Cicinelli E, de Ziegler D, Morgese S, et al. First uterine pass effect is observed when E2 is placed in the upper but not lower third of the vagina. Fertil Steril. 2004;81:1414-6.

39. Balasch J, Fabregues F, Ordi J, et al. Further data favoring the hypothesis of the uterine first-pass effect of vaginally administered micronized progesterone. Gynecol Endocrinol. 1996;10:421-6.

40. Miles R, Paulson R, Lobo R, et al. Pharmacokinetics and endometrial tissue levels of progesterone after administration by intramuscular and vaginal routes: a comparative study. Fertil Steril. 1994;62:485-90.

41. Atrini PG, Volpe A, Angioni S, et al. A comparative randomized study of three different progesterone support of the luteal phase following IVF/ET program. J Endocrinol Invest. 1995;18:51-6.

42. Blake EJ, Norris PM, Dorfman SF, et al. Single and multidose pharmacokinetic study of a vaginal micronized progesterone insert (Endometrin) compared with vaginal gel in healthy reproductive aged female subjects. Fertil Steril. 2010;94(4):1296-301.

43. Zegers-Hochschild F, Balmaceda JP, Fabres C, et al. Prospective randomized trial to evaluate the efficacy of vaginal ring releasing progesterone for IVF and oocyte donation. Hum Reprod. 2000;15:2093-7.

44. Bergh C, Lindenberg S; Nordic Crinone Study Group. A prospective randomized, multicentre study comparing vaginal progesterone gel and vaginal micronized progesterone tablets for luteal phase support after IVF/ICSI. Hum Reprod. 2012;27:3467-73.

45. Silverberg KM, Vaughn TC, Hansard LJ, et al. Vaginal (Crinone 8%) gel versus intramuscular progesterone in oil for luteal phase support in in vitro fertilization: a large prospective trial. Fertil Steril. 2012;97:344-8.

46. Farhi J, Weissman A, Steinfeld Z, et al. Estradiol supplementation during the luteal phase may improve the pregnancy rates in patients undergoing in vitro fertilization-embryo transfer cycles. Fertil Steril. 2000;73:761-6.

47. Griesinger G, Franke K, Kinast C, et al. Ascorbic acid supplement during luteal phase in IVF. J Assist Reprod Genet. 2002;19:164-8.

48. Ubaldi F, Reinzi I, Ferrero S, et al. Low dose prednisolone administration in routine ICSI patients does not improve pregnancy and implantation rates. Hum Reprod. 2002;17:1544-7.

49. Urman B, Meran R, Alatas C, et al. Low dose aspirin does not increase implantation rates in patients undergoing intracytoplasmic sperm injection: a prospective randomized study. J Assist Reprod Genet. 2000;17:586-90.

50. Tavaniotou A, Albano C, Smitz J, et al. Impact of ovarian stimulation on corpus luteum function and embryonic implantation. J Reprod Immunol. 2002;55(1-2):123-30.

51. Xu B, Li Z, Zhang H, et al. Serum progesterone level effects on the outcome of in vitro fertilization in patients with different ovarian response: an analysis of more than 10,000 cycles. Fertil Steril. 2012;97(6):1321-7.

52. Doldi N, Marsiglio E, Destefanu A, et al. Elevated serum P on the day of hCG administration in IVF is associated with a higher pregnancy rate in polycystic ovary syndrome. Hum Reprod. 1999;14:1601-5.

53. Hill MJ, Whitcomg BW, Lewis TD, et al. Progesterone luteal support after ovulation induction and intrauterine insemination: a systematic review and meta-analysis. Fertil Steril. 2013;100(5):1373-80.

54. Pirard C, Donnez J, Loumaye E. GnRH agonist as novel luteal support: results of a randomized, parallel group, feasibility study using intranasal administration of buserelin. Hum Reprod. 2005;20:1798-804.

55. Tesarik J, Hazout A, Mendoza-Tesarik R, et al. Beneficial effect of luteal phase GnRH agonist administration on embryo implantation after ICSI in both GnRH agonist and antagonist treated ovarian stimulation cycles. Hum Reprod. 2006;21:2572-9.

56. Brigante CM, Renzinin M, Dal Canto M, et al. Efficacy of luteal phase support with GnRH agonist: a preliminary comparative study. Fertil Steril. 2013;100(3):299.

57. Vander Linden H, Buckingham K, Farquhar C, et al. Luteal support for assisted reproduction cycles. Cochrane Database Syst Rev. 2011;(10):CD009154.
58. Fatemi HM. The luteal phase after 3 decades of IVF: what do we know? Reprod Biomed Online. 2009;19 Suppl 4:4331.
59. Devroey P, Bourgain C, Macklon NS, et al. Reproductive biology and IVF: ovarian stimulation and endometrial receptivity. Trends Endocrinol Metab. 2004;15(2):84-90.
60. Kolibianakis EM, Devroey P. The luteal phase after ovarian stimulation. Reprod Biomed Online. 2002;5 Suppl 1:26-35.
61. Kyrou D, Fatemi HM, Tournaye H, et al. Luteal phase support in normo-ovulatory women stimulated with clomiphene citrate for intrauterine insemination. Need or habit? Hum Reprod. 2010;25:2501-6.
62. Maher MA. Luteal phase support may improve pregnancy outcomes during intrauterine insemination cycles. Eur J Obstet Gynecol Reprod Biol. 2011;157:57-62.
63. Humaidan P, Papnikolaou EG, Kyrou D, et al. The luteal phase after GnRH agonist triggering of ovulation: present and future perspectives. Reprod Biomed Online. 2012;24:134-41.
64. Kerin JF, Broom TJ, Ralph MM, et al. Human luteal phase function following oocyte aspiration from the immediately preovular graafian follicle of spontaneous ovular cycles. Br J Obstet Gynecol. 1981;88:1021-8.
65. Smitz J, Devroey P, Faguer B, et al. A prospective randomized comparison of intramuscular or intravaginal natural progesterone as a luteal phase and early pregnancy supplement. Hum Reprod. 1992;7:168-75.
66. Miyake A, Aono T, Kinugasa T, et al. Suppression of serum levels of luteinizing hormone by short and long-loop negative feedback in ovariectomized women. J Endocrinol. 1979;80:353-6.
67. Beckers NG, Macklon NS, Eijkemans MJ, et al. Nonsupplemented luteal phase characteristics after the administration of recombinant human chorionic gonadotropin, recombinant luteinizing hormone, or gonadotropin-releasing hormone (GnRH) agonist to induce final oocyte maturation in in vitro fertilization patients after ovarian stimulation with recombinant follicle stimulating hormone and GnRH antagonist co-treatment. J Clin Endocrinol Metab. 2003;88:4186-92.
68. Duffy DM, Stewart DR, Stouffer RL. Titrating luteinizing hormone replacement to sustain the structure and function of the corpus luteum after gonadotropin-releasing hormone antagonist treatment in rhesus monkeys. J Clin Endocrinol Metab. 1999;84:342-9.
69. Daya S, Gunby J. Luteal phase support in assisted reproductive cycles. Cochrane Database Syst Rev. 2004;(3):CD004830.
70. Tavaniotou A, Albano C, Smitz J, et al. Effect of clomiphene citrate on follicular and luteal phase luteinizing hormone concentrations in in vitro fertilization cycles stimulated with gonadotropins and gonadotropin-releasing hormone antagonist. Fertil Steril. 2000;77:733-7.
71. Kolibianakis EM, Bourgain C, Platteau P, et al. Abnormal endometrial development occurs during the luteal phase of non-supplemental donor cycles treated with r-FSH and GnRH antagonists. Fertil Steril. 2003;80:464-6.
72. Ziad R, Suheil J. Luteal supplementation in in vitro fertilization: more questions than answers. Fertil Steril. 2008;89(4):749-58.
73. Yousef MA, Vanderveen F, Al-Inany MG, et al. Gonadotropin hormone releasing hormone agonist versus hCG for oocyte triggering in antagonist assisted reproductive technology. Cochrane Database Syst Rev. 2014: CD008046.
74. Humaidan P, Polyzos NB, Alsbjerg B, et al. GnRHa trigger and individualized luteal phase hCG support according to ovarian response to stimulation: two prospective randomized controlled multi-centre studies in IVF patients. 2013, 28(9): 2511-21.
75. Rosenwaks Z, Navot D, Veeck L, et al. Oocyte donation. The Norfolk program. Ann N Y Acad Sci. 1988;541:728-41.
76. Engmann et al. Fertil Steril. 2008;98:84-91.
77. Papanikolaou EG, Verpoest W, Fatemi H, et al. A novel method of luteal supplementation with recombinant leutizing hormone when a gonadotropin releasing hormone agonist is used instead of human chorionic

gonadotropin for ovulation trigger: a randomized prospective proof of concept study. Fertil Steril. 2011;95:1174-7.

78. Fatemi HM, Kolibianakis EM, Camus M, et al. Addition of estradiol to progesterone for luteal supplementation in patients stimulated with GnRH antagonists/rFSH for IVF: a randomized controlled trial. Hum Reprod. 2006;21:2628-32.

79. Lukaszuk K, Liss J, Lukaszuk M, et al. Optimization of estradiol supplementation during the luteal phase improves the pregnancy rate in women undergoing IVF-ET cycles. Fertil Steril. 2005;83:1372-6.

80. Ayoubi JM, Epiney M, Brioschi PA, et al. Comparison of changes in uterine contraction frequency after ovulation in menstrual cycle and in in vitro fertilization cycles. Fertil Steril. 2003;79:1101-5.

81. Mochtar MH, Van Wely M, Van der Veen F. Timing luteal phase support in GnRH agonist down-regulated IVF/embryo transfer cycles. Hum Reprod. 2006;21:905-8.

82. Nyboe AA, Popovic-Todorovic B, Schmidt KT, et al. Progesterone supplementation during early gestations after IVF and ICSI has no effect on the delivery rates: a randomized controlled trial. Hum Reprod. 2002;17:357-61.

83. Caspo AI, Pulkkinen MO, Wiest WG. Effects of lutectomy and progesterone replacement therapy in early pregnant patients. Am J Obstet Gynecol. 1973;115:759-65.

84. Schmidt KL, Ziebe S, Popovic B, et al. Progesterone supplementation during early gestation after in vitro fertilization has no effect on delivery rate. Fertil Steril. 2001;75:337-41.

85. Kohls G, Ruiz F, Martinez M, et al. Early progesterone cessation after in vitro fertiliza-tion/intracytoplasmic sperm injection: randomized controlled trial. Fertil Steril. 2012;98:858-62.

86. Attia GR, Zeitoun K, Edwards D, et al. Progesterone receptor isoform A but not B is expressed in endometriosis. J Clin Endocrinol Metab. 2000;85:2897-902.

87. Cahill DJ, Hull MG. Pituitary-ovarian dysfunction and endometriosis. Hum Reprod Update. 2000;6:56-66.

88. Donaghay M, Lessey BA. Uterine receptivity: alterations associated with benign gynecological disease. Semin Reprod Med. 2007;25:461-75.

89. Surrey ES, Silverberg KM, Surrey MW, et al. Effect of prolonged gonadotropin-releasing hormone agonist therapy on the outcome of in vitro fertilization-embryo transfer in patients with endometriosis. Fertil Steril. 2002;78:699-704.

90. De Ziegler D, Gayet V, Aubriot FX, et al. Use of oral contraceptives in women with endometriosis before assisted reproduction treatment improves outcomes. Fertil Steril. 2010;94:2796-9.

91. Berg PA, Navot D. The impact of embryonic development and endometrial maturity on the timing of implantation. Fertil Steril. 1992;58:537-42.

92. Jawar MP, Deshpande MM, Gadgil PA, et al. Histopathological study of endometrium in infertility. Indian J Pathol Microbiol. 2003;46:630-6.

93. Groenewound ER, Macklon NS, Cohlen BJ. ANTARCTICA study group. The effect of elevated progesterone levels before hCG triggering in modified natural cycle frozen-thawed embryo transfer cycles. Reprod Biomed Online. 2017;34:546-54.

94. Davar R, Janati S, Mohseni F, et al. A comparison of effects of transdermal estradiol and estradiol valerate on endometrial receptivity in frozen-thawed embryo-transfer cycles: a randomized clinical trial. J Reprod Infertility. 2016;17:97-103.

95. Labarta E, Mariani G, Holtman N, et al. Low serum progesterone on the day of embryo-transfer is associated with diminished on going pregnancy rate in oocyte donation cycles after artificial endometrial preparation: a prospective study. Hum Reproduction. 2017;32:2437-42.

96. Devine K, Richter KS, Widra EA, et al. Vitrified blastocyst transfer cycles with the use of only vaginal progesterone replacement with endometrium have inferior ongoing pregnancy rates: results from planned interim analysis of a three arm randomized controlled non-inferiority trial. Fertil Steril. 2018;109:266-75.

97. Lee VC, Li RH, Yeung WS, et al. A randomized double-blinded controlled trial of hCG as luteal support in natural cycle frozen embryo transfer. Hum Reprod. 2017;32:1130-7.

Hyperprolactinemia

Chaitanya Nagori

INTRODUCTION

Prolactin is secreted from lactotrophs of anterior pituitary. It is regulated by prolactin inhibitory factor (dopamine) secreted from hypothalamus. Hyperprolactinemia is one of the common causes of oligoanovulation. Prolactin secretion inhibits gonadotropin-releasing hormone (GnRh) secretion leading to decrease in follicle-stimulating hormone (FSH) and luteinizing hormone (LH) and so causes anovulation and amenorrhea.

EFFECT OF PROLACTIN ON REPRODUCTION

It acts directly on ovary by its action on aromatase enzyme causing menstrual irregularities. In follicular phase, higher levels affect follicular growth and anovulation. In luteal phase it affects the corpus luteum function. Increased level causes poor endometrial development.

Estrogen increases prolactin secretion and is commonly seen in polycystic ovary syndrome (PCOS) as estrogen level is high. High prolactin level inhibits GnRh secretion, which in turn inhibits FSH and LH release leading to anovulation. High prolactin level abolishes midcycle LH surge which is due to positive effect of rise in estrogen. This leads to luteal phase defect and recurrent pregnancy loss.[1]

CAUSES OF HYPERPROLACTINEMIA

Physiological

Rapid eye movement (REM) sleep, pregnancy, coitus, nipple stimulation, stress, etc. cause high prolactin levels in blood. The practical consideration is that if the breast is examined for galactorrhea, the blood test for prolactin should not be planned simultaneously with that. Similarly serum prolactin levels should not be asked for very early in the morning, immediately after waking up. Prolactin level is at peak after 5–8 hours of sleep. In both these conditions, prolactin level is raised. The collection of the blood sample for prolactin is therefore planned after 2 hours of waking up and before breat is examined for secretions.

Drug Induced

The drugs that are known to cause rise in prolactin levels are estrogen, methyldopa, phenothiazines, opiates, cimetidine, and oral contraceptive pills.

Pathological

The common causes are:

- idiopathic
- Prolactinoma
- Hypothalamo-pituitary tumors
- Polycystic ovary syndrome
- Hypothyroidism
- Renal failure.

About 30% of the patients with PCOS have hyperprolactinemia.[2] Hyperprolactinemia in PCOS patients do not require specific treatment for high prolactin levels, treating PCOS, will correct it. Similarly in hypothyroid patients, correction of thyroid problem automatically corrects related hyperprolactinemia.

PRESENTATION AND DIAGNOSIS

- Commonest presentation is galactorrhea.
- Oligoanovulation and infertility may be the cause for seeking medical advice.
- History of related drugs and illnesses should be ruled out.
- Hypothyroidism is to be excluded.
- Headache and visual disturbances are common in pituitary macroadenoma.
- Hyperprolactinemia without galactorrhea is because there is inadequate priming of breast due to estrogen.[3]

INVESTIGATIONS

Prolactin Level

Normal prolactin level is less than 30 ng/mL. There are three different types of prolactin. These are classified as little (80%), big, and big-big. The bioactivity of prolactin is mostly due to little prolactin. At times, blood prolactin levels may be high without galactorrhea or amenorrhea and no other symptoms. This is due to high levels of big and big-big prolactin, that have least bioactivity. It does not require any treatment.

Blood prolactin level of 100–200 ng/mL may be due to pituitary microadenoma. Level more than 200 ng/mL is due to pituitary macroadenoma and this is symptomatic. If ovulation is present then high level of prolactin should be ignored.

Computed Tomography and Magnetic Resonance Imaging

To diagnose microadenoma that is less than 10 mm and macroadenoma that is more than 10 mm, these are the investigations of choice.

Serum Thyroid-stimulating Hormone

Rule out hypothyroidism as increased thyroid hormone (TH) is associated with increased prolactin levels due to increased thyroid stimulating hormone (TSH).

TREATMENT

Dopamine receptor agonists are very effective in normalizing prolactin level. Commonly used drugs are bromocriptine and cabergoline.

Bromocriptine

It is started as 1.25 mg daily dose and is increased by 1.25 mg till maximum dose of 40 mg daily in divided doses till spontaneous menstruation occurs. Dopamine agonists can restore ovulatory cycles in 50–75% of cases. The same dose is continued till patient conceives in cases of hyperprolactinemia. Once normal level of prolactin is achieved, the test is repeated every 6 months.

Bromocriptine also reduces the tumor size in 3–6 months. So it is useful in symptomatic patients in pregnancy with prolactinoma. It is useful in nonoperable cases.

Cabergoline

It is more patient friendly than bromocriptine. It is administered in a twice a week dose and the results are comparable with bromocriptine. Initial dose is 0.25 mg twice a week and can be increased to 2 mg twice a week. It is effective in 70–80% of patients resistant or nontolerant to bromocriptine.[4] Gastrointestinal tract (GIT) and central nervous system (CNS) side effects are common and so increase in dose is always gradual. Common contraindications are hypertension, valvular heart diseases, and fibrotic diseases. Vaginal preparations, slow release oral tablets, and once a month preparations are under clinical trials. When used in infertile patients, pregnancy is achieved in almost 85% of cases. Quinagolide also gives equivalent results.

In cases of macroadenomas, surgery or radiation is required in persistent and resistant cases or recurrent prolactinomas. Patients who do not require pregnancy, microadenomas may be left untreated.

EFFECT OF HYPERPROLACTINEMIA IN FEMALE

- Oligoanovulation
- Decrease in FSH and LH secretion
- Increase in intraovarian androgens as it prevents aromatization
- Luteal phase defect.

TRANSIENT HYPERPROLACTINEMIA

Reduction in dopamine inhibitory effect raises prolactin and LH. Transient hyperprolactinemia is observed in normal prolactinemic patients with luteal insufficiency in 73% and galactorrhea in 80% of patients.[5]

This is commonly seen when clomiphene citrate is used for stimulation protocol. In these cases bromocriptine is given from day 5 of the cycle till ovulation. This improves the endometrial thickness and vascularity. In normoprolactinemic patient bromocriptine is not continued in luteal phase otherwise it may lead to luteal phase defect due to its effect on corpus luteum. The dose of bromocryptine is 1.25 mg twice a day from day 5 of cycle till ovulation. Here cabergolin can not be used as its effect lasts in the luteal phase and caused LPD. Here decreasing the prolactin level improved the secretion of FSH and also the quality of the follicle.[6,7] Rise of prolactin in these cases is because of high estrogen level and if bromocriptine is given to these patients, pregnancy rates up to 40% can be achieved as compared to in controls of 1%.[8]

Infertile women with galactorrhea and normal prolactin level responds well to bromocriptine.[9]

The explanation for normal prolactin with galactorrhea is that, biologically active form of prolactin is not detected in immunoassay. The second explanation is exaggerated nocturnal spikes of prolactin secretion, that are not recognized in random day time samples.[9]

CARRY HOME MESSAGE

- Hyperprolactinemia without symptoms may be because of "big prolactin".
- Hyperprolactinemia in PCOS requires treatment of PCOS only.
- Thyroid-stimulating hormone must be evaluated before treating hyperprolactinemia.
- Microadenoma does not require surgery.
- Galactorrhea without hyperprolactinemia requires treatment.
- Spikers should be treated with bromocriptine.

REFERENCES

1. Cunha-Filho JS, Gross JL, Lemos NA, et al. Hyperprolactinemia and luteal insufficiency in infertile patients with mild and minimal endometriosis. Horm Metab Res. 2001;33(4):216-20.

2. Isik AZ, Gulekli B, Zorlu CG, et al. Endocrinological and clinical analysis of hyperprolactinemic patients with and without ultrasonically diagnosed polycystic ovarian changes. Gynecol Obstet Invest. 1997;43:183.

3. Balen A, Jacobs H. Anovulatory infertility and ovulation induction, 2nd edition. Amsterdam: Elsevier; 2003. pp. 144-55.

4. Verhelst J, Abs R, Maiter D, et al. Cabergoline in the treatment of hyperprolactinemia: a study in 455 patients. J Clin Endocrinol Metab. 1999;84:2518.

5. Asukai K, Uemura T, Minaguchi H. Occult hyperprolactinemia in infertile women. Fertil Steril. 1993;60(3):423-7.

6. Yoshida K, Kayama F, Kimura Y, et al. The effect of occult hyperprolactinemia (OHP) on gonadotropin secretion system. Nihon Naibunpi Gakkai Zasshi. 1994;70(10):1101-14.

7. DeVane GW, Guzick DS. Bromocriptine therapy in normoprolactinemic women with unexplained infertility and galactorrhea. Fertil Steril. 1986;46:1026-31.

8. Ben-David M, Schenker JG. Transient hyperprolactinemia. A correctable cause of female idiopathic infertility. J Clin Endocrinol Metab. 1983;57:442-4.

9. Padilla SL, Person G, McDonough PG, et al. The efficacy of bromocriptine in patients with ovulatory dysfunction and normoprolactinemic galactorrhea. Fertil Steril. 1985;44(5):695-8.

Thyroid Disorders

Chaitanya Nagori

INTRODUCTION

Thyroid disorders in women are associated with menstrual disorders and impaired fertility. The restoration of euthyroid state after treatment shows definite improvement in menstrual disorders and fertility.[1] Formerly thyroid function tests were recommended for symptomatic women or with family history of dysfunction. This approach may miss 30–35% women with hypothyroidism. To screen all the patients, especially infertile and aged patients, for thyroid dysfunction is cost-effective and recommended by American Association of Clinical Endocrinologist.

HYPOTHYROIDISM AND REPRODUCTION

Normal thyroid-stimulating hormone (TSH) level is (0.45–4.5 mIU/L). Hypothyroidism is seen more often in females and increases with age.[2] Menstrual irregularities, spontaneous abortions, preterm deliveries, unexplained stillbirth and infertility are the common manifestations in a woman. Menorrhagia is due to anovulation, poor muscle tone, and platelet dysfunction.

Infertility

- Almost 70% of infertility in hypothyroid woman is due to anovulation.[3]
- Oligomenorrhea is the most common clinical presentation.
- It is found in women with unexplained infertility.
- Empirical treatment with thyroid hormones in euthyroid patients does not help in infertility management.
- Every woman after the age of 35 years should be screened for thyroid functions even though she is asymptomatic.

Mechanism of Action (Flowchart 18.1)

The exact mechanism of the effect of thyroid disorder on ovarian function is not known, but it has been postulated that thyroid hormone might have direct action on ovarian physiology through receptors in granulosa cells. Thyroid has got synergistic action with follicle-stimulating hormone (FSH) causing stimulatory effect on granulosa cells. Therefore, hypothyroid patients may have anovulation and may require higher doses for ovarian stimulation.

Flowchart 18.1: Mechanism of action of thyroid-stimulating hormone (TSH).

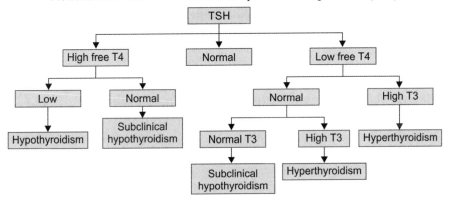

Normal level of thyroid has optimum effect on FSH modulated morphological differentiation of granulosa cells. So alteration in thyroid level will deteriorate ovarian function.[4] According to John Lowe, hypothyroidism can cause a picture similar to polycystic ovarian syndrome (PCOS) causing anovulation. Replacement of thyroid hormone can resolve the functional small cysts and anovulation. Study by Muderis et al. confirmed the above findings.[5]

Whenever TSH level is increased in hypothyroidism, there is increase in prolactin level that also causes anovulation. But here the treatment is thyroxine and not prolactin lowering drugs.[6]

So, high TSH and low T4 confirms the diagnosis of hypothyroidism and low TSH and high T4 or T3 confirms the diagnosis of hypothyroidism. Once the diagnosis is established the autoimmune disorder must be looked for. Antimicrobial antibody and antithyroid antibody and antithyroglobulin antibody are useful indicators of risk of progression.[7] But they rarely help as far as management is concerned. In patients with recent onset of hypothyroidism and hypothalamo-pituitary disorders, T4 should be assessed along with TSH. Transient changes

in TSH can be caused by glucocorticoids, dopamine, systemic illnesses, and psychiatric disturbances also. To decrease the miscarriage rate levothyroxine is given in patients with thyroid antibodies if TSH is > 2.5 mIU/L.

Treatment

With established diagnosis of hypothyroidism, there is always replacement therapy with 25–50 μg of thyroxine i.e. T4 to be given daily. The dose is increased by 25 μg daily after reassessment with biochemical and clinical examination after 4 weeks. With proper dosage, pregnancy rate can reach 64%.[8]

Subclinical Hypothyroidism

It is defined as TSH higher than the upper limit of normal range (4.5–5.0 mIU/L) with normal free T4 levels. During pregnancy upper limit is considered as 4 mIU/L but 2.5 mIU/L in first trimester. There is a fair evidence that treatment of subclinical hypothyroidism when TSH is more than 4 mIU/L is associated with improved pregnancy rate and decreased miscarriage rate.[9] Though there are some studies which also suggest that the TSH values between 2.5–5 mIU/L are not associated with adverse IUI outcomes. It has no signs or symptoms with normal T3 and T4 with

TSH between 7.5 mIU/L and 10 mIU/L. The treatment of subclinical hypothyroidism is still controversial for infertility. It is given to this group of patients as it has no negative effect and may improve fertility. The role of thyroid replacement on euthyroid patients in infertility has no proved value. But gonadotropin therapy and pregnancy may lead to subclinical hypothyroidism and may require thyroxine.[10]

But unless abnormal thyroid function can be documented by specific laboratory assessment, empiric treatment has no place. It does not help in infertile patients in euthyroid state.[11] But FASTER (First- and Second-Trimester Evaluation of Risk) trial does not show adverse effect on baby in subclinical hypothyroidism. Several studies recommend to maintain TSH between 0.5 mIU/mL and 2.0 mIU/mL.

Evaluation of Therapy

The goal is to maintain the TSH in lower half of normal range. The full response of TSH to changes in T4 is relatively slow. Minimum of 8 weeks is necessary between changes in dosage and assessment of TSH. Then further evaluation is done in 4 weeks.

HYPERTHYROIDISM

Mechanism of Action

Elevated thyroxine level leads to increased level of SHBG i.e. sex hormone binding globulin. So increased level of serum concentration of estradiol and testosterone is observed. The baseline levels of FSH and luteinizing hormone (LH) are also increased. There is attenuated midcycle LH surge, which causes oligoanovulation. It causes wide range of menstrual disorders from menorrhagia to amenorrhea.

Subclinical hyperthyroidism is as common as subclinical hypothyroidism.

The most common cause is of subclinical hyperthyroidism is the excessive doses of thyroxine.

Diagnosis

- *Clinical manifestations*: Tachycardia, exophthalmos, tremors, and enlarged thyroid gland.
- After the diagnosis, a possible cause may be diagnosed by ultrasound, radioactive iodine uptake, and antithyroid antibody.
- Screening is done by TSH assay.

Treatment

The goal is to establish a euthyroid state.

Medical Therapy

In infertile patients, medical therapy is recommended. The drugs of choice are carbimazole or propylthiouracil.

Dose schedule:
- *Carbimazole*: 10–20 mg 8 hourly
- *Propylthiouracil*: 100–200 mg 8 hourly
- *Methimazole*: 10–15 mg 8 hourly.

Common side effects are gastrointestinal (GI) symptoms, rashes, and agranulocytosis. It inhibits organification of iodide and decreases production of T4 and T3. The action is established in 2–4 weeks. Half-life of thyroxine is about 1 week and gland has large stores of T4. Maximum effect occurs at 4–8 weeks. Once the patient becomes euthyroid, the dose is to be titrated and gradually reduced to minimum of 5 mg daily and then once patient is euthyroid at that dose also, then the drug is discontinued. Symptomatic relief may be achieved by adding beta blockers, i.e. propranolol 40–60 mg 6 hourly or nadolol 40–240 mg daily.

It is better avoided in patients with asthma and cardiac failure. Relapse of hyperthyroidism can occur in 2 years. It can also be treated by surgery or irradiation, but pregnancy should be postponed for several months. Screening with highly sensitive TSH assay is a must in all cases of infertility.

CARRY HOME MESSAGE

- Hypo- or hyperthyroidism causes ovulatory dysfunction.
- Hypothyroidism can cause hyperprolactinemia.
- Treatment of subclinical hypothyroidism is controversial.
- Drugs for thyroid are of no value in euthyroid patients.

REFERENCES

1. Longcope C. The male and female reproductive system in thyrotoxicosis. In: Bravermann LD, Utiger RD (Eds). Werner & Ingbar's The thyroid, 6th edition. Philadelphia: Lippincott; 1991. pp 828-35.
2. Danese MD, Powe NR, Sawin CT, et al. Screening for mild thyroid failure at the periodic health examination. A decision and cost-effectiveness analysis. JAMA. 1996;276(4):285-92.
3. Goldsmith RE, Sturgis SH, Lerman J, et al. The menstrual pattern of thyroid disease. J Clin Endocrinol Metab. 1962;12:846-55.
4. Marou T, Hayashi M, Matsuo H, et al. The role of thyroid hormone as a biological amplifier of the actions of follicle-stimulating hormone in the functional differentiation of cultures porcine granulosa cells. Endocrinology. 1987;121(4):1233-41.
5. Muderris II, Boztosun A, Oner G, et al. Effect of thyroid hormone replacement therapy on ovarian volume and androgen hormones in patients with untreated primary hypothyroidism. Ann Saudi Med. 2011;31(2):145-51.
6. Madkar C, Balkawade NU, Dahiya PA. Thyroid Pituitary and Ovulation. In: Deshpande H (Ed). Practical management of ovulation induction. New Delhi: Jaypee Brothers Medical Publishers; 2016. pp. 46-7.
7. Rao AR. Hyperprolactinemia and thyroid disorders. Principle and Practice of Assisted Reproductive Technology, 1st edition. New Delhi: Jaypee Brothers Medical Publishers; 2014. pp. 8127-37.
8. Oravec S, Hlavacka S. Disorders of thyroid function and fertility disorders. Ceska Gynekol. 2000;65(1):53-7.
9. ASRM practice committee 2015, Subclinical hypothyroidism in the infertile female population: a guideline. Fertil Steril. 2015;104(3): 545-53.
10. Mandel SJ. Thyroid function during gonadotropin therapy. (abstract). Presented at the 10th International Congress of Endocrinology. San Francisco: The Endocrine Society; 1996.
11. Speroff F, Fritz MA. Reproduction and the thyroid. Clinical Gynecologic Endocrinology and Infertility, 7th edition. New Delhi: Jaypee Brothers Medical Publishers (p) Ltd.; 2005. pp. 803-23.

Index